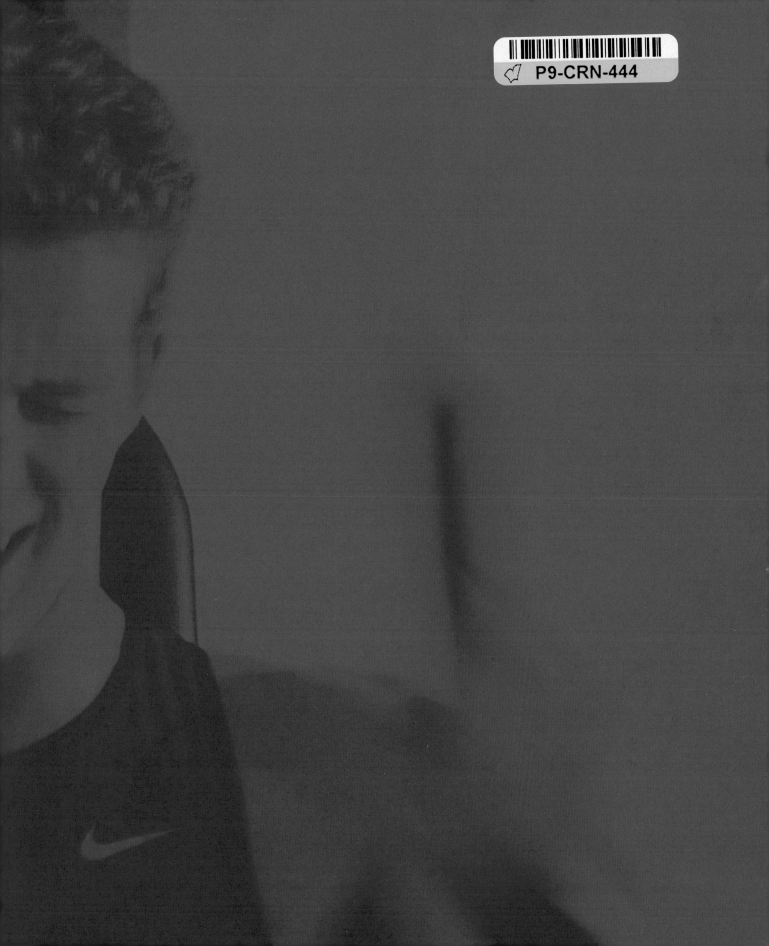

All around
Fitness

Copyright © 1998 Könemann Verlagsgesellschaft mbH
Bonner Straße 126, D-50968 Cologne

Art Direction and Design: Peter Feierabend
Project Coordinator: Kirsten E. Lehmann
Assistant: Miriam Rodriguez Startz
Layout: Erill Vinzenz Fritz
Production Manager: Detlev Schaper
Production: Mark Voges
Reproduction: TIFF Digital Repro, Dortmund

Copyright © 1999 for the English Edition
Translation from German: Sue Appleton, Paul Aston,
Dr. Colin B. Grant, Phil Greenhead, Timothy Jones, Fiona Müller
English-language Editor: Ilze Bezuidenhout
Managing Editor: Bettina Kaufmann
Assistant: Alex Morkramer
Typesetting: Oliver Hessmann & Thomas Lindner
Printing and Binding: Neue Stalling, Oldenburg

Printed in Germany
ISBN 3-8290-0438-9

10 9 8 7 6 5 4 3 2 1

Oliver Barteck

All around
Fitness

Photography:
Irmgard Elsner, Jürgen Schulzki

Contributing authors are:
Knuth Kröger, Alex Morkramer,
Simon Oswald, Dr. Gunnar Wöbke

KÖNEMANN

Contents

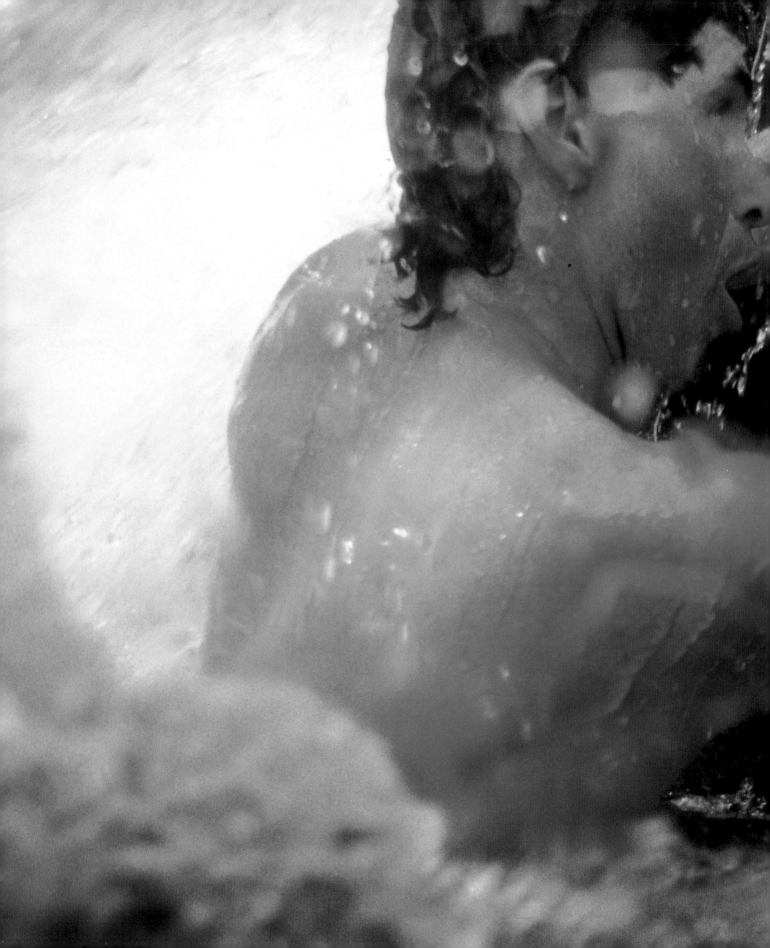

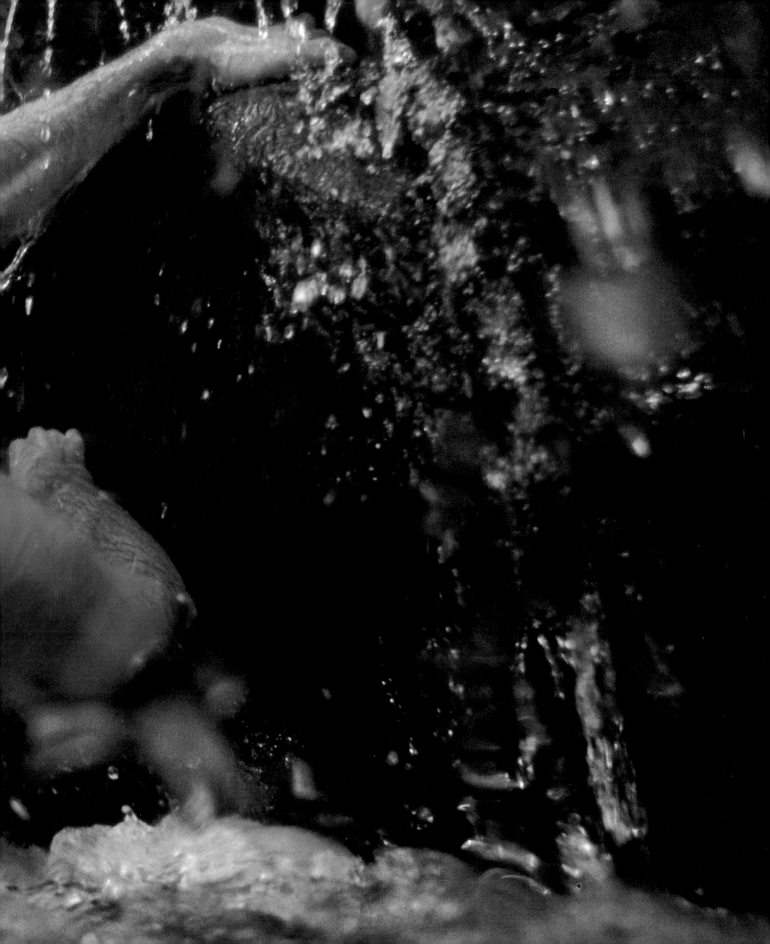

As a former competitive sportswoman there is one thing I know for sure: good training instructions can make the difference between success and failure – this does not only apply to the fight for Olympic medals but also to recreational sports – such as in mass sports. Anyone who actively participates in sport and wishes to improve his or her fitness can avail themselves of a multitude of possibilities.

Modern fitness centers do not only offer a wide spectrum of sports but, in many cases, also offer competent supervision. However, there are always situations in which you are either working on improving your fitness alone, for example at home, or in which a qualified trainer or teacher is not available. In this case it is useful to have a written instruction manual to offer assistance. However, if you look for specialized, easy-to-understand instructions you will quickly discover that such manuals are often difficult for the layperson to understand. Practical instruction manuals for the beginner, on the other hand, are often superficial and seldom impart the necessary knowledge.

All around Fitness fills this gap by presenting specialized easy-to-understand information and concrete illustrative material, so that the beginner can also quickly develop his or her comprehension of fitness training and planning. Furthermore it provides the advanced sportsman or woman with a comprehensive source of background tips and information. All in all, it offers optimal support for your fitness.

I wish you much pleasure and enjoyment.

Heide Rosendahl

Introduction

Is it not wonderful to watch children playing in their impetuous desire and compulsion for movement? Unfortunately, this natural desire and compulsion waste away with many "adults." Today's rapid technical progress has led to a lack of exercise, something that our ancestors never knew. The permanently increasing number of people who suffer for example from obesity or from back trouble indicates that many people ignore the demands of their body for physical exercise.

Once you have decided to do something to stop your natural physical need to exercise from getting rusty, this book can help you find a way to a life of fitness. Therefore, first of all, we shall explain what we understand by the term "to be fit."

Fitness training, as is practiced by around five percent of the population, originates in the bodybuilding movement. Even as bodybuilding slowly reached its peak in America in the 1950s and 1960s, the dynamic development of this sport is mainly coupled with the name of an Austrian, Arnold Schwarzenegger. His sporting success from the end of the sixties to the middle of the seventies led to more and more young men taking up weight training. In 1980 Arnold Schwarzenegger celebrated his sports comeback in support of his film career. From this point onwards public interest in muscle training has consistently grown. Gradually an increasing number of older people and women have become interested in using weights to train their bodies. During the 1980s and up to the 1990s the "Muscle Cellars" of the bodybuilders developed more and more into multi-functional fitness clubs, in which not only strength training but also the development of further sporting motor abilities of endurance, mobility, co-ordination and speed play an equal role. The members of a modern fitness club come from all walks of life and comprise a representative cross-section of the population.

The term "bodybuilding" today still conjures up the powerfully muscular image of Arnold Schwarzenegger. The word "fitness," however, is not related to such a precise image and derives originally from a kind of instruction manual for training sporting, motor abilities:

F requency

I ntensity

T ime

If you are "fit," then you have trained at an adapted frequency with a suitable intensity for an appropriate period of time.

The first chapter, the training guide, systematically answers the questions which result from the "fit formula" – including how the terms "suitable" and "appropriate" are to be understood. The structure of an optimal process for the management and monitoring of your individual training program should be given here. Proceeding from your present state of fitness, which can be determined by tests, you stipulate your personal targets yourself. Subsequently, a rough frame assists in the compilation of an individual training plan which is adapted to suit your personal requirements. Regular analysis of the training to date completes the training guide.

The next chapter presents the progress of an ideal fitness training unit. From warming-up to muscle-building, endurance training and mobility training to cooling down and regenerative measures, a wealth of useful information and insider tips are given on each important area of a comprehensive training program.

Some readers might like to start directly with the third chapter which deals with losing weight. However, it will quickly become clear that long-term weight reduction does not make sense unless it is accompanied by a suitable exercise program. Exercise represents one pillar of the successful loss of superfluous pounds. In addition, knowledge of a balanced diet, and the organizational and psychological components are of importance. All four components of a successful weight reduction program are examined more closely in Chapter 3.

In the fourth chapter those readers who are interested will find the opportunity to enlarge their comprehension of sport exercise processes on the basis of the fundamentals of anatomy. Particular importance is placed on the functions of the muscles and practical, relevant particularities of the passive exercise apparatus.

Finally, the fifth chapter once again presents exemplary training programs for various performance levels and targets. This chapter will give you stimuli on how to systematically tackle your own training program, also in the long term. This fitness manual should not replace your trainer but should rather enable you to become your own best and most important trainer, as nobody knows your body and your maximum strength levels better than you do yourself.

The fitness manual is conceived so that you can commence your exercise program immediately. The clearly laid out exercise catalogue enables speedy orientation so that you can quickly consult the manual, even at an advanced level. A detailed glossary and copies in the enclosure serve to facilitate the practical implementation of the illustrated know-how.

The publisher and the author both wish you lots of fun and every success in the utilization of the fitness manual as an exercise guide or as a reference book.

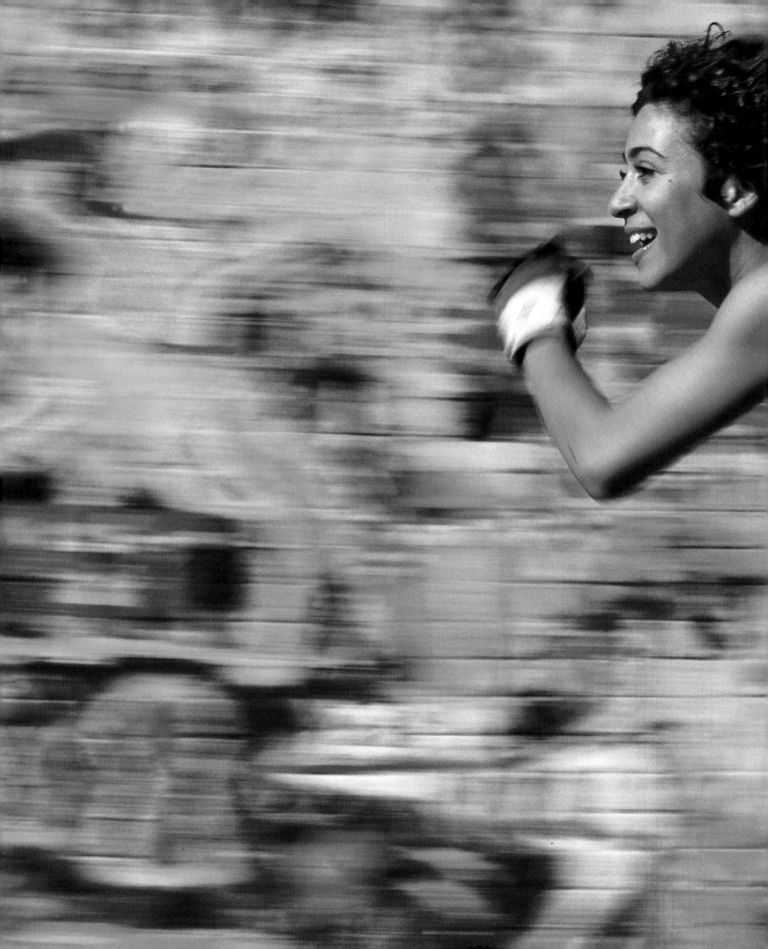

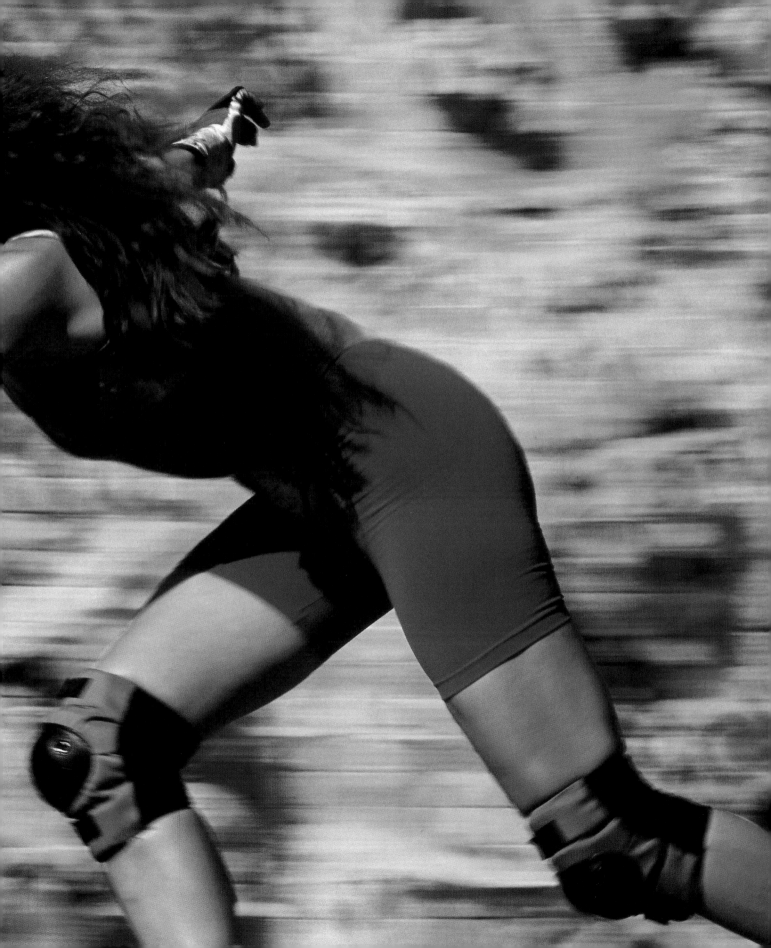

Training Guide

Almost everyone is fascinated by top-ranking athletes. Explosive movements shown in slow motion reveal a musculature which is so taut it seems as if it could tear apart, each fiber standing out under the skin. For a second, each one of us dreams of having such a body. But then you realize that such record performances not only demand a specific genetic predisposition but also a daily training program that is carefully planned – down to the last detail.

If one looks at the matter more closely, one discovers that the hereditary disposition of top-ranking athletes and that of men and women who play mass sports only differs to a slight extent with regard to physical fitness. If, however, one looks at the training program involved then visible differences are revealed. Top-ranking athletes not only, as a rule, commence training several years earlier, but also in most cases train together with an experienced trainer who is tuned in to their physical requirements. The training program is precisely planned in advance and is regularly examined to assess whether the desired results have accordingly been achieved.

The leisure athlete who wishes to increase his/her performance often has no training plan or imitates the training program of a successful athlete. The consequence is often unsatisfactory training progress or even injury due to overstraining with the exercise equipment or of the cardiovascular system. The dream of an optimal and generally applicable "special program" which has been proven in practical tests is therefore understandable. The unimaginable complexity and magnitude of the adjustment stages through which our body passes as a result of a training stimulus means that such a panacea is not possible. Regardless of whether you wish to start training to improve your strength, endurance, speed, mobility or coordination, your starting conditions differ from those, for example, of your neighbor or a top-ranking athlete.

The aim and purpose of a well-guided training program lies in the improvement of performance, whereby the term performance should not be equated with record performance. Naturally, as a leisure sports person you can take up training with the intention of reducing your weight or simply of improving your appearance. An optimization of performance already exists when you, for example,

can run nonstop at the same speed for five minutes longer than you could previously, or when you can do one more push-up than before.

Great progress has been made in the last few years in the science which examines to what extent the human organism can be trained. The human body with its biomechanical leverage conditions is explored in detail as are the biochemical metabolism processes during physical strain. Although some interesting questions in these sectors still have not been answered, much practical help has been derived from the knowledge gained which is primarily utilized by the competitive athlete. Naturally the training principles can be transferred to other people who practice sport in order to improve their performance.

Fitness Check

For each sector of your fitness program (strength, endurance, mobility, speed, coordination) you need to define your position. Besides training-related tests to determine the level of training required, your health should be checked by a physician if you:

- are over 35 years of age
- have not exercised for a long period of time
- are overweight
- suffer from limited mobility
- are taking medication (e.g. beta-blockers)
- suffer from acute or chronic illnesses of the respiratory tract
- suffer from metabolic disease, such as *diabetes mellitus*
- have an inflammation
- have a feverish illness
- have an infectious illness
- have organ damage or an injury
- have high blood pressure
- suffer from a joint disease (chronic, inflamed)
- have painful joints
- or feeling unwell.

If the prerequisites regarding health are fulfilled, then you can begin to set the guidelines of your training program. At the beginning of an optimal training guide your actual physical condition should be determined – as it were your starting point – followed by the determination of targets, the so-called target conditions. Only then can a training plan be compiled which will accompany you from the start start to finish. Finally, regularly examine your training success in order to be able to react to any deviations from the plan and to take corrective measures as necessary. The following illustration shows how the four elements combine to form an effective training guide.

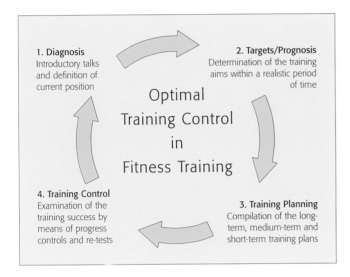

1. Diagnosis/ Actual Physical Condition

In order to be able to develop a program that is tailor-made for you, it is necessary for you to take your measurements. The information for determining your actual physical condition does not only refer to height, waist measurement etc., but data relating to the person, health and performance must also be determined.

- Person-related data: age, gender, type of constitution, weight, proportional body fat, physical measurements, photos, …
- Health-related data: blood pressure, medication taken, orthopedic disease, metabolic disease, acute disease, consequences of an accident, …

- Performance-related data: endurance tests, mobility tests, strength tests. Speed tests are seldom necessary as coordination is trained with correctly performed high-quality exercises.

"Two left hands" in most cases only means a lack of exercise! References to sections which train coordination can also be found under endurance sports.

A test – regardless of whether mental or physical – should always provide a picture of the current level of fitness. For example, if your grade in a math test is unsatisfactory, then the result could be considerably better when the test is repeated a week later, when you have interpreted the test results correctly and have initiated a deliberate program to correct your weaknesses.

In the physical sector a similar procedure is possible. If you test your general endurance and receive a comparable rating which lies 20% under the rating for average fitness, then you can develop a carefully directed strategy (program) which will lead you from an untrained performance level to an average performance level. The test (actual physical condition) consequently forms the basis for achieving a forecasted target condition through planning the current performance level. During the course of the execution of such a plan one must constantly examine whether the performance development results according to plan (analysis) in order to enable corrective measures to be taken as necessary.

In particular the performance-related data does not only enable comparison with a person who has an average standard of training, but above all enables comparison of one's own fitness over a given period of time. The test is repeated every six weeks, the test results then show whether and to what extent the performance has been improved in the previous weeks.

Physical Data

Body weight

For many people the scales decide whether they are happy with their figure or not, whereby a so-called ideal weight or at least normal weight is often aimed at. The best-known formula calculates this standard weight on the basis of height as follows:

- Normal weight: Height in centimeters minus 100
- Ideal weight for women: Normal weight minus 15%
- Ideal weight for men: Normal weight minus 10%

The formula, developed by Broca, reflects an ideal whose relevance in accordance with what we know today can only be applied to a limited extent. Although "more precise" calculation methods have in the meantime become accepted, the impression given by your reflection in the mirror should primarily be of greater relevance than what the scale tells you. However, many people find it helpful to be able to make a comparison to certain standard ratings.

These ratings also include the so-called *Body Mass Index (BMI)*, the proportional *body fat* and also to a certain extent the *Waist to hip ratio.*

Body Mass Index (BMI)

The BMI takes into consideration the dependence of body weight on the body surface area, which, in the opinion of recognized experts, supplies a far more useful standard than the calculation formula of Broca. BMI = current weight (kg) ÷ body height (in m)^2. Example: a man who weighs 70 kg and is 1.70 m tall has a BMI of: $70 \div 1.7^2 = 24.22$.

BMI = Weight (kgs) ÷ Height (in m)^2 Convert weight and height into metric system (1 lb=0.45 kg; 1 ft=0.3 m) **BMI Rating**	Women	Men
Underweight	<19	<20
Normal weight	19–24	19–25
Overweight	>24	>25
Adipose (obese)	>30	>30
Highly overweight	>40	>40

You can interpret your individual rating on the basis of the following table. The following ratings are only of limited relevance when the water distribution deviates highly, that is, caused through illness, as well as for children and senior citizens.

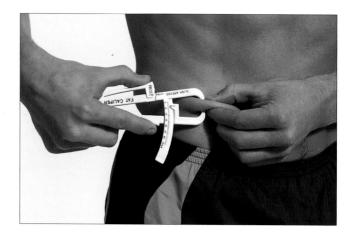

Proportional body fat

The proportional percentage of body fat complements the relevant statement made by the ratings derived from the body weight and height. Although the distribution of fat is of utmost importance, a conclusion can be derived from the following standard age-dependent ratings, at least when great deviations exist in one direction or the other. The proportional body fat can be measured in various ways: the *fat caliper measurement,* or the *infrared measurement* or the so-called *bio-electric impedance analysis* (BIA), – until recently you always needed a qualified assistant to carry out these measurements. However, lately a measurement procedure has been developed on the basis of BIA, which is used in the same way as bathroom scales and is considered sufficiently exact. This method uses a weak, harmless current which is sent through the body. Conclusions can be drawn on the basis of the flow speed of the current with regard to the

Proportional Body Fat Standard ratings for proportional body fat		
Age	Men	Women
17–29 years of age	15%	25%
30–39 years of age	17,5%	27,5%
over 40 years old	20%	30%

composition of the tissue. When the aim of the training program is weight reduction, the proportional body fat is to be classed higher in its relevance than body weight, as primarily fat need to be reduced.

Waist to hip ratio

If, by means of the method quoted, you discover a relative proportional body fat rating which is considerably higher than the standard rating, it is not always dangerous from a health point of view. Through a simple test which you can carry out at home, it is possible to estimate better the risk of heart disease.

For the Waist to Hip Test you should measure the size of your waist above the navel. Do not hold your stomach in but remain easy and relaxed. Furthermore measure your hips at the widest point. Divide the waist measurement by the hip measurement. If the result lies under 0.9 for men and under 0.8 for women then the risk of heart disease is not higher in comparison to the average rating.

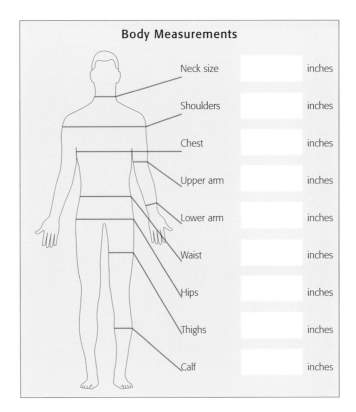

Body Measurements

Neck size		inches
Shoulders		inches
Chest		inches
Upper arm		inches
Lower arm		inches
Waist		inches
Hips		inches
Thighs		inches
Calf		inches

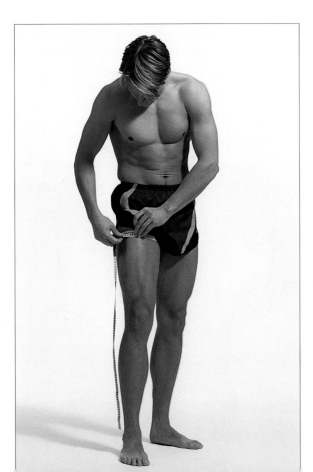

Body Measurements

Once you have determined your waist and hip measurements, it is a good idea to record further measurements. When you repeat these, you will get a reliable picture of whether and how much your figure has changed. Even if taking measurements is somewhat old-fashioned, it is still a very precise method which does not require any assistance. Make sure you always take measurements in the same place and in a relaxed condition; neck size, shoulders, chest, upper arm, lower arm, waist, hips, thighs and calf size.

Photos

A highly effective diagnosis tool that increases motivation is a photo of yourself with very little clothing (bikini or swimming shorts). Have photos taken from the front and from the side. These photos will always remind you of how you once looked. If you have new photos taken after a certain period of time you can compare them, which is far more precise than comparing your current reflection in the mirror with the initial photos.

Types of Constitution

In many areas of daily life different talents and predisposition are seen as interesting and attractive. However, in most cases this does not apply to our different basic types of figures – also known as types of constitution (after Sheldon). Often fate is challenged when one tries to change one's body type by any means possible. It should , however, be made clear that you can never change a "Fred Astaire" type into an "Arnold Schwarzenegger." Equally a "Rubens type" can never become a "Twiggy type." Therefore, before you start a battle that you can never win, you should instead try to make the best of your type. It is anyway questionable whether one should perceive as certain type is worth striving for, as opinions of which type is currently *in* regularly change. In any case, the constitution types described below seldom occur in pure form but almost always occur as an intermediate type.

The leptosome/ectomorphic type

The leptosome type has the following main features:

- tall and slim
- pelvis is wider than the shoulders
- highly mobile joints (hyper-mobility)
- little muscle development (often with poor posture)
- low blood pressure
- high pulse at rest
- on the whole weak circulation (low endurance)
- cold hands and feet, dizziness after quickly standing up
- highly active nervous system
- low metabolism effectiveness (more difficult to put on weight)

The characteristics of the ectomorphic type for the performance of sports, which require strength, strength endurance or endurance, are more unfavorable in comparison to mesomorphic and endomorphic types. Naturally these performance components can be considerably improved through training, and precisely due to these poor conditions, they should in particular be trained.

With regards to their figures, ectomorphic types are often envied by other people. Ectomorphs (leptosomes) *make poor use of nutrition* which means they can eat as much as they want and seldom become overweight.

The athlete/mesomorphic type

The mesomorphic type differs from the other types based on the following characteristics:

- muscular and robust physique
- shoulders are wider than the pelvis
- the fitness of the muscles and the circulation system is very good
- low blood pressure and pulse at rest for active mesomorphic types
- inactive mesomorphic types have higher blood pressure and pulse at rest
- not sensitive to cold
- as a rule good posture
- normal digestion
- fat deposits as a result of inactivity and over-eating arise more in the center of the body

The mesomorphic type can increase his/her fitness considerably with relatively little training as a result of these favorable conditions. Due to the quick ability to improve the muscular

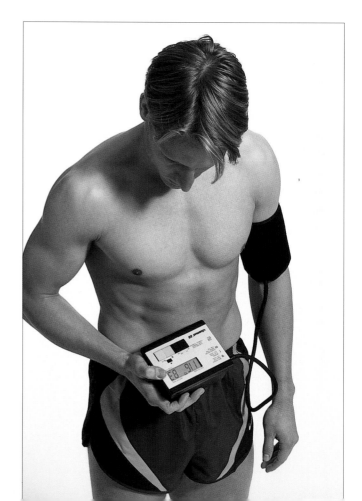

performance and the low capability of the muscles to be lengthened, however, the risk of injury is higher. It is therefore recommended that during training much time be devoted to the maintenance and improvement of the capability of the muscles to be lengthened.

The figure of the active, mesomorphic type, respectively of the athletic type corresponds on the whole to the ideal beauty of the 1980s and the 1990s. Many people consequently attempted to adjust their appearance to match this ideal, even if they are rather more the ectomorphic or endomorphic constitution type which has a very different physique. These attempts are naturally of a limited nature. Those people who refuse to recognize this fact are consequently often permanently frustrated by the continual, more or less unsuccessful struggle to achieve their dream image.

The pyknic/endomorphic type

The endomorphic type mainly differs from the other constitution types based on the following characteristics:

- tends to have fat and a curvaceous body shape
- shoulders are as wide as the pelvis or somewhat wider (mostly concealed by overweight)
- more even weight spread than the other two types
- with regard to physical performance components, lies between the two other types
- posture also lies between that of the ectomorphic type and the mesomorphic type
- good conditions for strength and endurance performance
- good nutrition resorption and slow digestion result in easy weight gain
- low pulse at rest, normal blood pressure (for active pyknics)

The endomorphic type possesses good conditions for the improvement of strength, endurance and mobility. Depending on the circumstances, however, a very high body weight can have an impeding effect. Besides high-quality nutrition suited to the body's requirements, emphasis should be put on endurance training in order to keep the body weight within certain limits.

The endomorphic type has the type of figure which is least envied considering the beauty ideals of today. However, from the above-stated main characteristics it can be seen that at least the active endomorphic type possesses the best health and sport conditions. If the endomorphic type uses his/her genetic potential in a positive way, then being even a few pounds overweight cannot do him/her any damage or injury.

Health-Related Data

In general the interpretation of health related data is and remains a matter for a physician. If, during the start check, you find there is any reason which would make it advisable to consult a physician, then you should not hesitate to make an appointment for a physical check-up immediately. If there are any limitations health-wise, then it is imperative that you get the OK of a specialist before you take up regular sport training. If you do not visit a doctor, then at least you still have a small chance that a strained physical condition will be noticed by your trainer. But, if you train alone, the danger of overstrain or even injury is a foregone conclusion.

Normal blood pressure	120/80 mm Hg
Normal systolic pressure	100 + age (up to max. 160 mm Hg for senior citizens over 60)
Mild hypertonicity	diastolic pressure: 90–104 mm Hg
Moderately severe hypertonicity	diastolic pressure: 105–114 mm Hg
Severe hypertonicity	diastolic pressure: >115 mm Hg
Hypertonicity limit	140–159/90–94 mm Hg
Hypotonicity	<105/65 mm Hg

The initial tests which are often carried out in fitness clubs also include the measurement of blood pressure. It is really surprising how many people have high blood pressure and first learn of it at the gym. If you can determine your blood pressure at home (see photo), then you can examine whether or not your rating is normal on the basis of the following table. *Hypertonicity* means that the rating is too high and *hypotonicity* means that the rating is too low.

Strength Test

The maximal strength test method

As strength plays the dominant role in Olympic weight-lifting, the methods in the training field are related predominantly to maximal strength. Regardless of whether *strength endurance, hypertrophy, speed strength* or strength should be trained, the actual physical condition is determined by the range of *maximal strength.* This makes sense for athletes whose competitive fitness primarily depends on their maximal strength. However, the development of maximal strength should not be a priority for the fitness athlete. Nonetheless, the maximal strength method provides a good model for controlling the strain intensity over a period of several weeks, as it determines a step-by-step increase in the strain within that period. How does it work?

After warming up, a weight is selected for the exercise to be performed, with which exactly one repetition can be completed and not be repeated a second time. The maximum weight determined in this manner forms the basis for calculation for the following weeks of training. The following classifications are then made:

Training target maximal strength
Strain range: 75–100% of the tested maximum performance
Number of repetitions: 1–6
Number of sets: 5–8
Breaks between the sets: 2–5 minutes

Training target speed strength
Strain range: 50–70% of the tested maximum performance
Number of repetitions: 6–10
Number of sets: 4–6
Breaks between the sets: 1–4 minutes

Training target strength endurance
Strain range: 25–50% of the tested maximum performance
Number of repetitions: 20 to over 30
Number of sets: 3–5
Breaks between the sets: "worthwhile breaks," that means the pulse rate returns to 130.

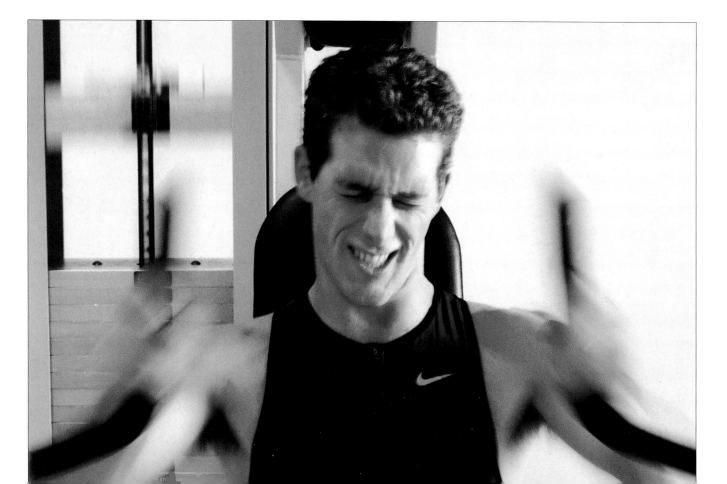

Individual Performance Chart Method (IPC Compilation)

The variouss components of the maximal strength method are not all optimally suitable for the athlete who wishes to train his/her fitness and who primarily not just aims to improve his/her maximal strength. Although the implementation of these components in the training plan provides a variation in the intensity of the training, as the resistance – regardless of the respective test weight – increases continuously over a period of several weeks, whereby the waviness of the biological adjustment processes is taken into consideration (see "Strain control in accordance with the IPC method"). However, the risk of injury during the test, through maximum weight, is comparatively high and the range of exercises with which a maximal strength test can be carried out is relatively limited (it is difficult to imagine a maximal strength test for isolated, single joint movements).

Overview of the execution of the IPC method		
Step 1	Selection of the training target and the corresponding number of repetitions, and the exercises	Strength endurance: 15–25 repetitions Hypertrophy: 10–12 repetitions Maximal strength: 5–8 repetitions
Step 2	IPC test with the corresponding number of repetitions: 1. general warming up 2. special warming up 3. one test set with the prescribed number of repetitions	Hypertrophytraining, e.g.: Bench presses, 10 repetitions with 175 lbs Flyings, 12 repetitions with 35 lbs Horizontal rowing, 10 repetitions with 110 lbs etc.
Step 3	Translation of the test results into the training plans	Selection of the training intensity on the basis of the rough frame (see "Strain control in accordance with the IPC method")

As a result, an alternative test method was developed more than ten years ago by the BSA Academy, a German training institute in the fitness sector, which has the advantages of the classic test method but which also avoids some of its disadvantages: the individual performance chart method (IPC method). The idea which led to its development is fairly simple: as there are athletes with mainly fast-twitch muscle fibers, athletes with mainly slow-twitch muscle fibers and various intermediate types, a considerably more individual strain control is achieved when precisely that strain range which should subsequently be trained is tested. Consequently, if strength endurance is to be trained, then maximal strength endurance is tested. The same applies to hypertrophy and strength. In principle each exercise in the training plan is simply tested with the number of repetitions aimed at in the best possible quality of movement.

If the disadvantages of the maximal strength method are compared with the properties of the IPC method, one can see that as a result of the individual approach of the IPC test, all disadvantages of the classic test method can be avoided. The risk of injury through a maximal strength test can be ruled out. The problem of no longer being able to test certain exercises also does not arise. An isolated movement which, for example, can be applied in muscle development training is not tested with a maximum repetition but with a precisely planned number of repetitions with a corresponding quality of movement. Even the most serious disadvantage of the maximal strength test – the lack of consideration of the different muscle compositions of people – is avoided, as precisely those performance components of the musculature are tested which are subsequently trained.

The practical implementation of the individual steps of the IPC method can be seen in the table above. An assistant should always be available to secure the weight during execution of the tests.

Endurance Test

Please note that if you suffer from one of the following circumstances, the endurance test should in general not be executed or should only be executed under medical supervision:

- acute and chronic disease of the respiratory tract
- feverish illness
- infectious illness
- high hypertonicity
- organ damage or injury (e.g. of the heart or lung)
- inflammation
- taking medication (e.g. beta-blocker)
- feeling unwell

The endurance test which is probably most often mentioned in sports literature is the so-called Cooper Test. The aim of the test is to cover as long a level distance as possible in a quick nonstop run within a period of 12 minutes, although walking is allowed for a time when the athlete feels overstrained. As far as is possible, however, one should not stand still. The distance covered is recorded and compared with the Cooper Test Table. This table shows the current performance level.

This test has the advantage that it can be carried out without assistance, provided that a suitable running track and a stopwatch are available. A disadvantage is that the test requires a certain experience of running and that the test results can be falsified through the test person's capacity not being deployed to the fullest or through premature exhaustion. In addition, this test is only recommended for advanced athletes as his/her capacity should be deployed to the maximum. In case of discomfort (pain, dizziness, nausea, etc.) the endurance test should be stopped immediately.

A further endurance test which can be carried out without any assistance is the Harvard Step Test (see *Fixx*) for which you ideally need a heart rate meter, a stopwatch and a step or bench. If you do not have a

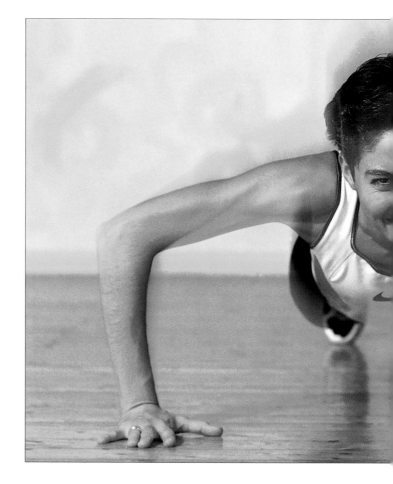

Cooper Test		Distance in miles, M = male, F = female			
Age		20–29	30–39	40–49	50–59
very good	M	1.64–1.75	1.56–1.68	1.53–1.64	1.44–1.57
	W	1.34–1.44	1.30–1.38	1.24–1.33	1.18–1.29
good	M	1.50–1.63	1.45–1.55	1.40–1.52	1.30–1.43
	W	1.22–1.34	1.18–1.29	1.11–1.24	1.06–1.17
average	M	1.31–1.48	1.30–1.45	1.24–1.38	1.16–1.30
	W	1.11–1.22	1.06–1.17	0.98–1.19	0.93–1.05
weak	M	1.21–1.30	1.17–1.30	1.13–1.23	1.–1.16
	W	0.96–1.19	0.94–1.05	0.88–0.97	0.83–0.92
very weak	M	<1.20	<1.17	<1.13	<1.02
	W	<0.96	<0.94	<0.88	<0.83

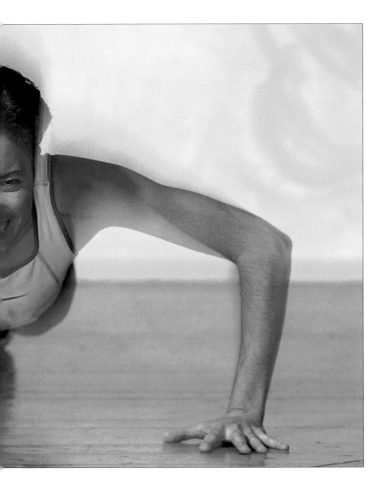

Harvard Step Test

Height	Step height
<4ft. 9in.	1 ft.
<5ft. 3in.	1ft. 2in.
<5ft. 7in.	1ft. 4in.
<5ft. 9in.	1ft. 7in.
>6 ft.	1ft. 6in.

pulse a + 3000 divided by pulse b + 3000 divided by pulse c = endurance index. For example, if your pulse on completion of the strain is 160 (pulse a), after one minute is 120 (pulse b) and after two minutes is 100 (pulse c), then the following endurance index is calculated:

3000 divided by 160 = 18.75
3000 divided by 120 = 25.00
3000 divided by 100 = 30.00
Endurance index = 18.75 + 25.00 + 30.00 = 73.75

With the help of the index below, the results of the endurance test will enable you to plan your training and to estimate whether you should train in the lower or upper pulse range recommended.

pulsimeter, you can also test your heart rate by feeling your carotid artery with your fingertips. The height of the bench or step should depend on your own height.

For this test you should step up and down on the bench in two-second intervals for a period of four minutes. It does not matter whether you alternate the leg with which you step up or whether you execute the whole set with the same leg. After four minutes, you immediately measure your heart rate (pulse), and then again after exactly one minute and again at two minutes after completion. You therefore have three figures which you then insert in the following formula: 3000 divided by

Endurance index (evaluation)

	under 35 years of age	over 35 years of age
<50	insufficient	unsatisfactory
51–60	unsatisfactory	sufficient
61–70	sufficient	satisfactory
71–76	satisfactory	good
77–85	good	very good
86–90	very good	excellent
>90	excellent	absolutely first-class

Mobility Test

Although no training guide and planning is customary for mobility training as is for muscle-building or endurance, it is nevertheless necessary to determine your actual physical condition. Depending on how you use your body in your day-to-day life, not only do certain strength conditions of the muscles result which are necessary for the movement of a joint, but also certain mobility conditions.

In particular a sedentary way of life forces certain muscles into a shorter state, while others are forced into a longer state. If we change our posture, the shortened muscles and the joints which they surround, pull us into an undesired flexed position. The opposite muscles can barely oppose this tension, as they have constantly been in a longer state during the period of sitting, and therefore tend to become slack. While the weakened muscles require particular strengthening, the muscles which have a tendency to shorten should be regularly stretched. Whether your muscles also need strengthening and stretching should first of all be examined.

The muscle function tests described cannot replace medical diagnostics if you have orthopedic problems. These tests are also defined as "semi-objective" procedures and are not an exact measurement of mobility. They are, however, sufficiently precise for someone who wishes to train his/her fitness and who wishes to gain information on the mobility of his/her musculature. You will require the assistance of a second person for the execution and interpretation of the results of the muscle function tests, who should also be familiar with the precise conditions of the tests. Ideally, the test should be carried out by a fitness trainer who has had experience of these tests. You will also require a somewhat higher, stable bench or a stable table as well as a tape-measure. All tests are carried out without warming-up previously.

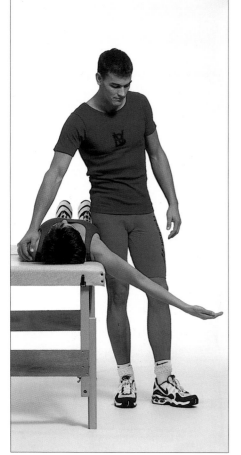 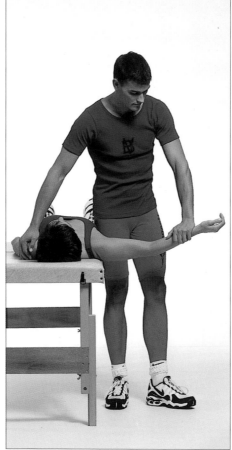

Chest musculature *(m. pectoralis major)*

- Initial position: The test person lies on a bench on their back. Their body is positioned with the body length along the edge of the bench so that the arm, on the side of the body to be tested, can hang freely over the edge.
- Test execution: The examiner or the trainer can stabilize the body by holding down the opposite shoulder or the thorax.
- Assessment: The angle which is formed between the arm which is stretched out sideways and the body level supplies information on the extent of the mobility of the greater pectoral muscle *(m. pectoralis major)*.
- Evaluation: The upper arm falls below the horizontal = good.
  The upper arm does not reach the horizontal fully, only after light pressure has been applied = slightly shortened.
  The upper arm turns inwards, whereby the shoulder moves upwards = highly shortened.

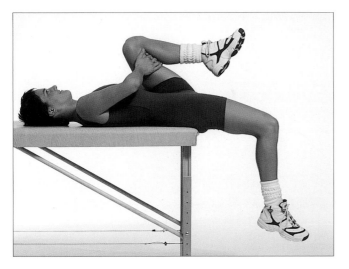

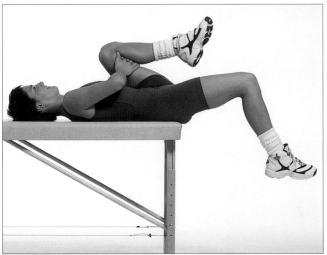

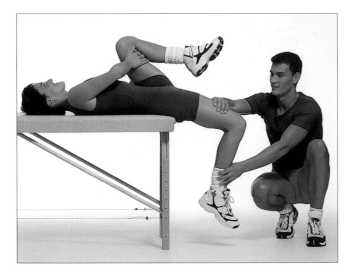

Hip flexors *(m. iliopsoas)* **and rectus thigh muscle**

- Initial position: The test person lies on his/her back on a couch or on a box whereby the buttocks touch the front edge. One leg is held with both hands by the person being tested in the hollow of the knee and drawn up to the chest at an angle. This serves to stabilize the pelvis. The leg that is to be tested hangs loosely flexed over the end of the couch.
- Test execution: The test to determine the mobility of the lumbar ilium muscle takes place in the initial position.
- Assessment: The angle, which is described by the angle of the thigh of the leg to be tested to the table edge, shows the capability of the lumbar ilium muscle *(m. iliopsoas)* to be lengthened. This muscle connects the pelvic bone to the thigh bone and therefore bridges the hip joint.

In order to be able to make a statement on the mobility of the rectus thigh muscle *(m. rectus femoris)* which pulls over the hip and knee joints, the lower test leg is moved towards the bench by the examiner or trainer while, at the same time, the thigh is held in the horizontal position. The angle between the lower leg and the thigh, which is achieved when the examiner applies light pressure, shows the extent of the mobility of this muscle.

- Evaluation lumbar ilium muscle:
  >0° = greatly shortened
   0° = slightly shortened
  <0° = good

- Evaluation rectus thigh muscle (lower leg bent):
  up to 90° = good
        90° = slightly shortened
       >90° = greatly shortened

Biceps of thigh *(m. biceps femoris)* –
Hamstring group

- Initial position: The test person lies on their back on a bench, table or on the floor, the arms are placed at their side beside the body. The examiner uses one hand to stabilize the opposite hipbone or the thigh.

- Test execution: The examiner holds the lower leg of the leg to be tested in their free hand and moves the leg in a out-stretched position upwards.

- Assessment: The height of the out-stretched leg is decisive, without any eva-sive movement of the pelvis, pain due to stretching, trembling or flexible injury in the musculature being noticeable.

- Evaluation:
    >90° = good
    90°–80° = slightly shortened
    <80° = greatly shortened

- Possible mistakes: When the hamstring muscles have a small capability to be lengthened, the pelvis reacts with a compensatory movement or the legs are not both stretched out.

Repeat the tests at regular intervals to determine the actual physical condition, at the latest every three to six months in order to be able to recognize any change in your rating immediately.

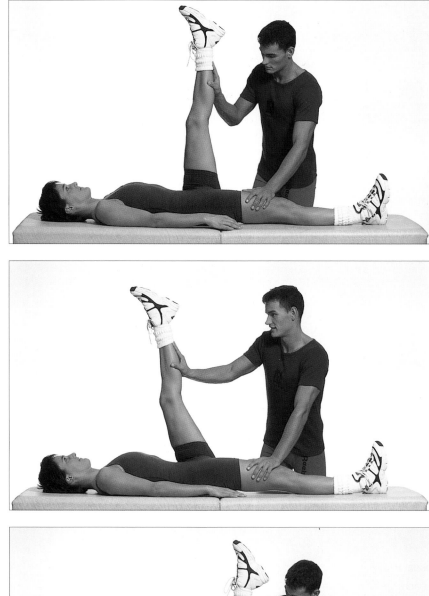

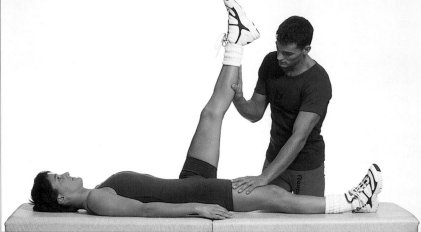

2. Prognosis/Target

In numerous surveys in various fitness centers the most common wishes of beginners recorded include: to reduce weight, to combat back problems, to become stronger and to build up stamina, etc. Often the desire remains unfulfilled because no target is defined ("20 pound weight loss") and no deadline (e.g. by the end of the year) is fixed. But it is only the extent and the period of time that changes a wish into a target. It seems that many people shirk away from defining their wishes because then the wishes become quantifiable. This, however, is the biggest advantage of setting up definite goals.

With a definite goal in mind, you will be able to establish the necessary framework for achieving it. If arriving at your goal requires exercising three times a week, you will have to allow yourself the adequate time to do so. With every intermediate goal you reach, motivation and the will not to give up will grow and help you to make it to the final goal. In order to reach every single intermediate stage and your final goal, you have to pay attention to setting up a realistic time frame. Even if it is theoretically possible to loose 20 pounds of body weight in six weeks, it is not advisable if you aim for a constant loss of weight.

Ideally, it is best to have the support of an experienced trainer who could help you with weight reduction, building up muscles or strength, improvement of cardiovascular fitness and the stabilization of your body posture. He can realistically assess which targets can be made in a certain period of time, taking into account your personal natural aptitudes and your body data. If you do not have a coach, the following numerical values in the table can give you a rough outline.

The values refer to an increase in weight by increasing the muscle tissue and is calculated from the beginner's level, assuming favorable conditions. If conditions are not as favorable, noticeably lower values are reached. There are exceptions where the peak values are surpassed due to exceptional natural ability and favorable training conditions. The progress to be made after the third year of training within the given scale is largely due to hereditary disposition. In general, the additional possible muscle growth reduces year by year until the genetic limit is reached.

With regards to weight reduction, between half a pound to one pound of body fat can be reduced – under favorable conditions – in one week in a healthy way. Not taking small variations into account, the body weight can be reduced relatively steadily to a "normal" value. Substantial weight loss can, of course, be effected relatively easily, but they consist mainly of muscle tissue and water. If you act in such an extreme manner, the reduction of body weight will often stagnate because the metabolism slows down before the desired fat reduction has taken place.

With regards to increases in strength and cardiovascular fitness, a prognosis in numerical values is even more difficult. If someone starts off with a slight deficit in strength or stamina, it should be possible to reach average or normal values within the

Muscle growth per training year		
	Women	Men
1st year	up to 7 pounds	up to 11 pounds
2nd year	up to 5 pounds	up to 7 pounds
3rd year	up to 2 pounds	up to 5 pounds
… year	1–2 pounds	2–5 pounds

first six months of training. If the deficit is more substantial, an approach to the average takes up to one year. People who are already in average or better shape should base their target on the previous training cycles. Here again – as in muscle training – the beginner's possible success rate is significantly higher than the success rate you can achieve later. A decreasing progress rate should therefore be taken into account when fixing specific goals. As far as suppleness is concerned, specific targets are also possible. Especially if the muscles' functional analysis shows shortening in one of the muscle groups, you should add about six months with special flexibility exercises to your training schedule so that those deficits can be balanced.

3. Training planning

Supercompensation/over-training

Training means exertion that leads to a reduction of energy reserves and thus to a reduction in performance. This reduction can only be stopped and compensated for if the organism has enough opportunity to recuperate. It is therefore necessary to rest. A sensible training schedule not only contains an appropriate exertion phase but also sufficient time for recuperation. Exertion and recuperation work together.

The real success of training is an improvement in performance which is due to the fact that – if the preceding training stimulus was strong enough – the effect of the exertion is not only compensated but compensated beyond the original level of performance (in specialist terminology: it is "supercompensated").

If the next training stimulus occurs in the phase of supercompensation (Fig. 1, Phase 3), the result is a steady increase in per-

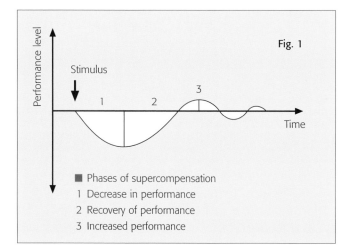

Fig. 1

■ Phases of supercompensation
1 Decrease in performance
2 Recovery of performance
3 Increased performance

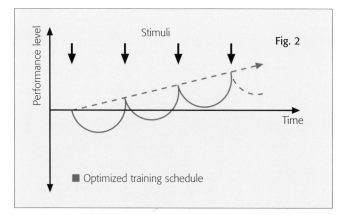

Fig. 2

■ Optimized training schedule

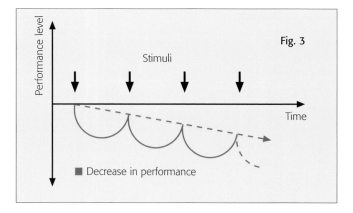

Fig. 3

■ Decrease in performance

formance (Fig. 2). As there are no measuring methods available that allow an exact determination of the period of supercompensation, it is the central task of an optimized training schedule to do this. This task is – among other things – complicated by the fact that the exhaustion caused by training is subject to numerous variables, e.g. the amount of training, number of sets and repetitions, duration of intervals, weights, etc. Moreover, the recovery period for the different muscles after a training stimulus varies, so that a small muscle may be already ready for training again while a larger muscle has not yet completely recovered.

To plan training sensibly, it is advisable to take into account and keep as many variables as possible constant over a limited training period. Thus, the exhaustion during this period is caused by training intensity measured against the amount of weights moved. If all other variables are constant, and no progress is made, only the intensity of the training has to be changed and the effect of the training progress tested.

Fig. 3 shows the result of not waiting for the adequate time after exhaustion: If the next training stimulus takes place before complete recovery, the starting level for the next training exhaustion automatically decreases. If this happens several times, the performance decreases. The first step to fight such a state of overtraining is a break of several days. After the break, it is easy to see if the original performance has returned. A good indicator for the assessment of overtraining is not only a stagnating or decreasing of performance, but also an increased pulse at rest. Moreover, there is a higher risk of injury.

Periodization in Strength Training

In order to avoid overworking the body and to make steady progress, it is advisable not to concentrate the exercising on one area for longer than four to six weeks. A regular change of the training schedule in this pattern is called periodization. This means that one mesocycle corresponds to one period of several weeks. A single training unit is called a microcycle. The so-called macrocycle is a longer planned period and contains several mesocycles, e.g. one year or six months of training.

With regard to weight training a mesocycle is a training schedule that is designed to improve the main areas of muscular endurance, hypertrophy or strength, using the principle of periodization. Below is a description of the different areas.

Muscular endurance

Muscular endurance is called for in the 400-meter sprint. The training of muscular endurance requires a certain set duration and a certain number of repetitions. Equally important is the duration of the break. When an advanced stage of fatigue is reached the muscle develops *lactic acid* that causes the characteristical burning in the muscle. One of the main effects of the muscular endurance training is to increase the tolerance towards the hyperacidity of the muscle. For that, various acid buffers are created which are able to neutralize part of the lactic acid. Therefore, it takes the muscle longer to show an acid reaction and the muscles continue working for several additional seconds or repetitions before refusing to continue.

Hypertrophy

According to current findings, the growth of the *muscle cell* is caused by a long and sufficiently intensive tension stimulus. The high-energy *phosphate compounds* in the muscle cell are exhausted down to a minimum. This causes the cell nucleus to produce new *protein chains* that increase the muscle cross-section in the form of muscle filaments.

Maximal strength

The maximal strength of a muscle depends, apart from the size of the muscle cross-section, mainly on how many *muscle fibers* can be used simultaneously in a movement. The cooperation between *nerves* and *muscles* determines the power efficiency of the muscle.

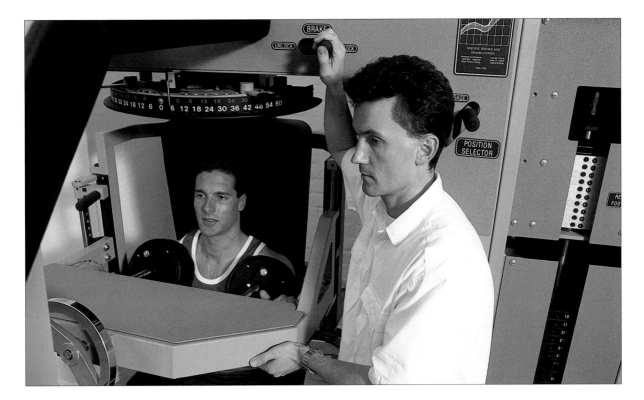

Periodization in Endurance Training

In endurance sports the approach to training success control comes from competitive sports. Here too the leisure-time athlete can profit from adopting certain basic training principles of the professional athlete. Whereas in weight training the weight and the number of repetitions are good indicators for the quantity of exertion, in endurance training there is a comparatively more exact way of measuring exertion: the *heart rate* (*HR*, see picture on right-hand page; exact measurement of heart rate with a chest sensor). Even when at rest, the heart rate tells us something about the person's state of fitness. When under stress, additional interesting aspects develop. To make specific recommendations for the training heart rate, it is advisable to know the maximum heart rate. It can be found out by using various tests that lead to a maximum strain on the cardiovascular system. Thus this cannot be freely recommended to the occasional athlete.

The theoretical maximum heart rate can be determined by the following formula: "Maximum heart rate (MHR) = 220 minus age."

On the basis of this formula, the optimal pulse range for cardiovascular training is between 70 and 85 per cent of the maximum heart rate, for fat metabolism training between 60 and 70 per cent, depending on age. In endurance sports different stress methods can be defined. The training theory distinguishes between:

- *Endurance Method*
- *Interval Method*
- *Repetition Method*
- *Competition Method*

In leisure-time sports the endurance method and sometimes the interval method are mainly used. Repetition and competition methods mean a training load similar to that in competitions with a very high or maximum exertion. They can therefore not be recommended for the leisure-time athlete.

The endurance method is characterized by an effective exertion that continues over a longer period of time without interruption. It is applied automatically by most of the leisure-time athletes with more or less training effect, provided the intensity of the exertion remains within the optimal pulse rate respective of age.

The interval method alternates between exertion and rest intervals. During the rest interval only an incomplete recovery takes place. The endurance training devices in modern fitness training centers allow interval training by means of the so-called hill programs. This can especially be recommended for the advanced endurance training athlete as a supplement to the endurance method. Taking into account that endurance athletes use the endurance method for 80 to 90 per cent of their total training, it should also be of major importance to the leisure-time athlete.

Age	MHR per minute	60% of the MHR per minute	65% of the MHR per minute	70% of the MHR per minute	75% of the MHR per minute	80% of the MHR per minute	85% of the MHR per minute
20	200	120	130	140	150	160	170
25	195	117	127	137	146	156	166
30	190	114	124	133	143	152	162
35	185	111	120	130	139	148	157
40	180	108	117	126	135	144	153
45	175	105	114	123	131	140	149
50	170	102	111	119	128	136	145
55	165	99	107	116	124	132	140
60	160	96	104	112	120	128	136
65	155	93	101	109	116	124	132
70	150	90	98	105	113	120	128

Strain Control by Means of the IPC Method

Apart from the periodization of weight training or a training schedule designed with changing content as a mesocycle with four to six weeks, there is another method to avoid overworking and over-training and to achieve regular training success. This method has been mentioned when describing the strength test and shall be discussed in detail here: the controlling of exhaustion intensity by means of the IPC method.

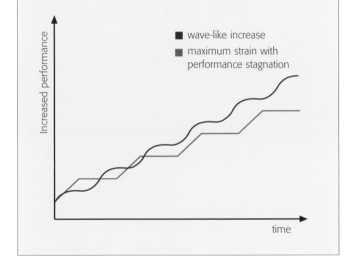

Planned wave-like increase in exertion in comparison to constant maximum exertion with respective performance stagnation

- ■ wave-like increase
- ■ maximum strain with performance stagnation

Increased performance (vertical axis) / *time* (horizontal axis)

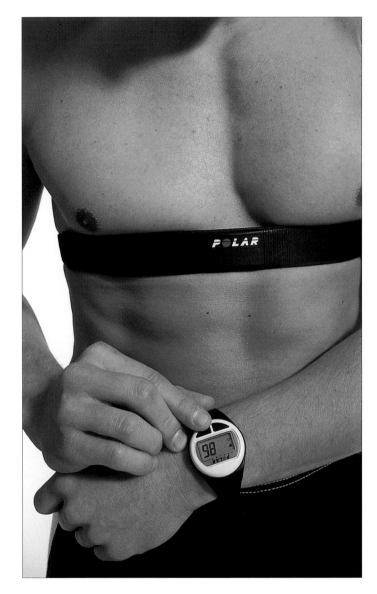

Irrespective of whether you are a leisure-time or a top athlete – if one tries to always exercise with 100 per cent of their available reserves, he will sooner or later realize that this is not the optimal method. Either the performance stagnates or the athlete even injures themselves. In order to understand why the straightest path is not always the quickest, it helps to have a look at other biological processes. You will then realize that all natural processes are subject to a certain rhythm, e.g. womens' monthly cycle, the phases of the moon, the tides, etc. The graph above shows the difference between the attempt to force a regular increase in performance and the deliberate wave-like approach to a higher efficiency level by planned variation of the exertion intensity.

Almost every serious athlete varies the training intensity in the way described, irrespective of the discipline, i.e. they work their way forward in a certain rhythm from a low exertion levels up to a higher intensity step by step. This wave-like increase of the exertion intensity should be considered in the training control of the leisure-time athlete, so that he will be able to exercise in a state of supercompensation throughout the year. On the following page the rough outline for an optimum training plan according to the IPC method is applied in such a way that all training variables, e.g. numbers of repetitions and sets, exercises, etc., remain constant for a training period of four to six weeks. Only the intensity of the strain (weights) is increased for the respective performance level on the basis of the current test result in the course of those weeks (e.g. advanced between 70 and 90 per cent of the test weight). This systematizes the search for the period of supercompensation that the strained muscle needs after training stimulation and makes it easier to identify. In case of a lack in training progress, the intensity is the only "set screw" that needs to be manipulated. The basic principle of the IPC method is: *Optimum for maximum.*

The rough schedule shown below has been developed on the basis of the experience and knowledge of many athletes and training scientists, and is meant to save the leisure-time athlete a couple of unpleasant and superfluous experiences. It is not a specific program from a particular top athlete, but the rough schedule can instead be adapted to individual requirements by several variables:

- It enables a periodisation of the training contents on a four to six week rhythm.
- The level of exertion can be controlled by the intensity of the training. The intensity is newly determined for each training period.
- The athlete is classified according to experience and performance demands.

For the practical use of the rough schedule see chapter *Programs*.

It makes no difference if you are just starting off with weight training or if you have already been exercising for quite some time – the rough pattern allows you to step in at any point. For the

Rough schedule for the optimum training schedule according to IPC method

	Introductory	Beginners	Intermediate	Advanced	Competitive training level
Time level in months	up to 1.5	1.5–6	6–12	12–36	36 and more
Training system	whole body +	whole body +	whole body + and split in two*	split in two*	split in two and three*
Training frequency	2	2	2–3	3–4	4–6
Number of exercises per muscle group	1–2	1–2	2	2–3	2–4
Number of sets per exercise	1–2	1–2	2	2–3	3–4
Repetitions per set	10–12	min. 8, max. 15	min. 8, max. 20	min. 5, max. 25	min. 5, max. 25
Intensity in % of IPC	low	50–70 #	60–80 #	70–90 #	80–100 #

beginner the first six weeks are for orientation, i.e. you first learn the exact technique for the relevant exercises, the correct rhythm of movement and the correct breathing. Only after that introductory phase can you test your muscular endurance. Thanks to the test in the field of higher numbers of repetitions the risk of injury is minimized. People with previous experience of other sorts of training should have their first test in IPC with regard to muscular endurance. Once you have started with this kind of training control, you will also train hypertrophy and maximal strength in the training cycles that follow. Due to the regular testing, you always have an overview of your current performance level which does not only increase your control of the training success but also your motivation.

The individual performance levels of the rough schedule for the optimal scheduling of training as a result of the IPC method are classified according to the duration of the training experience. This sounds plausible straightaway. Nevertheless, even at this stage, a classification that differs from the rough schedule can be necessary. The following comments show why the different frameworks of the individual exhaustion and performance levels should be kept.

Two examples: A twenty-year-old gymnast who has exercised intensively since his sixth year but has never been to a fitness center will certainly feel completely unchallenged after a few weeks with regard to the amount of the training as well as the intensity. A fifty year old manager, who has exercised for five years, but cannot manage to exercise more than twice a week due to professional and family commitments, cannot be classified as a

"serious athlete" regarding frequency. In such cases an experienced coach should adapt the classification. Thus, the gymnast would be able to pass the individual performance levels quicker, while the manager could be upgraded in her training intensity, but could also stick to the framework of the experience level.

One can easily understand that a beginner will not exercise as frequently and extensively as an advanced athlete. Training that is frequent and extensive at the same time can not only lead a beginner to over-training but also to a lack of training success. If a training stimulus is too early regarding the rest curve, this will cause an overload in which an increase of strength or muscles is not possible. It is also obvious that an untrained person should not and cannot exercise too intensively. If one determines the training weights that a beginner should use, one easily gets the impression that he will not feel challenged most of the time in view of such a controlled training.

Example for determination of training weights for beginners

Tested exercise	Leg presses	
Training target	Muscular endurance training with 15 repetitions	
Testing result	15 repetitions with 110 pounds	

Training weights for two sets and 15 repetitions		
1st week	55 pounds	50 per cent of IPC test weight
2nd week	60 pounds	55 per cent
3rd week	65 pounds	60 per cent
4th week	70 pounds	65 per cent
5th week	75 pounds	70 per cent

In order to understand why in the first months of weight training one should exercise below the possible strain level, i.e. to use less weight than possible, it is necessary to compare the adaptability of muscles to the adaptability of tendons, ligaments and cartilage (see graph on following page).

Why does a muscle adapt to a strain stimulus much quicker than, for example, a cartilage tissue or a tendon? As the muscle is supplied with blood by the vascular system up to the individual muscle cell (= muscle fiber) and thus receives fresh oxygen and

Explanations of the table on the left:
+ The whole body training system trains all of the larger muscles in the body directly or indirectly in one training unit.
* If split-training, not all muscle groups are worked in one unit but are split up into two or more units. One distinguishes an A program and a B program. This means if you exercise four times a week as an advanced with a double split, the A program exercises could contain, for example, abdominal, legs, back, biceps, and the B program lower back, chest, shoulders, triceps.
 # The intensity figures do not refer to the one maximum performance but to the maximum performance respective of the exercised number of repetitions.

new nutrients in a quick rhythm, regeneration after an exhausting strain can be induced and carried out relatively quickly. The cartilage tissue (of an adult) or the tendons, however, are not actively supplied with blood. The fiber cartilage of the intervertebral discs, for example, has to rely on a steady change of pressure and suction to be adequately nourished. In an immobile condition it takes much longer to get new nutrients to this cartilage. This explains the frequent overloading injuries and those injuries that occur with athletes training with weight who are too

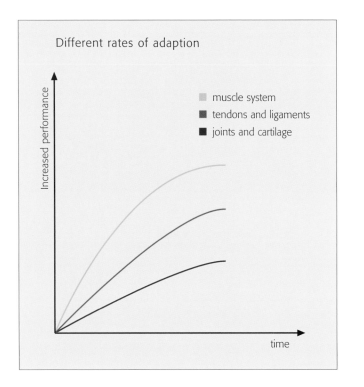

Different rates of adaption

Increased performance

- muscle system
- tendons and ligaments
- joints and cartilage

time

ambitious and motivated and whose target during the first year of training is mainly muscle growth. Especially during this phase, the training scheduling with the rough schedule of the IPC method can be of help to prevent injuries. Only when the passive locomotor system has adapted to the increasing weight strain, an increase in intensity will be effected which strains the muscle in the last weeks of a partial cycle up to the limits of its capacity. Correct technique is, of course, adhered to in those weeks of intensive strain. A training partner can be of use here.

Questions on the IPC method

Although the concept of the Individual Performance Diagnosis Method is logical and very convincing, especially in practical application, questions often arise when putting it into practice. The most important questions are answered below:

Question: "What do I do if I am unexpectedly forced to interrupt my training for a shorter period of time (about a week)?"

Answer: "Normally, if interrupted for one week or less, the training can be continued with the intensity of the last training week before the break. If interrupted a little more than that, it would be advisable to go another week backwards with respect to training intensity."

Question: "What shall I do if I cannot avoid an interruption of several weeks?"

Answer: "Independent of the training cycle in which the interruption takes place, it is recommendable to start with a new training cycle after the break. The testing weight must, of course, be newly determined."

Question: "What do I do if I want to build up strength, for example for better performance in another sport, but if I do not want to build up additional muscle mass. Can I nevertheless make sensible use of the rough schedule of the training scheduling?"

Answer: "To a certain extent the maximum strength that can be reached is bound to the muscle cross-section. Nevertheless, it is possible to acquire an optimal exploitation of strength for a certain muscle volume. In addition, the possibilities for building up muscles definitely depends on nutrition. The strength can be improved at a constant muscle cross-section by establishing priorities in training. For this, the muscle building cycle should either be trained with clearly lower intensity or not at all, i.e. the muscular endurance and power cycles should alternate."

Question: "Is it sensible for me as a woman to exercise with a system that has, amongst others, building muscles and an increase in strength as targets?"

Answer: "The answer is mainly due to your personal target. The targets mentioned most often in modern fitness centers include shaping up of the body and back stabilization which normally requires building up the muscles as well as increasing the strength. For women, even if this increase does not take on the extent of that of a man with a similar target, it nevertheless means regular exercising to get the respective results. Here a well thought-out system like the IPC method can at least save time and frustration or injuries."

Question: "Do I have to do a new IPC test for each of the new training cycles?"

Answer: "Of course, as the last test results were meant for another training cycle with partially different exercises and the last test was effected at a stage when the performance level was lower."

Question: "If I use a split program, do I have to use a separate testing day for each different training day?"

Answer: "Yes, this is advisable because otherwise the fatigue at the end of an individual testing day would result in lower testing weights and therefore training weights."

Question: "Is the testing day not a wasted training day?"

Answer: "No, because as you try to determine the 100 per cent limit, it is highly intensive training. Often, after a testing day, sore muscles occur which can be credited to very intensive strain."

Question: "I cannot exercise more than twice a week because I do not have time. Nevertheless, I would like to improve continually and, after the respective training experience, train with the intensity of the advanced level. Is this goal at all possible?"

Answer: "After at least one year of training with the IPC method, the passive locomotor system of your body will have adapted enough to be able to compensate for the higher training intensities."

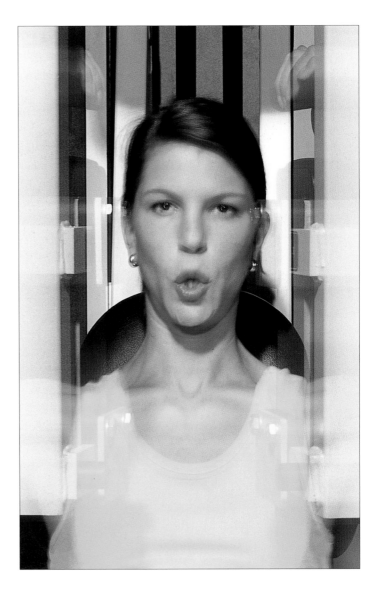

For athletes who exercise constantly but do not want the effort of scheduling training control and therefore do not want to proceed according to the IPC method, there is the possibility to use two of the most important basic principles underlying the method. A periodization of the strain between muscular endurance, hypertrophy and weight training as well as a wave-like control of the training intensity is possible. For periodization, the regular alternation of the strain parameter in a rhythm of four to six weeks is – if need be – enough. The intensity can roughly be classified as light, medium and heavy to very heavy, according to feeling. So if the performance is not tested, one can exercise lightly during the first two weeks of the new training, work out at a medium level for the next two weeks, and train heavily to very heavily for the last two weeks of the cycle. This is only recommendable after one year of training experience, to make sure that you do not overload the passive locomotor system in the last two weeks. Of course, many of the advantages are lost when measuring strain by feeling, but at least the risk of injury and the danger of overloading can be reduced as well as the risk of stagnating in the training progress for a long time.

4. Training Control

The introduced concept of training scheduling needs to be supplemented with what is widely described as training control. The term controlling seems more adequate in the sense of an evaluation of existing data and control of future developments. Even if there is an exact diagnosis and a realistic target, it is always possible that the training schedule which has been drawn up for a mesocycle can only partially be put into practice. This can be subject to several reasons, for example illness, injury, professional needs or other reasons, which can all cause a training interruption. Or perhaps some intermediate goals could have been reached, others not. Here it is necessary to adapt the training schedule for the next mesocycle accordingly.

If you regularly exercise without external influences, you may notice that the training targets that have been planned do not challenge you enough or are too much. The analysis then is similar to an altimeter in a plane: if the altitude differs in either direction, up or down, a correction is necessary so that it will not multiply in one of the directions. A possible reason for extreme discrepancies between the forecasted results and the real results can also be due to mistakes when the tests were conducted.

The Training Diary

Reasons for not achieving intermediate goals can be ascertained more easily by means of a training diary rather than by reconstructing possible disturbances from memory. The training diary should, beside the data of the training schedule, contain details about nutrition, additives, resting intervals, sleep, special events, etc. An appointment with the dentist or preparing for an examination can influence training results, for instance.

The example given is for your own records. You will find a copy for use in the appendix. According to your individual goals, it can be supplemented by further details like nutritional data, measurements or the things you consider important for the assessment of your training. By early adaptation of the training schedule to special circumstances, you can avoid training standstills and aim at further continuous improvements. Possible adaptations include among others: changes of training intensity, changes in the exercise order, repeated tests and resulting new training schedules.

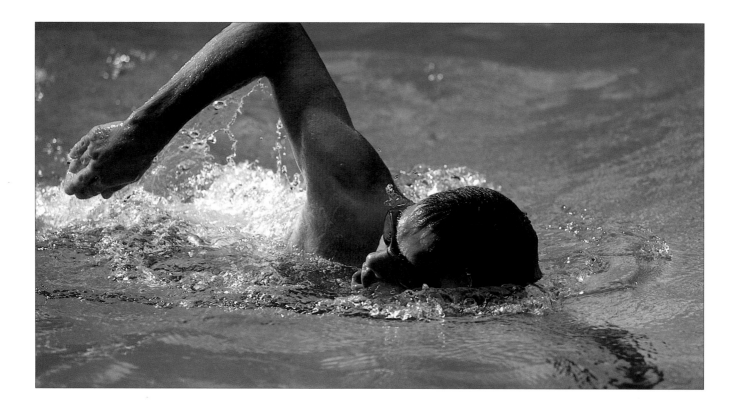

Training

| | Date | **May 27** | | Body Weight | **166 pounds** |

Muscle Area	Exercise	Sets	Repetitions	Weight per Set		
Trunk	Abdominal Crunches	3	15	/		
Legs	Leg Presses	3	15	120	120	120
Chest	Chest Presses	3	16	52.5	52.5	52.5
Shoulder	Lateral Raises	2	15	7.5	7.5	

Training Duration **40 min**

Aerobic Activities

Training Device/Kind of Sport	Duration	Strain in Watt/Level	Starting Pulse	Intermediate Pulse	Termination Pulse	Recreation Pulse
Bicycle	10	125 Watt	68	130	143	/
Stepper	30	Level 7	95	146	139	103

Total Training Duration **40 min**

Rest Intervals

From	To	Duration	Comments
23:30	5:00	5.5 h	
	Total	5.5 h	

Training Control – Summary

- Before you start, find out if taking up fitness training is a risk to your health.
- Determine your starting position in terms of strength, endurance and flexibility, speed and coordination.
- Draw up realistic training targets for yourself taking your body data into account.
- Plan your training for longer periods (e.g. six to twelve months).
- Divide the long-term training schedule into partial cycles (mesocycles) of four to six weeks.
- Alternate the mesocycles of your strength training schedule regularly between the focus on muscular endurance, hypertrophy and strength (maximal strength).

- Alternate the respective training schedule for the individual endurance sports regularly between *short-term, medium* and *long-term endurance.*
- Increase training intensity in your strength training and endurance in the course of a mesocycle. Start each first phase of a new partial cycle with relatively low intensities.
- Check regularly if your training is still in line with your main targets. If not:
  - change your next mesocycle in time
  - repeat the initial tests already described regularly
  - and execute further in-between tests at the end of each mesocycle to evaluate your training.

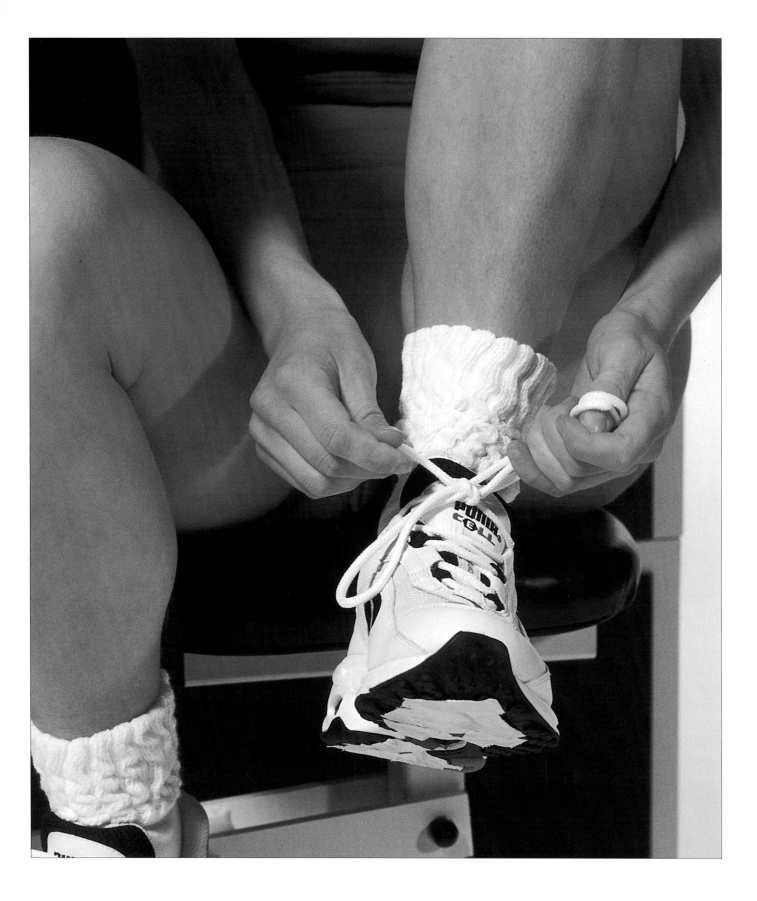

TRAINING SESSION

The Training Session

The average leisure-time athlete trains one-and-a-half-hours twice a week. This investment in time must be exploited to the fullest extent. All the elements, which contribute towards an effective training program, must be taken into account and coordinated. Of course, there are considerable exceptions to these average values, but even for athletes who spend considerably more or less time on their training the given guidelines are relevant. The breaking up of a training session into different sessions with specified aims, such as endurance training, strength, etc., is especially relevant for athletes who spend more time than average training. If you aim to improve the whole of your physical performance, the training units should build up logically and then you will achieve the best possible results.

The perfect training session:
1. Warm-up
2. Strength training
3. Endurance training
4. Mobility training
5. Cool down
6. Regenerative measures

It does not matter how short or long your training session is, there is no avoiding a thorough warm-up. The following text explains the changes and stages your body goes through in this phase as well as providing practical advice for your warm-up session.

Your body is ready to perform at the end of the warm-up session. Now is the time for weight training. Your long- and short-term energy store that your body needs for weight training is still full. The success of your weight training depends to a large degree on the efficient cooperation of your brain, nervous system and muscles. The efficiency of weight training after an endurance training unit is noticeably less. Due to fatigue, the danger of injury is also increased, and for this reason endurance training should definitely be done after weight training.

In order to achieve measurable improvement in endurance and for your body to adapt, a training period of at least one hour per week is recommended. This hour should be divided into two half-hour sessions or at most five 12-minute training units per week. If, for example, you train three times per week, your weight lifting should be followed by endurance training for 20 minutes. For the optimal improvement in heart circulation, you should plan a total time of three hours per week, which you should divide into between three and six training sessions.

You should also spend enough time on the development of your suppleness. Important for effective training is that, after weight training, you train the suppleness of your muscles in the same session. Thus you avoid leaving your muscles partially contracted and also avoid permanent shortening of the muscles. You can do this in a separate unit after endurance training, or as described in the chapter on "Mobility," or do a stretching exercise for the trained muscle between each weight training exercise. Another alternative is to end the endurance training with the cool-down and finish the training session with stretch exercises.

In the warm-up and cool-down phases you should reduce your bodily functions down to their normal speed. In the appropriate chapter you will find a description of how the cool-down phase can mark the turning point between training induced exhaustion and recuperation of physical resources. Recovery which started with the warm-up can be continued with regenerating measures. By using this method, your body will be capable of achieving improved training results sooner.

Even if you are only doing weight training or if your aim is simply to become stronger, you should warm up and cool down, work on your suppleness and finally enjoy a recovery period at the end of your session.

Warm-Up

The frequently neglected but nevertheless extremely important warm-up prepares the body for the exercise to come and helps it to perform without the danger of injury. The following advantages are attributed mainly to warm-up.

• General improvement of performance potential
• Improved physiological performance potential
• Improvement of physical coordination
• Reduction of injury danger

However, warm-up is not simply warming up. It can be divided into three phases.

• General warm-up
• Individual warm-up
• Special warm-up

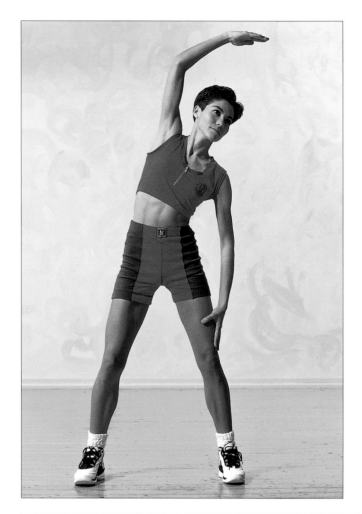

The general warm-up should improve the circulation, increase the body temperature and stimulate the sweat production. Due to the increased body temperature, the blood and lymph fluid in the muscles thin and becomes fluid, elasticity of the muscles is increased and the danger of injury reduced. The increased circulation improves the supply of oxygen and energy to the muscles, which results in an improvement in performance. The general warm-up phase should last between eight and 12 minutes with low to middle exertion and can be done in a fitness center, for example, on the exercise cycle, stepper or treadmill. The general warm-up should not be neglected when you are outdoors. Running or cycling, for example, should be done with low exertion for ten minutes. A low to middle rate of exertion should be kept up, in other words, the heart frequency over a period of about ten minutes is gradually increased as exertion is increased. A 40-year-old athlete should at the end of a warm-up session have increased the pulse rate to 120 to 140 beats per minute (160–180 beats per minute minus age in years). Do not stretch out the general warm-up phase longer than 12 minutes, because then general fatigue and energy loss can start to take place which can impede the training to follow.

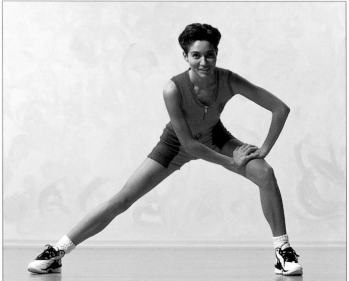

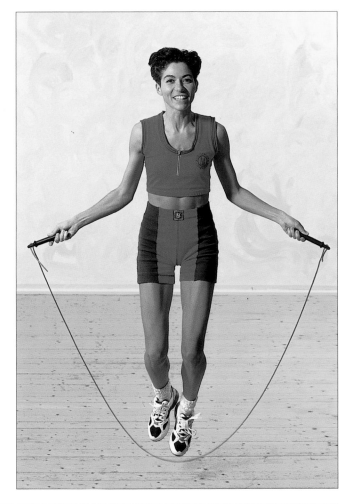

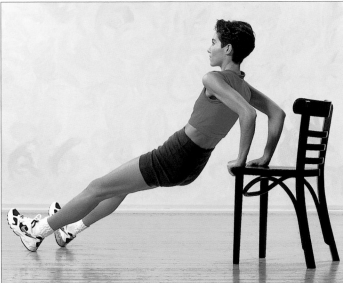

The individual warm-up is suited to the individual's personal requirements and preferences. All elements such as capabilities, limitations such as old injuries, age, etc. must be taken into account. An athlete who has shortened certain muscles should stretch them in the warm-up phase and exercise the appropriate joints. Generally those who have no physical limitations can also stretch the muscles which they will later train and the joints which will be used.

The special warm-up for weight training should specifically prepare the muscles, the joints and the cartilage for the exertion to follow. The synovial fluid is produced in large amounts during warm-up, which not only reduces friction but also enhances the cartilage elasticity. The cartilage absorbs the synovial fluid. In addition the cartilage thickens, increasing its puffer capacity and surface area, which leads to a better distribution of pressure. The coordination between the nervous system and the muscles is also substantially improved through a special warm-up. The simplest way to warm up the muscles that will be specifically trained, is to do the planned exercise with a substantially lighter weight and with more repetitions. For example: if you want to do ten bench presses with 120 pounds, your special warm-up should entail 20 repetitions of 60 pounds, after a break of about 90 seconds again 15 repeats with 90 pounds, and then after an additional break, the training unit of 120 pounds and 10 repetitions.

Theoretically, we should add the mental warm-up to the three phases. The athlete concentrates on the coming training session and makes the transition from the mental preoccupation with small and larger everyday problems to the selflessness of repetitive exercise. Successful athletes visualize their training program during their mental warm-up, that means they imagine the coming training. A high jumper sees the complete movement including the final jump by intensely visualizing the real movements, in combination with slight physical suggestions. The best high jumpers say that they are unable to successfully complete a jump attempt if they are interrupted in this concentration phase. The mental preparation is not only to be recommended for the professional athlete but also for the leisure-time athlete whose performance improvement can be helped and the danger of injury substantially reduced.

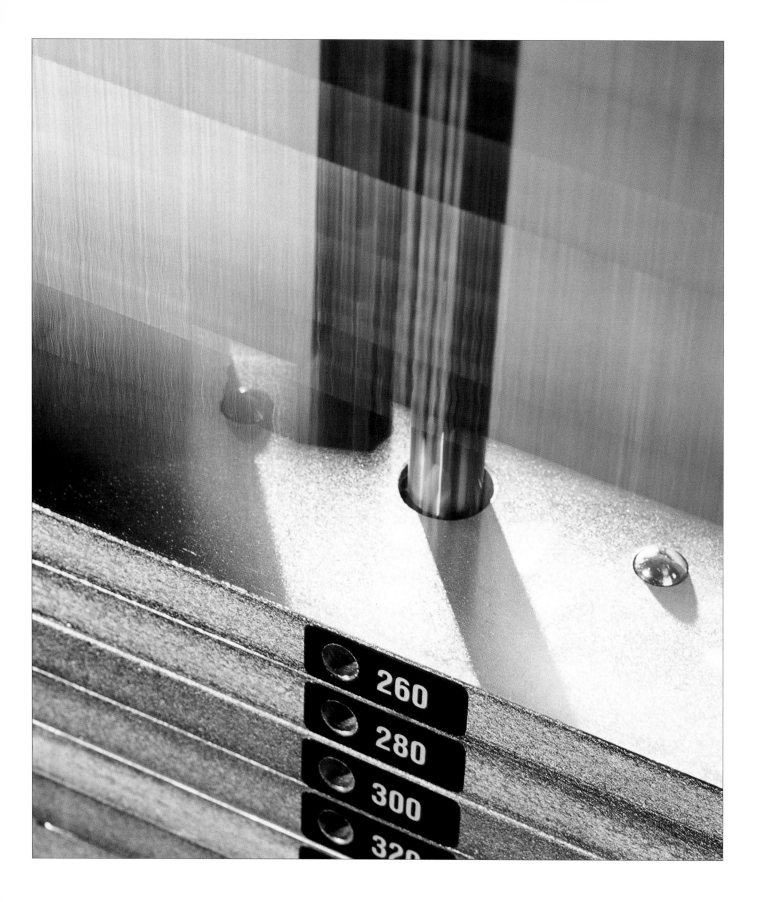

260

280

300

320

STRENGTH TRAINING

Strength Training – How Does It Work?

Mechanically seen, every muscle, muscle cell and muscle fiber has only one purpose: to contract. The muscles work according to an absolute principle, in other words a single muscle fiber either contracts with the full power at its disposable or it does not contract at all. When the stimulus that comes from the nervous system is done arbitrarily and is strong enough, it leads to a total contraction of the muscle. If the stimulus is too weak, however, the muscle will only be passively moved. The part of the musculature that allows movement of the limbs is called the skeletal muscle. In contrast to the cardiac muscle tissue or so-called smooth musculature, which can be found in veins or in the digestive system, the skeletal musculature, also known as diagonal musculature, is controlled by willpower.

The supporting frame of a body, the skeleton, is composed of approximately 210 single bones which are connected to each other by moveable joints. The joints are bridged by at least two muscles that are joined to the bones by tendons. If the muscle contracts due to an order from will, the power is transmitted through the nerve to the moveable bone. Once the muscles have moved together as close as possible, the working muscle, also called the *agonist,* cannot change the movement any more because it can only contract actively but not release. To separate these muscles, an opposite power is necessary. This power is provided by the muscle on the opposite side of the joint. This muscle which can counter the movement of the agonist is called the *antagonist.*

If several muscles in a joint contract in the same direction, they support each other with their combined strength and they are referred to as *synergists.* The joining point between the muscle and bone through the nerve is called the base or origin. The origin is generally nearer to the middle of the body and an unmovable joining point, whereas the base is generally further away from the body's middle and is joined to moveable parts.

Every single one of the over 400 skeletal muscles can move a joint in a specific way. This movement depends on the specific construction of the joint as well as the exact position of the base and origin of the muscle.

You can find further details in the chapter "Anatomy". In order to choose a particular exercise to train a muscle or a group of muscles it is only necessary to know which function the muscle carries out, that means with which joint and in which way a

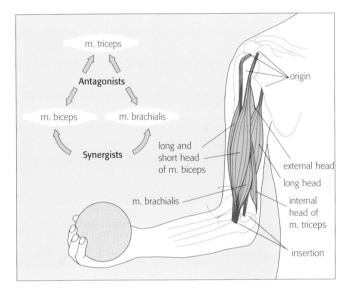

A muscle (agonist) with opponent (antagonist) and fellow players (synergist) are displayed by bending the arm and the arm musculature.

movement is carried out. Thus, the best exercise for a muscle group can be chosen and additionally you know which muscles are involved in the movement. In principle the muscles which have the shortest joining distance between the approaching bones are those principally responsible for the movement. The better these muscles are stretched in advance, that means, the longer the contractible length of the muscle is, the more effective the chosen exercise will be.

Avoiding and Combating Weakness

On the following pages, as in the whole strength catalogue of exercises, you will find many references that require an understanding of the muscle's functions. You can supplement your knowledge by looking at the illustrations in the *Anatomy* chapter. The most important advantage of knowing more about the way the muscle to be trained works is that after some weight training experience, you will not only move a weight in a particular direction – externally – but you will also consciously determine which particular muscles – internally – contract. You will notice the difference right away because your ability to consciously move and control each muscle and your awareness of your whole body will be greatly enhanced in every respect. Additionally, you will also use your muscles consciously in everyday life so that your posture will improve.

Beneath the skeletal muscles you find, among other things, muscles that are responsible for posture, as well as muscles which fulfill the primary dynamic functions.

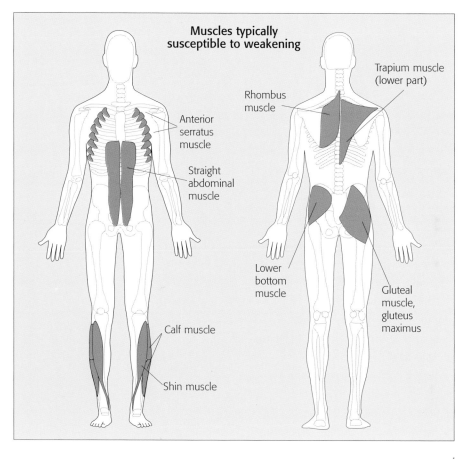

Muscles typically susceptible to weakening

Anterior serratus muscle

Straight abdominal muscle

Calf muscle

Shin muscle

Trapium muscle (lower part)

Rhombus muscle

Lower bottom muscle

Gluteal muscle, gluteus maximus

The posture muscles are called the *tonic musculature,* the dynamic muscles are referred to as the *phasic musculature.* With one-sided, incorrect or too excessive training, pressure is increased in the tonic musculature while accordingly the muscle shortens, whilst the tension in the phasic muscle sinks and is weakened. The resulting imbalance is referred to as muscular *imbalance.* In the chapter *Mobility,* you will find detailed descriptions of which muscles tend to shorten and how to stretch them effectively. In this chapter, however, we are going to deal with the phasic musculature – the muscles which are most susceptible to weakening (see drawing).

Even though the weakening of the muscles can be minimized by specific weight training or physical strengthening exercises, it is recommended that you are indeed aware of the dangers and either eliminate them altogether or at least minimize them to a substantial degree. The following factors can cause a range of problems in the body's muscular balance:

- General lack of exercise
- One-sided working position (e.g. hairdressers, photographers, dentists, etc.)
- Often sitting for long periods of time, especially in furniture not suited to the body's requirements
- Shoes that are not orthopedically suitable
- Born with orthopedic disabilities
- Psychological pressure/stress

Due to the modern lifestyle many people are forced to sit several hours per day. As a result, the muscles which are lengthened and stretched tend to weaken, for example the buttock muscles. In addition, the mobility apparatus is often over-burdened and weakened through one-sided sport. For athletes from different disciplines there are tips on how to avoid one-sided exercise by using complementary exercises in the chapter *Programs.*

Terminology

When you talk to a weight-lifter about their sport, you will soon realize that there is special terminology. Below you will find a introduction to weight-lifting terminology .

Positive Movement Phase or *concentric muscle work:* The phase of a movement that strengthens muscles, in which resistance is overcome, such as when a weight is lifted; it is a positive movement phase or concentric muscle work.

Negative Movement Phase or *eccentric muscle work:* The phase of a movement to strengthen muscles, when the pressure is yielded to, such as when a weight is lowered; it is a negative or eccentric movement phase.

Static muscle work: The muscle contracts against resistance, without the base of the muscles and origin coming into close contact with one another.

Dynamic muscle work: The muscle overcomes the resistance, which means it contracts and the base of the muscle and origin come into close contact with one another.

Repetition: The movement cycle from the starting position when the muscle is long over the middle position in which the trained muscle is short, to the last position or rather the starting position, is called a repetition. The repetition is composed of a positive and a negative phase.

Set or session: A continuous series of several repetitions is known as a set, series or repetition series. For the training aims of endurance, hypertrophy and strength, the repetition is a set of between five and maximal 25 repetitions, for a health-orientated fitness program, as described in the chapter *Training Guide.*

Isometric muscle tension: In isometric tension the muscle tension is increased whilst the muscle remains the same length, thus statistic muscle work.

Isotonic muscle tension: The tension that is developed within the muscle remains constantly high, whilst the muscle length changes. This kind of muscle tension is difficult to achieve because every movement that works against resistance involves different leverage, which leads to variations in tension. Because training to build up muscles works best when the pressure in the muscle is held at a regular high level as constant as possible, modern training equipment has a somewhat kidney-shaped wheel called a cam. This design feature should balance out the changing tension caused by the variations in the leverage.

Auxtonic muscle tension: Here the muscle tension changes with the muscle length. This kind of tension in the muscles is provided through the varying leverage during a movement. Auxtonic muscle tension occurs during all of the practical and daily dynamic physical movements, totally independent of whether a weight is moved or only a part of the body.

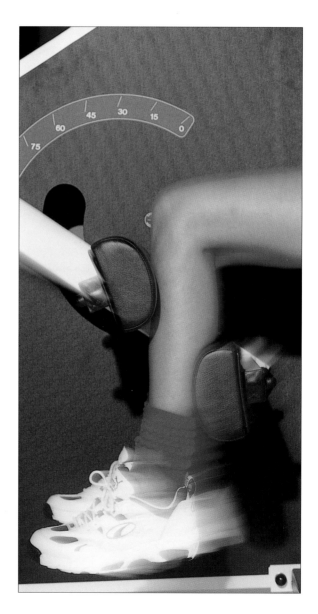

General Guide

Golden Rules

Before using training equipment or dumbbells, you should check the following safety precautions:

- Is the right weight (disc) on and are the weights securely fixed?
- Is the right sitting, lying, standing position set up?
- Is there enough space to move freely?
- Are the weights on an adjustable barbell equal on both ends?
- Are the bar plates secured with locking screws?
- Are there any visible technical faults, for example a worn band, a frayed rope or cable?

Watch your breathing when training, breathe out when lifting the weight (when the muscles contract). Breathe in when lowering the weight (when the trained muscle is long again).

The most important rule when training with weights is, always to control the movement of a weight, that means without jerking movements or swinging. It should be possible to stop the exercise at any given point without hesitation. This rule guarantees not only the full use of the muscle, but protects in the best possible way from over-training and injury.

The choice of exercises for muscle training and the correct execution of these exercises place much emphasis on protecting the joints involved. Some exercises could easily be carried out over longer periods of time than described; this however, would mean that the joint is put under unnecessary pressure. The protection of the joints and the passive kinesthetic system must always have priority in fitness oriented training – more so than the training effect on the muscles concerned. Only when minimal strain can be guaranteed for the passive kinesthetic system can the exercise be built up in order to let the muscles profit fully from the exercise.

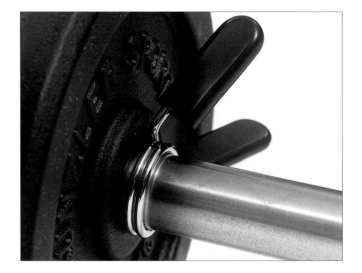

Equipment Guide

There are different kinds of weights suitable for weight training. The following are the most common:

- Equipment with detachable weights
- Equipment with air pressure
- Equipment with oil pressure
- Free weights (barbells, dumbbells)
- Elastic stretch bands in different materials (e.g. chest expanders made of steel springs, or rubber strips, tubes and rubber-bands)
- Parts of the body or the total body weight.

Although the way the muscle works remains the same, the stress curve varies according to the different machines used. For

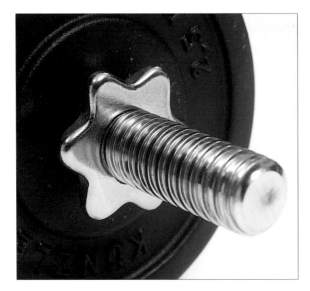

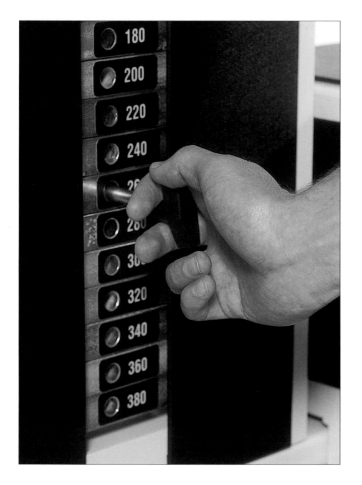

whereas with a barbell or dumbbell this part of the exercise can be easier than that part in the middle when the force of gravity is at its strongest. Modern training equipment transmits the chosen weight via a cam to the athlete's muscles. Due to its special construction the cam keeps the tension relatively constant throughout the whole movement.

The various training effects of different equipment makes it sensible to combine and vary the different types of machines used in your training. Thus the muscles in different target areas can be trained optimally. That means, in effect, that the effort produced by the muscles is spread evenly throughout the whole movement. Furthermore the training aims of endurance, hypertrophy and strength also benefit from this.

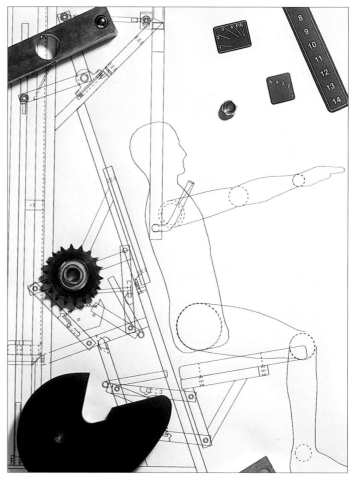

example, the leverage rules in normal gravity play a role in exercises with free or partially free weights, the pressure that a muscle is subjected to through elastic stretch bands or variable resistance machines are considerably different.

Tubes or rubber-bands, which are used to intensify the effect of the exercise are available in different flexibilities. They are color-coded for better identification and allow a quick change of resistance without time intensive changing of the discs. Apart from that, the bands are light and easy to transport, for example, in order to continue training while on vacation or a business trip. The movement involved in an exercise using a stretch band varies greatly from that done with a barbell or dumbbell. While the resistance to the movement done with a barbell or dumbbell is relatively regular, the resistance created using a stretch band builds up from the beginning to the end of the exercise. Here, the highest point in the movement is therefore also the hardest,

Explanation of the Exercise Catalogue

Shoulder and shoulder girdle musculature, elbow musculature

S 1 Dumbbell side laterals, single joint.
S 2 Dumbbell alternative front raises, single joint
S 3 Dumbbell bent-over laterals, single joint
S 4 Seated dumbbell overhead presses, multi-joint
S 5 Seated overhead presses, multi-joint
S 6 Upright rows, multi-joint
S 7 Dumbbell shrugs, single joint
S 8 Lat machine pulldowns behind the neck, multi-joint
S 9 Front lat machine pulldowns, multi-joint
S10 Machine rows, multi-joint
S11 One-arm dumbbell bent-over rows, multi-joint
S12 Bench presses, multi-joint
S13 Incline presses, multi-joint
S14 Vertical chest press, multi-joint
S15 Dumbbell pullovers, single joint
S16 Pec deck flyes, single joint
S17 Flat-bench dumbbell flyes, single joint

Wrist musculature

S31 Barbell wrist curls palms facing up, single joint
S32 Dumbbell wrist curls palms facing up, single joint
S33 Barbell wrist curls palms facing down, single joint
S34 Dumbbell wrist curls palms facing down, single joint

Hip joint musculature

S49 Leg adduction machine, single joint
S50 Leg abduction machine, single joint
S51 Multi-hip adductor, single joint
S52 Multi-hip abductor, single joint
S53 Multi-hip glutes, single joint

Ankle joint musculature

S54 Standing/seated calf machine toe raises, single joint

Spinal musculature

S35 Floor crunches, multi-joint
S36 Twisted crunches, multi-joint
S37 Crunches machine, multi-joint
S38 Machine seated twists, multi-joint
S39 Hip lifts, multi-joint
S40 Machine lower-back movements, multi-joint
S41 Back hyperextensions, multi-joint
S42 Hyperextensions reverse, multi-joint

Elbow musculature

S18 Barbell curls, single joint
S19 Seated dumbbell curls, single joint
S20 Standing dumbbell curls, single joint
S21 Scott-curl, single joint
S22 Concentration curls, single joint
S23 Preacher curls, single joint
S24 Pulley pushdowns, single joint
S25 One-arm dumbbell tricep extensions, single joint
S26 Dumbbell kickbacks, single joint
S27 Close-grip bench press, single joint
S28 Machine dips, single joint
S29 Lying barbell triceps extensions, single joint
S30 Lying dumbbell triceps extensions, single joint

Hip, knee and ankle musculature

S43 Squats, multi-joint
S44 Front squats, multi-joint
S45 Leg presses, multi-joint
S46 Leg extensions, multi-joint
S47 Lying leg curls, single joint
S48 Seated leg curls, single joint

The explanation on this double spread should simplify the use of this exercises catalog. It should prove especially useful when, after some training experience, you want to compile your own program suited to your own capabilities. The joints are sorted into the categories of primarily and dynamically used muscles. The comment single joint/multiple joints indicates if the movement takes place in one or more joints at the same time. However, exercises which are labeled as single joint can directly involve and shorten muscles which span more than one joint. For example exercise K 18 which is listed as single joint, one of the muscles mainly involved in the movement, namely the biceps muscle *(m. biceps brachii)*, spans the shoulder as well as the elbow joints. However, the movement in this exercise only takes place in the elbow joint. The reference single joint is simply to help you control the correct exercise movement, because here the movement should be carried out externally only in one joint. If this single joint exercise is carried out on a exercise machine with a fixed pivot point, care should be taken that the turning point of the body is in line with that of the machine. Thus unnecessary pressure on the joints involved can be avoided.

General Set Up of the Exercise Catalogue

The exercises described in the following exercise catalogue are classified according to the muscle groups and joints they belong to. The body is sorted from top to bottom, from the shoulder and neck area to the ankle joint muscles. In particular, the multiple joint exercises defy categorization and a definite order. With squats (S43), for example, three joint axis – hip, knee and ankle joints are in dynamic action. Additionally, almost the complete torso and back musculature is statically used for stabilization. In the case of such exercises, an order for the sets has been chosen according to the main dynamically affected muscles.

The unit system that is used on the following pages will later help you to develop a balanced individual training plan. Each exercise is described in the following basic style:

Variation:
Here you find variations on the basic exercise, which you can use to vary your training. Some of the illustrated variations are more suitable for experienced weight lifters and are marked as such. Usually the same muscle is put under pressure but at a slightly different angle or with a different power curve.

Tips:
The tips are not only for beginners but also offers a great practical help to advanced athletes. Sometimes it is a small detail which can substantially increase the value and quality of an exercise.

Muscle body front and back view:
The red marked muscle areas give a quick guide to the muscles that are exercised.

S number and name of the exercise:
The numbering allows a quick abbreviation that is useful when making a note of exercises in your training plan.

Main muscles involved:
The information listed here, in conjunction with the chapter *Anatomy*, can help the interested reader to understand the contextual function of the exercise. It also helps you to compile a balanced program, thus you can choose exercises to help the phasic muscles which are prone to weakening.

Starting position:
Here the basic position for specific exercises is described. Especially emphasized are tips that help you avoid training incorrectly.

Performing the exercise:
The execution of the exercise is described in detail including the positive and negative movement phases. As always, much emphasis has been placed on safety. The effectiveness of the exercise on the target muscle is also listed.

S26 One-Arm Dumbbell Tricep Extensions

Main muscles involved:
This exercise trains all three parts of the triceps (*m. triceps brachii*).

Starting position: Stand in the basic position with your feet parallel. One hand rests on your hip; the other arm, slightly bent, should be raised as vertically as possible. Hold a dumbbell in your hand with the wrist in a straight line with your forearm. The palm should face forwards.

▶ Performing the exercise: Keeping the upper arm vertical, lower your forearm by bending at the elbow until the upper arm and forearm form an angle of about 45°. Then lift your arm smoothly back to the starting position. After you have done the exercise on one side, perform it on the other side in the same way.

Variant: If you are advanced and can stabilize the middle part of your body well, you could perform the exercise with a dumbbell in each hand, simultaneously.

ⓘ Tip: Use a Scottbench or a preacher curl machine and sit on it the wrong way around. Your back is supported approximately up to the bottom edge of your shoulder blades, so that you cannot come into contact with the back rest while lowering the dumbbell, as would be the case with a normal adjustable exercise bench.

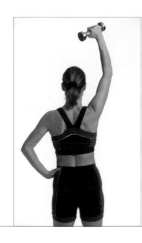
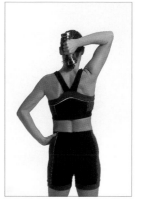

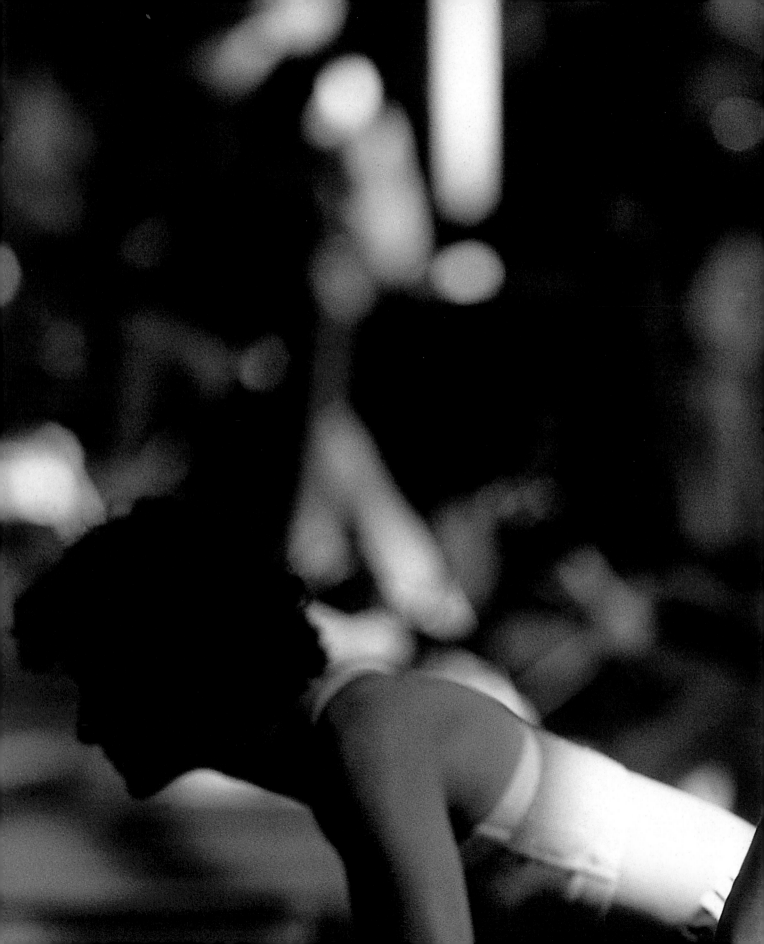

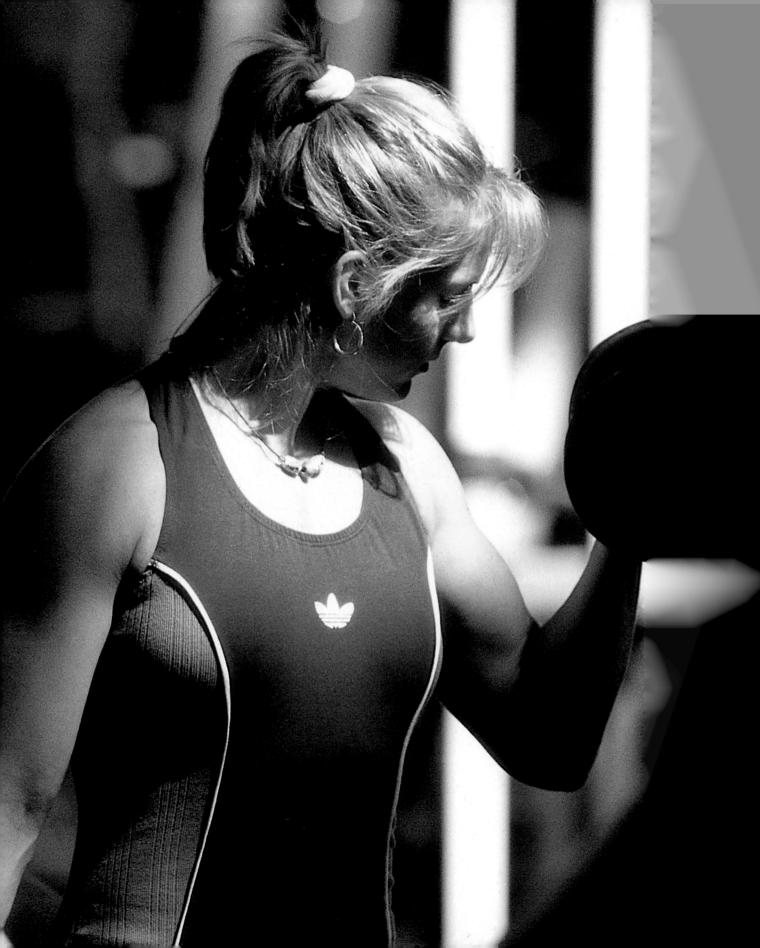

Dumbbell Side Laterals

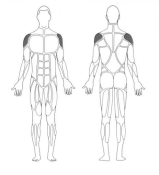

Main muscles involved:

Dumbbell side laterals train primarily the deltoids *(m. deltoideus)*, especially the side head of muscle.

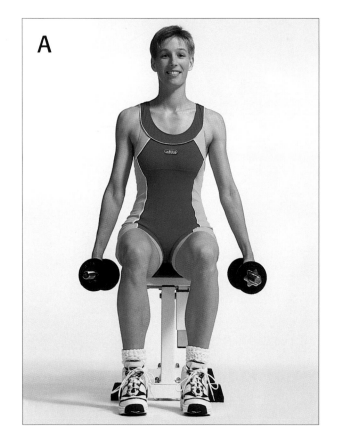

A

Starting position: Sit in the basic position with your arms bent slightly. Hold a dumbbell in each hand, with your palms facing one another. In the starting position, the distance between your hands and thighs should be about four inches. If you exercise while your back is supported, movement of the upper part of your body is automatically avoided. The exercise is thus carried out only by the intended muscle, which often means that a lighter weight is used.

▶ Performing the exercise: Lift your arms evenly in a semicircle to your shoulders. Keep the arms exactly in line with your body and your wrists in line with your forearms. Your arms must be slightly bent throughout the whole movement. Lift your elbows to the same level as your wrists. Do not raise your arms above your shoulders, as this would excessively strain the upper part of the trapezius and not achieve the intended effect of the exercise. If you straighten your arms by locking your elbows, strain is put on the elbow joints.

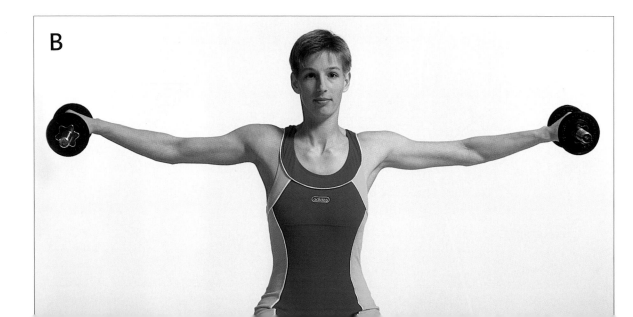

B

VARIANT

A

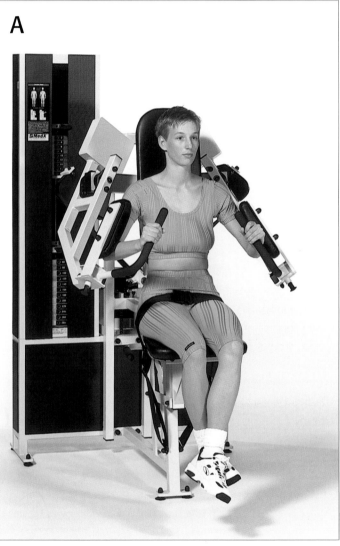

B

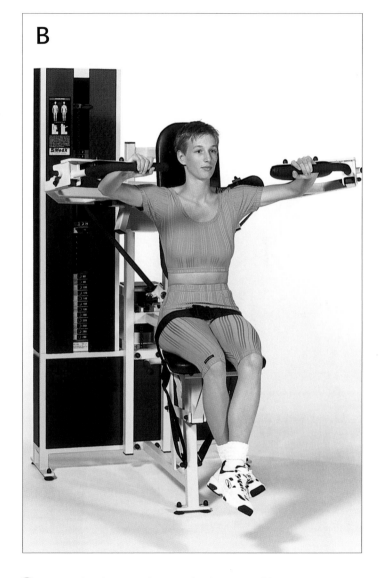

Variant: This exercise can also be done on a machine. Adjust the height of the seat so that your shoulder joints are at the same level as the pivotal joint of the machine. Do not transfer the strength via your hands onto the lever arms, rather via the padding at your elbows.

Tip: To develop a feeling for the best possible movement, imagine emptying a coffeepot with a big rounded movement of the arm. That way the upper arm turns inward into the shoulder joint and the side of the shoulder muscle is particularly used.

Dumbbell Alternate Front Raises

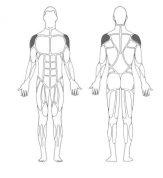

Main muscles involved:

This exercise trains primarily the deltoids *(m. deltoideus)*, especially the front head of the muscle.

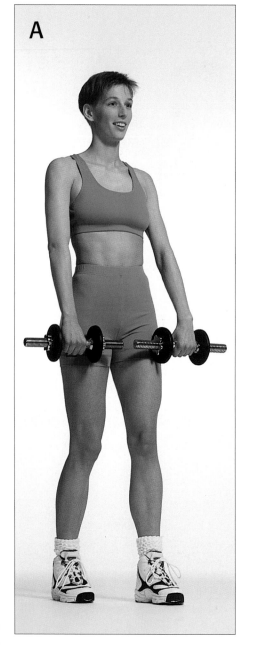

A

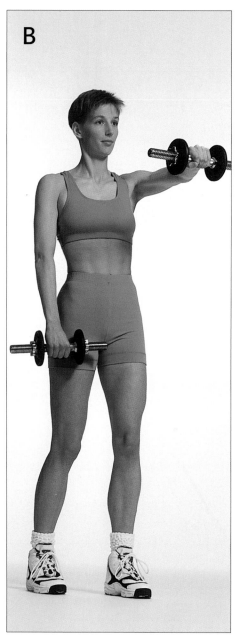

B

Starting position: Stand in the basic position with your feet parallel. Your hands must be in line with your arms in front of you, palms facing inwards. Your wrists should be straight, and your head should be held to form the natural extension of your spine.

▶ Performing the exercise: Take turns in lifting up each arm. Remember to keep your arms slightly bent, and maintain the basic tension. Your arms should be shoulder-width apart. Alternate raising one dumbbell and lowering the other. In the end position, the back of your hands should point upwards.

Variant: You could also raise and lower the dumbbells simultaneously to eye level. The upper part of your body will then lean forward a little. It is better to start this exercise in the basic position with one foot forward.

⚠ Tip: If you want to avoid the upper part of your body moving, lean with your back against a wall, your feet about a foot's length away from it.

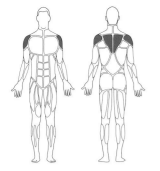

Dumbbell Bent-Over Laterals

Main muscles involved:
Primarily the back head of the deltoids *(m. deltoideus)*, greater rhomboids *(m. rhomboideus major)* and the middle part of the trapezius are trained.

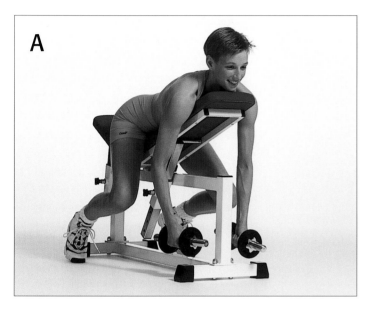

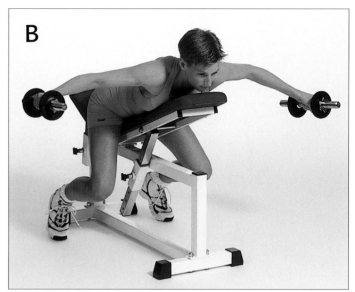

Starting position: Ideally you should lie on your stomach on an incline bench (about 30°). If the backrest of the bench is longer than the upper part of your body, place your forehead on the bench. Otherwise, stabilize your head with the strength of the muscles in the natural extension of your spine. Hold a dumbbell in each hand in front of you. In the starting position your hands should be under the bench, about four inches wider apart than your shoulders, with the palms facing one another. Your arms should be slightly bent.

▷ Performing the exercise: Raise both arms simultaneously and evenly in a circular movement to shoulder level. The arms, always slightly bent, stay in the shoulder axis throughout the movement. The upper part of your body should remain on the bench throughout the exercise.

Variant: If an incline bench is not available, you can also do the exercise standing up. Your legs should be visibly bent and the upper part of your body leaning forward at the same angle as in the above-mentioned variation. This technique requires that you build up a good basic tension in your body, otherwise the upper part can easily move.

🕛 Tip: For this exercise you should use light weights initially. By using heavy weights, the exercise will train bigger and stronger muscles, such as the latissimus dorsi or the upper part of the trapezius, which are not supposed to be trained.

Seated Dumbbell Overhead Presses

Main muscles involved:

This exercise trains the upper head of the deltoids *(m. deltoideus)*, as well as the triceps *(m. triceps brachii)* and the upper part of the trapezius.

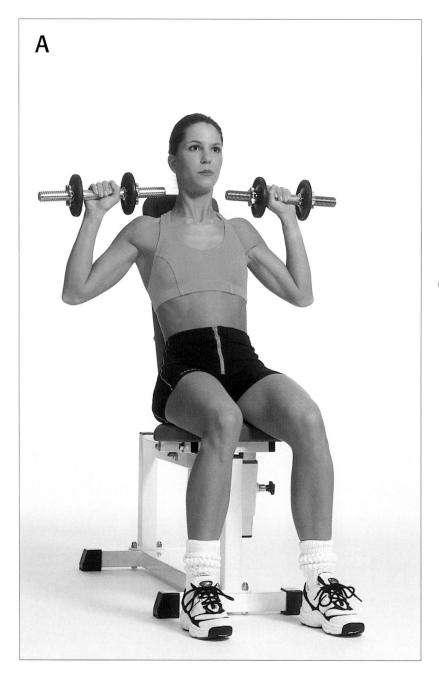

A

Starting position: Sit on a bench that has a backrest with an angle of 90°. Support the upper part of your body and head firmly on the backrest, while your legs are as wide apart as your shoulders. If the backrest is not high enough to support your head, then hold it as the natural extension of your spine. Hold a dumbbell of equal weight in each hand at ear level. Palms facing forward, your hands should be four to eight inches away from your shoulders. Your arms and the dumbbells form a right angle with your shoulders.

▷ Performing the exercise: Stretch your arms upwards evenly and parallel. The movement of the dumbbells should be rounded. In the end position your hands are in line with your shoulders, and your arms slightly bent.

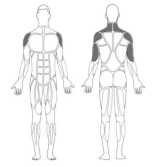

Seated Dumbbell Overhead Presses

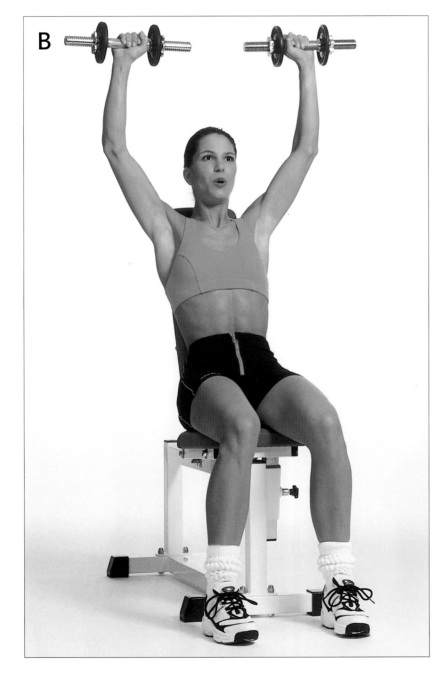

B

Variant: Hold the dumbbells about eight inches in front of you at the same level as in the starting position. The hands are exactly in front of the shoulders, with the palms facing inwards. While stretching your arms upwards, turn into the shoulder axis. By turning your hands, the end position will be the same as in the basic exercise. This variation is only advisable for the more advanced athlete because the coordination is quite demanding. It is named "Arnold-presses" after its inventor, Arnold Schwarzenegger.

! Tip: Exercise in front of a mirror to check that you are moving your arms evenly. If a bench with a backrest is not available, do the exercise standing up. Remember to stand in the correct position with your feet parallel, and to maintain the basic tension in your body.

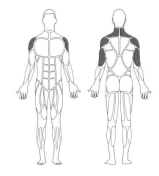

S5 Seated Overhead Presses

Main muscles involved:
This exercise trains the same muscles as in S4.

Starting position: Lean against the backrest of the machine with your whole back. Depending on the machine, adjust the height of the seat or the grips so that, in the starting position, your hands are at about the same level as your shoulders. Your palms should face inwards. Your arms are at your sides, slightly in front of your body. Keep your wrists locked, as an extension of your forearms. Lean your head against the backrest. If possible, your feet should touch the ground, otherwise cross your ankles.

▷ Performing the exercise: Push the grips upward in an even movement. Keep your arms bent in the highest position. Be aware of the basic tension in your stomach and back throughout the whole movement, and keep leaning against the backrest. Remember to keep your wrists in line with your forearms.

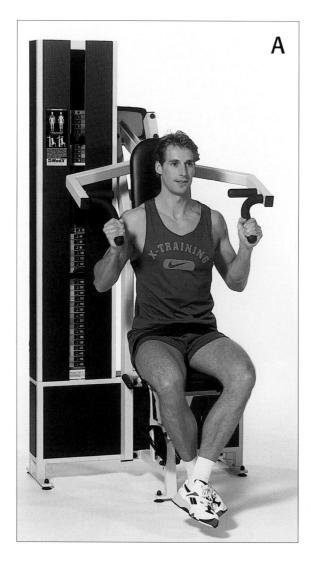

A

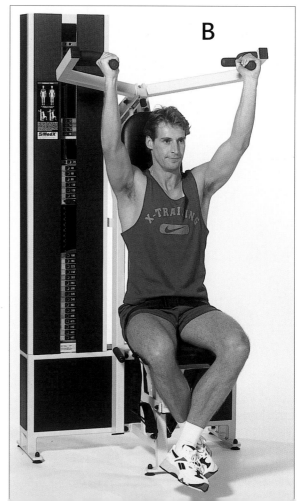

B

VARIANT

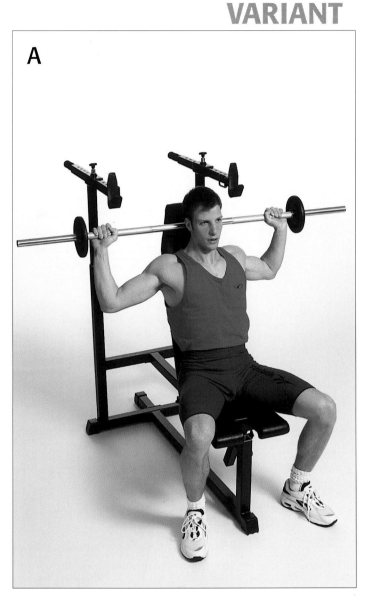

A

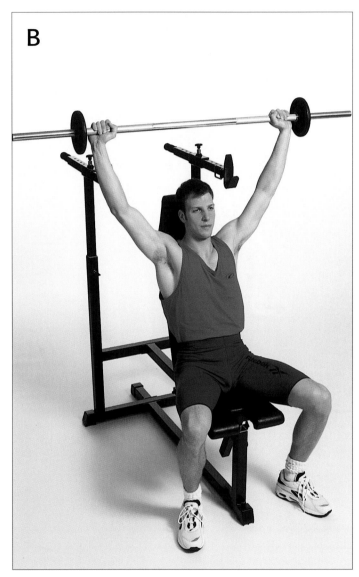

B

Variant: You can also do the exercise with a barbell on a squat rack that has the back rest in an upright position. Grip the barbell in such a way that the forearms form a right angle with the upper arms, when they are parallel to the floor. The wrists must be an extension of the forearms. Your back and head should lean against the backrest completely. Do not lower the barbell any further behind your head than to ear level, while your head remains the natural extension of your spine.

🛈 Tip: If you feel uncomfortable in your shoulder joints during this exercise, however, do K4 – Seated Dumbbell Overhead Presses instead.

Upright Rows

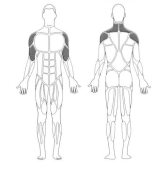

Main muscles involved:

This exercise trains the upper part of the trapezius, deltoids *(m. deltoideus)*, greater rhomboid muscles *(m. rhomboideus major)* and biceps *(m. biceps brachii).*

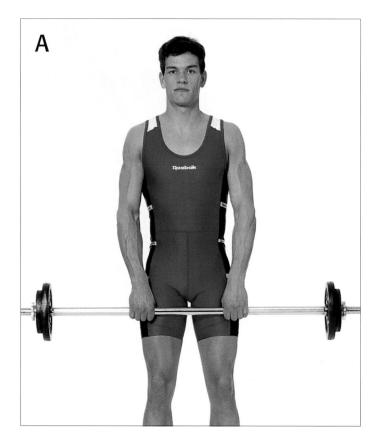

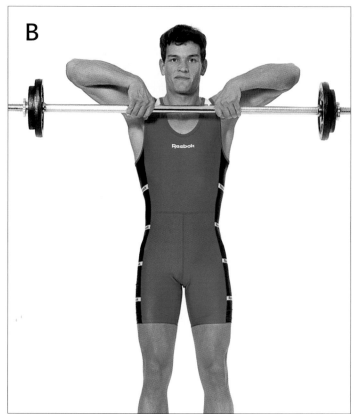

Starting position: Stand upright in the basic position with your feet parallel. Your slightly bent arms hang in front of your body, holding a barbell or an EZ-curl bar. Your palms face towards your legs; your arms are shoulder-width apart.

▶ Performing the exercise: Pull the barbell upwards in a straight line, close to your body but not touching it. Your elbows should move outwards, always above your hands and the barbell. In the end position, your hands should be at about the level between your chin and your chest, and the elbows at ear level. The barbell is lowered in exactly the opposite way, that is, your elbows are lowered last.

Variant: This exercise can also be done using a pulley, either with a straight or a bent bar. The technique is the same as using a barbell.

❗ Tip: In order to develop a feeling for the best possible movement, imagine your elbows being pulled up and outwards with a rope.

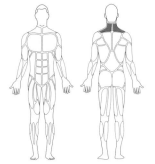

Main muscles involved:
This exercise mainly trains the upper part of the trapezius.

Starting position: Stand in the basic position with your feet parallel, holding a dumbbell in each hand at the side of your body with arms slightly bent. Your palms should be facing one another. Let the weight of the dumbbells pull your shoulders down as far as possible.

▷ Performing the exercise: Raise your shoulders simultaneously and evenly in a straight line, as if to touch your ears with your shoulders. The arms remain bent at the same angle as in the starting position, that is, your shoulders move up exactly the same distance as the dumbbells. Return to the starting position by moving the dumbbells down slowly and evenly.

Variant: You can hold the dumbbells so that the back of your hands faces forward. This way the arm turns a little more in the shoulder joint, which leads to the shoulder blades turning outwards a little, resulting in a different effect.

⚠ Tip: The more advanced athlete can make slight circular movements in either direction. This may be more difficult to coordinate, but it trains the muscles more intensively.

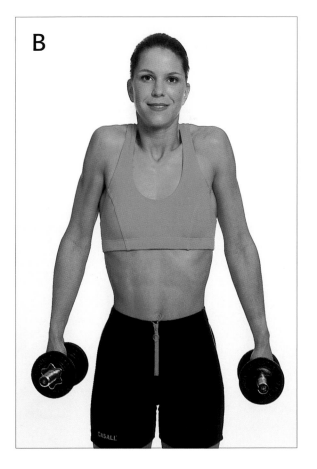

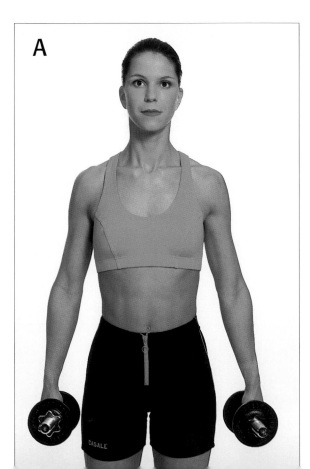

Lat Machine Pulldowns behind the Neck

Main muscles involved:

This exercise primarily trains the latissimus dorsi with the following muscles supporting it: the lower and middle part of the trapezius, greater rhomboid muscles (*m. rhomboideus major*), ...

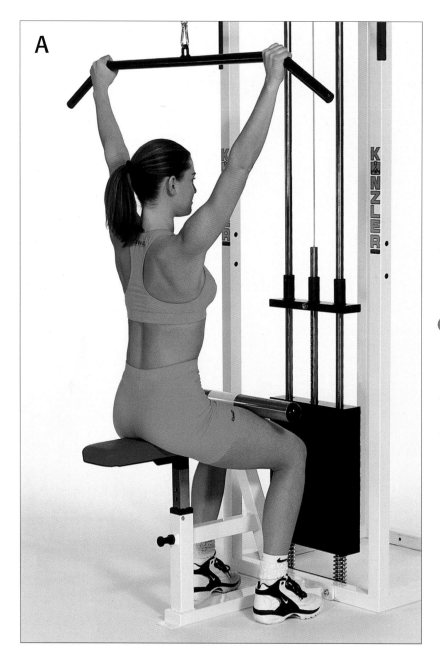

A

Starting position: Sit facing the pulley that exercises your back muscles. Your feet should rest on the ground. When using heavier weights, your legs should be fixed under a variable bar. Your pelvis should be positioned higher than your knees. Keep your head to form the natural extension of your spine, while the upper part of your body forms a right angle with the seat, and is exactly under the pulling bar. Grip the bent pulling bar behind the bends at the same distance from the middle, palms facing the machine. Your arms should be slightly bent and the shoulders raised a little.

▷ Performing the exercise: Pull the bar down behind your head to your shoulders in an even movement. Ideally you should move neither the upper part of your body nor your head. Pull down your shoulders at the same time as your arms. When moving the arms back into starting position, you should raise the shoulder girdle.

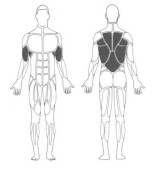

... teres major and minor *(Mm. teres major et minor)*, the lower part of the infraspinous muscle *(m. infraspinatus)* and the biceps *(m. biceps brachii)*. The erector muscle of the spine *(m. erector spinae)* is strained statically.

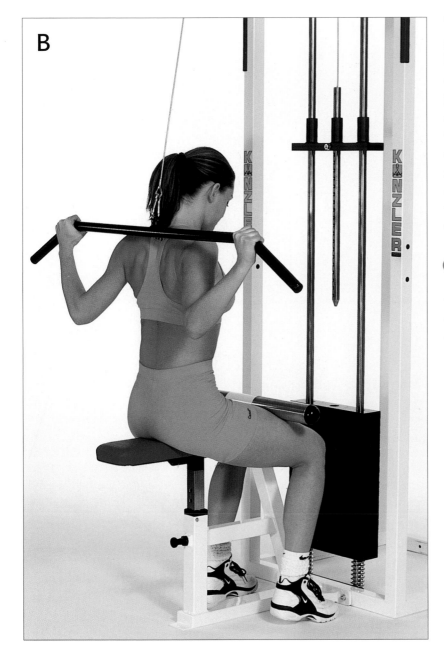

B

Variant: You can alter the distance of your grip. In the basic exercise the grip should be such that the forearms form a right angle with the upper arms, which are parallel to the floor. Varying the grip by approximately four inches on each side changes the effect of the exercise. There are special handles allowing a variation in grips. If, for instance, your palms face one another when gripping the T-shaped bar, the muscles are challenged in different ways.

⚠ Tip: If, due to a lack of mobility of the shoulder girdle, you are not able to pull the bar behind your head without moving your head forward or leaning forward, then do the front lat machine pulldowns as described in K9.

Front Lat Machine Pulldowns

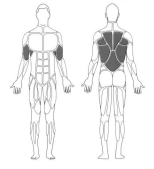

Main muscles involved:

In the different variations the same muscles are trained as described in S8. Due to the various grips each muscle is trained to a different degree.

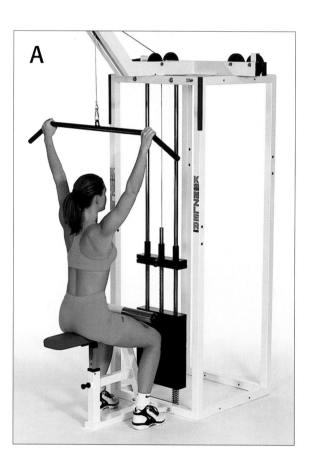

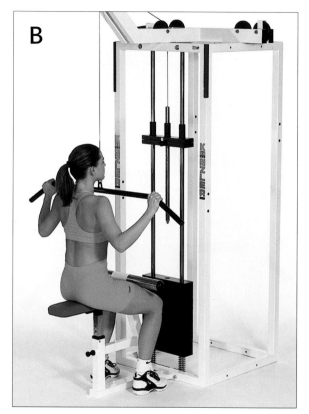

▶ Performing the exercise: Pull the bar towards your body in an even movement, as if to pull it through your body. The bar touches the upper chest. Pull your elbows outwards and your shoulders back and down. The bar moves back to starting position in the same way, without changing the angle of the upper part of your body.

Starting position: Sit facing the pulley that exercises the back muscles. Your feet should be placed firmly on the floor, while your knees are lower than your pelvis, and your legs pushed under a bar, if necessary. The upper part of your body should lean backwards a little, while your head forms the natural extension of your spine. Your pelvis is positioned exactly under the pulling bar, whereas your shoulders lean slightly backwards. Grip the pulling bar evenly behind the bend; your shoulders should be slightly raised to the front.

Variant: You can also do this exercise with a narrow grip, with the palms facing towards your body, or with a short bar where the palms face one another. In this variation the biceps are more involved, and the latissimus dorsi are also stretched more intensively.

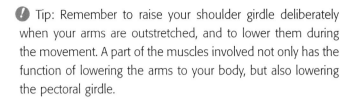 Tip: Remember to raise your shoulder girdle deliberately when your arms are outstretched, and to lower them during the movement. A part of the muscles involved not only has the function of lowering the arms to your body, but also lowering the pectoral girdle.

VARIANT

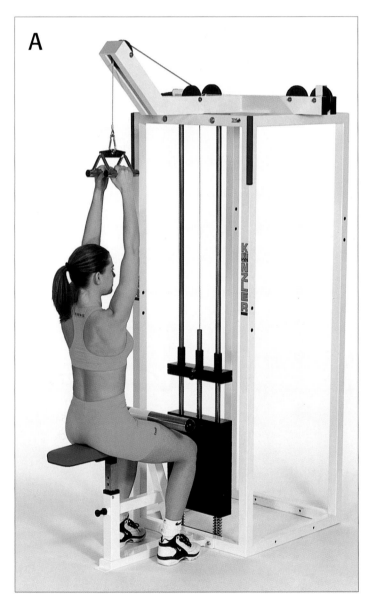

A

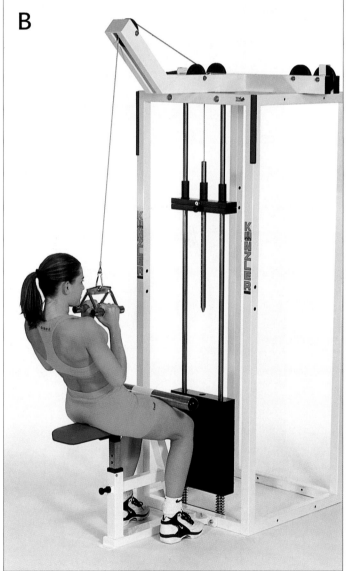

B

Main muscles involved:

Together with the latissimus dorsi, mainly the middle part of the trapezius and the rhomboids are exercised. In addition, the major muscles mentioned in S8 play a supporting role. The back of the head of the deltoids *(m. deltoideus)* is also exercised.

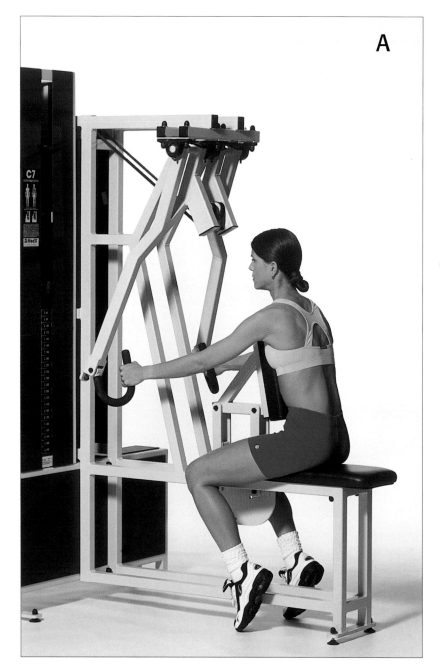

A

Starting position: Sit on a rowing machine with adjustable seat and chest pad. The whole width of the trunk should be supported by the chest pad. Place your feet on the floor, if possible. Your knees should be lower than your pelvis. Grasp the grips below shoulder height, with your palms facing one another and with your arms slightly bent. For the starting position, your shoulders should be drawn forward as far as possible. Hold your head to form the natural extension of your spine.

▷ Performing the exercise: Without tensing up, pull your arms back close to your body. Your shoulders should also move back along with your arms. In the end position, your shoulder blades are drawn together as closely as possible. Then push the grips as far away from you as you can, not only extending your arms, but also bringing your shoulders forward again. In the process, your shoulder blades are pulled away from one another.

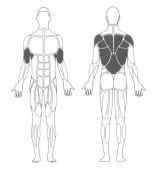

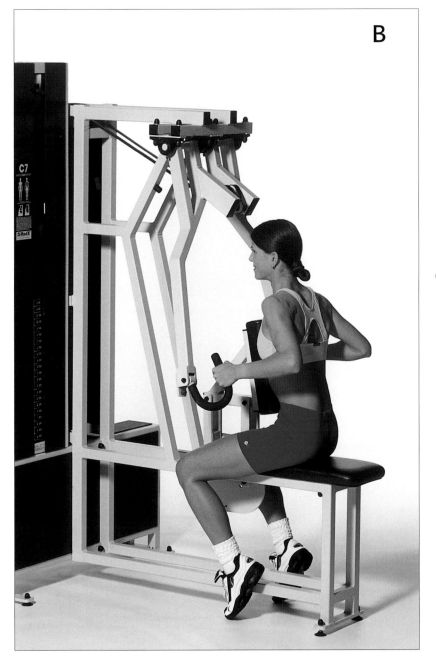

B

Variant: This exercise can be varied in several ways simply because of the different ways in which various machines are built. There is, for example, a difference in the demand put upon the muscles in the case of machines where the grips are positioned parallel to the ground, just below shoulder level. Here, the elbows are not pulled back close to the body, but back and out instead. With this variation the latissimus dorsi is not trained so intensively, while all the other muscles mentioned are exercised more.

⚠ Tip: With the following types of machines, make absolutely sure that your legs are sufficiently bent: machines with a long bench, machines where the feet are placed on two small supports in front of the body, where the grips are attached to cables, and where there is no chest pad. Otherwise the pelvis tends to be pulled back by the thigh flexors, which leads to the lumbar region being put under too much strain. In order to protect your back when using these machines, it is important to keep the upper part of your body completely still while doing the exercise.

Main muscles involved:
Rowing with a dumbbell exercises the groups of muscles described in S10.

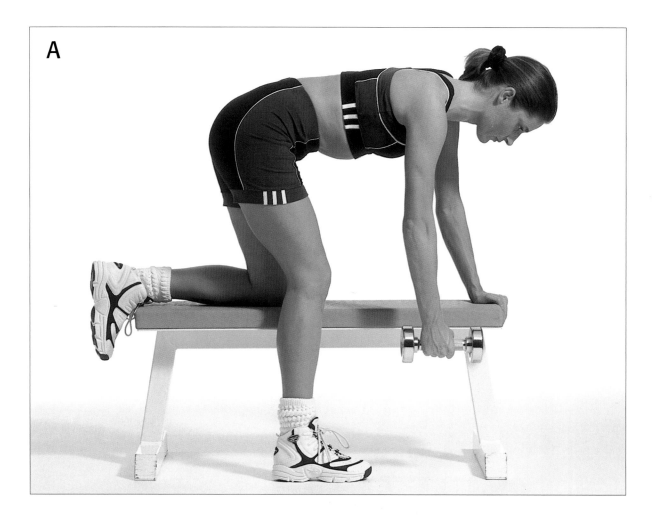

A

Starting position: Support your left leg on one end of an exercise bench and place your left hand on the other end. The upper part of your body should be parallel to the ground or slanted slightly upwards, in which case the shoulders should be somewhat higher than the pelvis. Your right leg should be slightly bent and support your body on the side. Hold a dumbbell in your right hand with the palm facing inwards. Bend your right arm slightly with the shoulder pulled downwards. Your head should form a natural extension of your spine. Shoulders and hips should be parallel to one another.

▷ Performing the exercise: Lift the dumbbell close to your body. Your elbow moves backwards and upwards, and your shoulder is raised as high as is possible without contorting the upper part of your body. The forearm should point vertically downwards throughout the movement. When bringing the dumbbell back to its original position, the arm should again be kept close to the body with the shoulder being drawn downward as far as it goes. After you have performed a set in this position, swap sides and exercise the other side of the body as well.

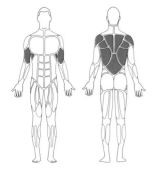

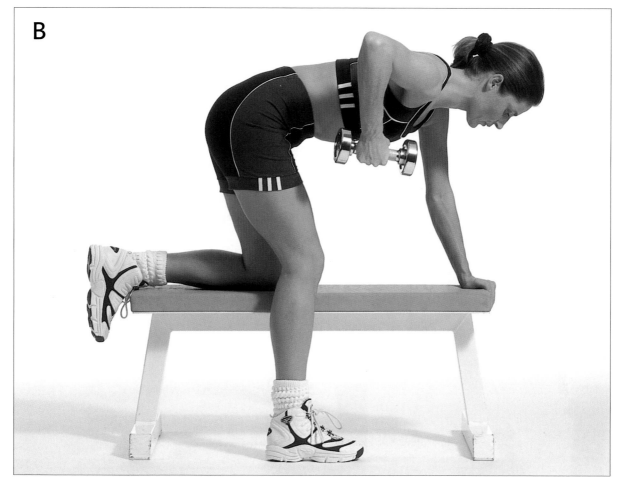

B

Variant: You can also lift a much lighter weight than that used for the basic exercise by moving your elbow outwards, keeping your upper arm in line with your shoulders. While doing this variation, the back of your hand should point forwards. Lift until your hand is at shoulder height and your shoulder is raised as high as possible. This variation exercises the latissimus dorsi less; all the other muscles involved participate much more.

Tip: If an adjustable exercise bench is available, place the back rest at an angle of about 45° to help perform this exercise correctly. Rest your knee on the seat and your forearm on the tilted back rest. In this way, your body is much better stabilized and it will be considerably easier for you to keep your shoulders parallel to your pelvis, thus avoiding any damaging contortion of the lower back.

Main muscles involved:

This exercise mainly trains the greater pectorals *(m. pectoralis major)*. In addition, the front head of the deltoids *(m. deltoideus)*, triceps *(m. triceps brachii)* and lesser pectorals *(m. pectoralis minor)* are also exercised.

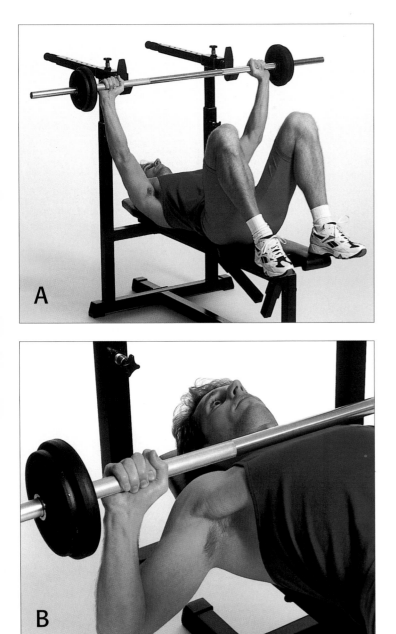

A

B

Starting position: Lie on your back on a flat bench with your knees bent and your feet placed near the end of the bench. Look straight up at the ceiling. Your eyes should be directly under the bar of the barbell. Your hands should grasp the bar far enough apart so that the forearm forms a right angle to the upper arm when the upper arm is parallel to the floor. The barbell support rack should be high enough for the arms to remain slightly bent in the starting position. Keep your wrists firm and in line with your forearm; your palms should face your feet.

▷ Performing the exercise: Lift the barbell from the support rack with a smooth movement and lock it above your chest with slightly bent arms. Now lower the weights smoothly down to chest level. The barbell should touch your chest gently, approximately in the center of your breastbone. Then lift it again without any jerking; upon completion of the exercise the arms should again be slightly bent.

Variant: If you vary the distance between your hands by about four inches in either direction, the muscles involved in this exercise will be trained to differing degrees. This is particularly the case with the greater pectorals *(m. pectoralis major)* and the triceps *(m. triceps brachii)*.

❗ Tip: To take the strain off the lower back you can bend and cross your legs, especially if you have a shortened iliopsoas. Do this exercise only with a training partner; this will reduce the risk of accident or injury considerably. When helping to secure the weights, make sure you are standing firmly to avoid straining your back or injuring yourself.

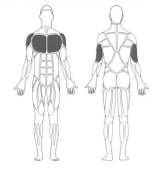

Main muscles involved:
Incline presses exercise the same groups of muscles as in S12. The upper part of the greater pectorals *(m. pectoralis major)* is more involved.

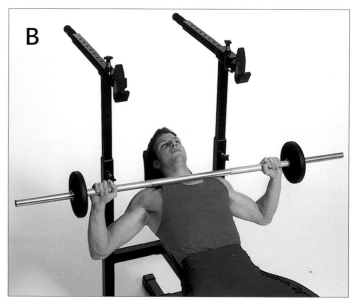

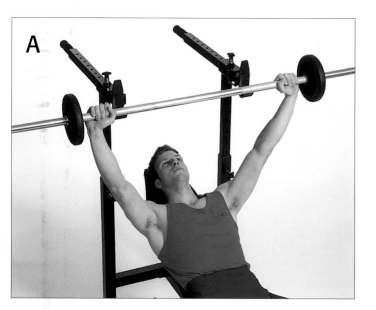

Starting position: Lie on an incline bench with the back rest tilted at an angle of 30° to 45°. Support your legs either on the ground or on the platform provided for this purpose at the lower end of the bench. Take hold of the barbell with your hands apart as described under bench presses. When doing incline presses, your eyes should be more or less under the bar of the barbell. Tense the stomach and lower back muscles. The support rack for the barbell should be at a height where the arms are slightly bent before lifting it out.

▶ Performing the exercise: Lift the barbell from the support rack and lock it vertically with slightly bent arms above the upper part of your pectorals. Lower the barbell slowly until it touches your pectorals lightly, then raise it again by extending your arms. Upon completion of the exercise, the arms should again be slightly bent. Make sure that your wrists remain in a line with your forearms the whole time. Maintain the tension in the middle of your body.

Variant: Vary the distance between your hands by about four inches in either direction to change the amount each muscle involved is trained. Adjust the back rest between 30° and 45° to exercise different parts of the greater pectoral muscle *(m. pectoralis major)*.

❗ Tip: If you do not have an adjustable bench with a platform at the end, or if the bench is so high that it is not possible for you to press your feet against the floor, place an exercise bench across the end of the bench and put your feet on it.

Main muscles involved:

This exercise trains mainly the greater pectoral muscle *(m. pectoralis major)*. In addition, it exercises the front head of the deltoids *(m. deltoideus)*, triceps *(m. triceps brachii)* and lesser pectorals *(m. pectoralis minor)*.

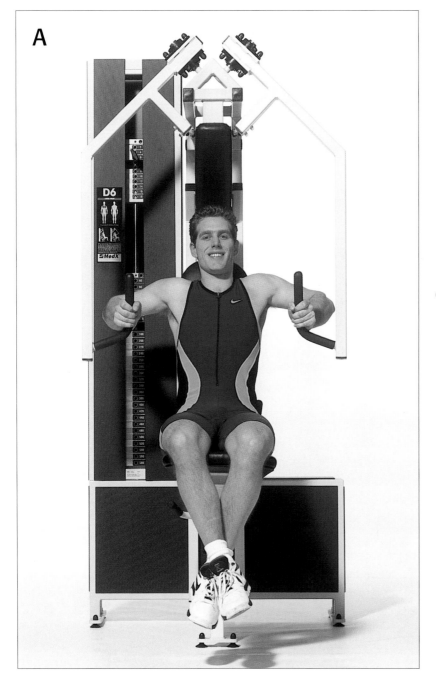

Starting position: Adjust your seat so that your shoulders are a few inches above the grips; in other words, the grips should be about halfway up the breastbone. Put both feet on the ground, provided that the seat is low enough. If not, cross your lower legs. The upper part of your body should be completely supported by the back rest and your head should form the natural extension of your spine. Your arms should be slightly bent when you pull the grips towards each other in front of your body; your palms should face one another.

▷ Performing the exercise: Pull your arms slowly and evenly back towards your body. Your elbows should remain slightly below shoulder level. Stop moving your arms back when your hands are in line with your chest as seen from the side. Now begin straightening your arms smoothly and without any sudden movements, bringing the grips back to the starting position with the arms still slightly bent.

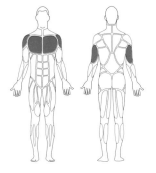

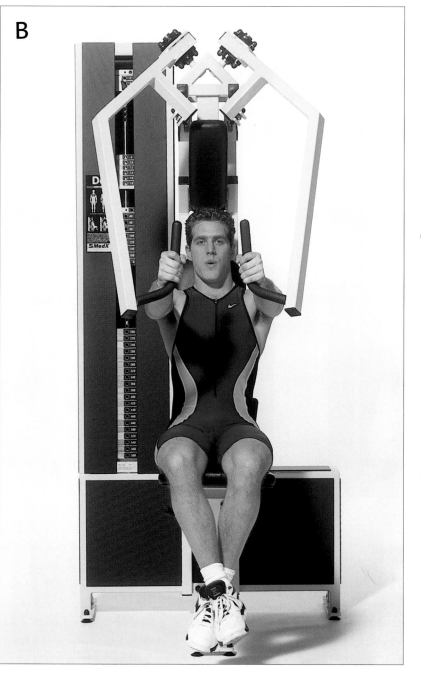

B

Variant: With many chest press machines you can do this exercise with your palms facing downwards. Here it is often possible to vary the distance between the hands as well. For the basic exercise they should be so far apart that the lower and upper arm form a right angle halfway through the exercise. If you place your hands about four inches further apart in either direction, your pectorals and triceps will be exercised more intensively.

⚠ Tip: Modern chest press machines are mostly equipped with a start help. With this, the weights can be brought into the starting position using the strength of your legs. This especially protects the shoulder joints, which could otherwise come under unnecessary strain when first lifting the weights due to the lack of preliminary tension in the muscles and the unfavorable angle. If the chest press machine does not have such a start help, have a training partner assist you for the first repetition of the exercise and thus the first time you lift the weights.

Pullover

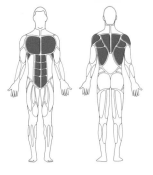

Main muscles involved:
With the pullover exercise almost all the muscles in the upper part of the body are trained directly or indirectly: both the latissimus dorsi and the greater pectoral muscles *(m. pectoralis major)...*

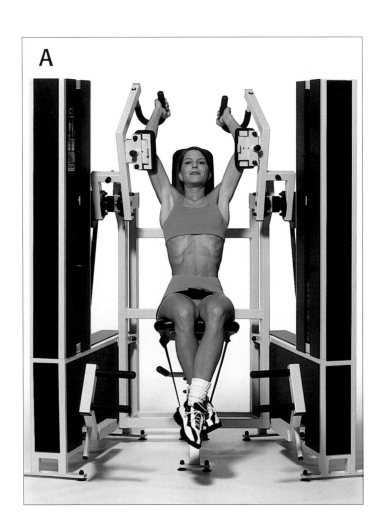

A

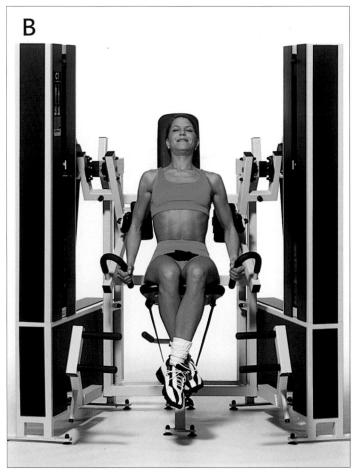

B

Starting position: When you train with a pullover machine, make sure that the height of the seat is adjustable. Position the seat so that your shoulders are in line with the machine's axis of rotation. If it is possible to fasten your pelvis with a belt you should always do so, even if your training weight is low. The upper part of your body should be fully supported by the back rest throughout the exercise. Rest your head on the head rest, keeping it to form the natural extension of your spine. If the equipment has a start help, use it to bring the grips far enough forward to be able to hold them comfortably. Depending on the type of equipment, the elbows either rest on a pad or are free. In the starting position, the upper arms form a vertical extension of the upper part of the body.

... the straight abdominal muscle *(m. rechtus abdominis)*, trapezius, greater rhomboids *(m. rhomboideus major)* and triceps *(m. triceps brachii).*

VARIANT

▶ Performing the exercise: Pull your arms down in a semicircular motion in front of your body, keeping them slightly bent. At the finish, your upper arms should be somewhat behind your body. From here bring your arms slowly and evenly back to the starting position.

Variant: This exercise can also be carried out while lying on your back on a flat exercise bench. Hold a dumbbell with both hands at one end and bring your arms into a starting position almost vertically above your body, keeping your arms slightly bent. Now lower the dumbbell in a semicircular movement back behind your head, the arms remaining constantly bent at the same angle. The end position is reached when the upper arms form the extension of the body. From here the arms and dumbbell are brought back to the starting position in a smooth curve.

❗ Tip: If you want to involve your triceps more, you can bend your arms sharply while lowering them and straighten them again in the movement upwards.

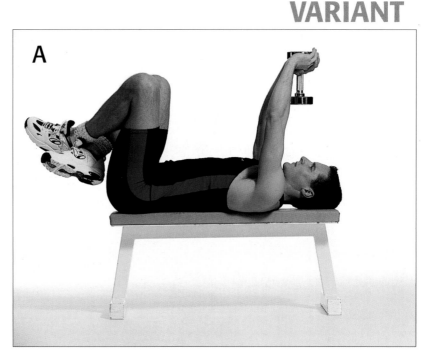

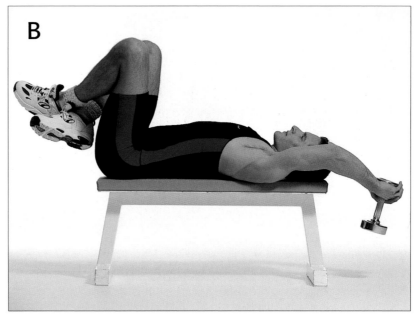

Pec Deck Flyes

Main muscles involved:

This machine trains both the greater and lesser pectorals *(Mm. pectoralis major et minor)* more or less in isolation. In addition, it exercises the front head of the deltoids *(m. deltoideus).*

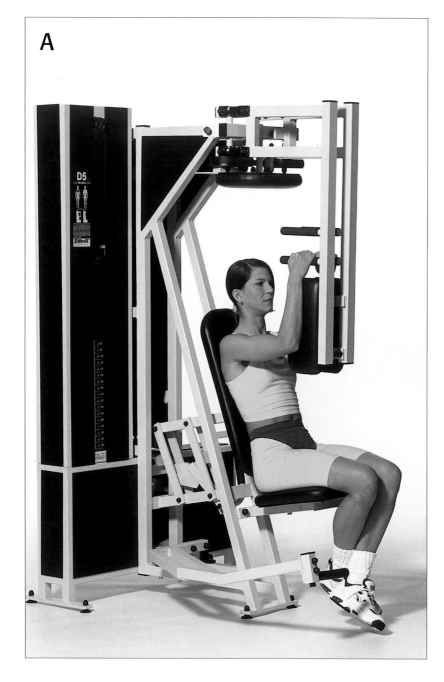

A

Starting position: Sit with the whole upper part of your body supported by the back rest. If the back rest is not long enough to support your head, position your head so that it forms the natural extension of your spine. Place your feet on the floor or, if this is not possible, cross the lower legs. If the machine has a start help, operate it with your legs so that the arm grips can be pulled towards one another in front of the body without resistance. Hold the grips in such a way that your forearms are vertical and your upper arms parallel to the floor. You can achieve this position by adjusting the height of the seat accordingly. For the starting position, hold the grips pulled tightly together in front of the body. Depending on how the machine is built, the strain is taken by the inner side of the forearm and the elbows.

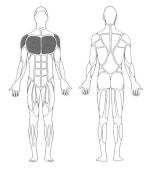

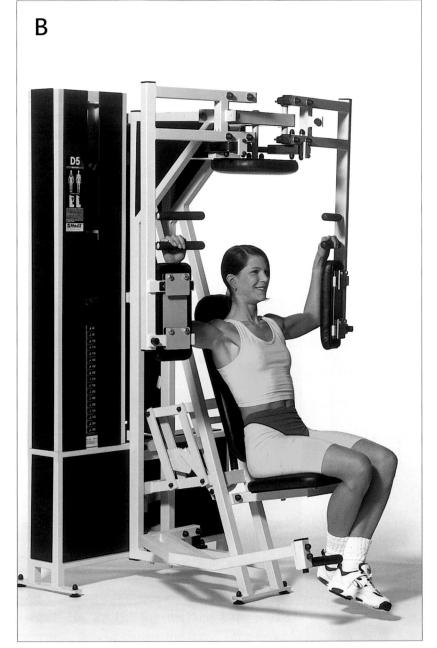

B

▷ Performing the exercise: Open your arms slowly and simultaneously. In the end position the arms are at the sides of the body. From here bring the grips smoothly and without stopping back to the starting position, where they should touch briefly exactly in the middle in front of your body.

Variant: With some equipment you can hold the grips only with your hands. In this case, the elbows are raised to just below shoulder level, and the forearms and upper arms are held parallel to the floor. In this way the strain on the shoulder joints can be reduced if the shoulders are sensitive. Otherwise the exercise corresponds to the basic form.

❗ Tip: Maintain the tension in the contracted position for one or two seconds in order to intensify the effect of the exercise.

Seated Dumbbell Curls

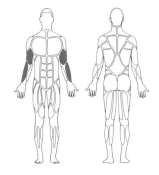

Main muscles involved:

This exercise trains the biceps *(m. biceps brachii)*, the brachial muscles *(m. brachialis)* and the brachioradial muscles *(m. brachioradialis)*.

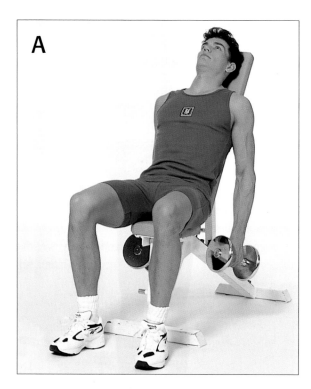

A

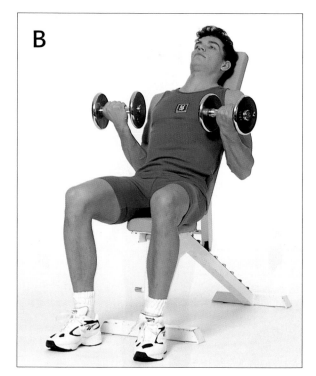

B

Starting position: Sit on an incline bench with the upper part of your body and your head supported by a back rest tilted back at about 30°. Hold two dumbbells of equal weight, one in each hand, with your palms facing one another. Because of the slant of the backrest, your slightly bent arms should be behind the axis of your body.

▶ Performing the exercise: Lift the dumbbells in an even, parallel motion close to your body. The upper arm should remain more or less vertical to the floor, while the forearm, turned at the elbow joint, moves upwards. In the course of the upward movement, the elbow should rotate 45° outwards. At the end of the movement, the backs of your hands should face forward. When lowering the weights, the palms again turn to face one another.

Variant: For variety you can also perform the exercise by alternating sides: in other words, when lifting one arm, lower the other and vice versa.

❗ Tip: To make the turning outwards or supination of the forearm more difficult, you can make the inner side of the dumbbell heavier than the outer. This, of course, only works with dumbbells where you can put the discs (weights) on yourself. This trick exercises the biceps *(m.biceps brachii)*, which has among its functions the supination of the forearm, even more intensively.

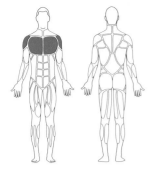

B

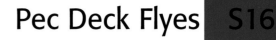

▷ Performing the exercise: Open your arms slowly and simultaneously. In the end position the arms are at the sides of the body. From here bring the grips smoothly and without stopping back to the starting position, where they should touch briefly exactly in the middle in front of your body.

Variant: With some equipment you can hold the grips only with your hands. In this case, the elbows are raised to just below shoulder level, and the forearms and upper arms are held parallel to the floor. In this way the strain on the shoulder joints can be reduced if the shoulders are sensitive. Otherwise the exercise corresponds to the basic form.

❗ Tip: Maintain the tension in the contracted position for one or two seconds in order to intensify the effect of the exercise.

Flat-Bench Dumbbell Flyes

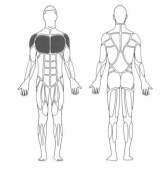

Main muscles involved:
This exercise trains the same groups of muscles as in S16.

Starting position: Lie on your back on a flat exercise bench. Bend your legs and place your feet on the end of the bench. Hold a dumbbell in each hand vertically above your shoulders, keeping your arms slightly bent. Your palms should face one another and your wrists should be straight.

▶ Performing the exercise: Lower each dumbbell out to the side in a semicircular movement. During the downward movement the arms should bend more. The dumbbells should not reach behind the axis of your shoulders. Depending on your flexibility, you can lower the dumbbells to shoulder level or a few inches below. From the lowest point, lift the weights without jerking in an even movement back to the starting position.

Variant: If you use a bench with an adjustable back rest, you can exercise the chest muscles from different angles. In tilted positions up to approximately 45°, the upper part of the greater pectoral muscles *(m. pectoralis major)* is exercised more intensively.

❗ Tip: Use a narrow bench for this exercise so that the shoulder blades can be pulled closer together and the upper arms are not hindered in their downward movement by the protruding edges of the bench. In this way the pectorals are stretched better, thus making the contraction at the end of the movement more effective.

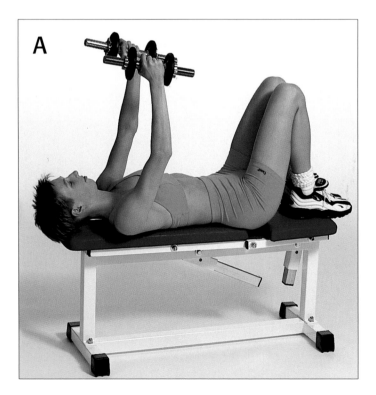

A

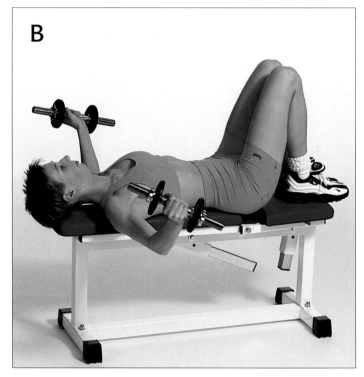

B

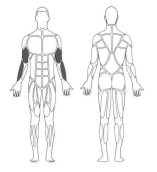

Main muscles involved:
Barbell curls primarily train the biceps *(m. biceps brachii)* and the brachial muscle *(m. brachialis)*.

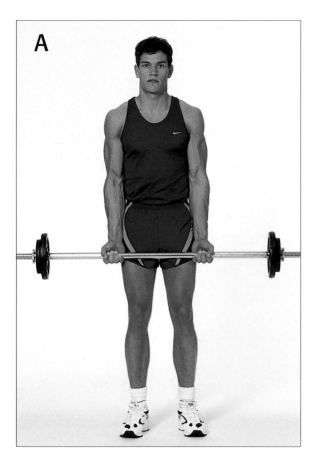

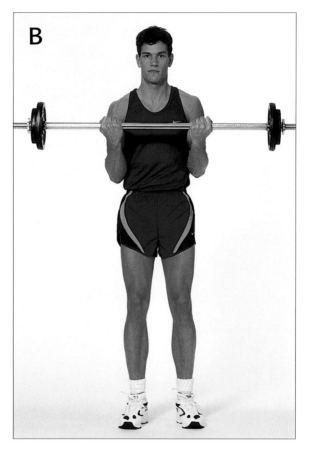

Starting position: Stand in the basic position, feet in line with your shoulders, arms at your sides and slightly bent. Hold the barbell with your hands shoulder-width apart, palms facing the front. Make sure that your wrists are straight and that your head position is correct.

▶ Performing the exercise: Lift the barbell in a semicircular movement. The elbows act as an axis and remain in one position, resting at your sides. Stop lifting when the group of muscles responsible for bending the arm have reached maximum tension, without moving the upper arms forward.

When lowering the arms again, the elbows should again remain close to the body. The arms always remain slightly bent, even in the lowest position.

Variant: Instead of a straight barbell, use an EZ-curl bar, holding it behind the second bend from the middle.

❗ Tip: If you tend to involve the upper part of your body in the exercise, simply lean your back against a wall. Your feet should be parallel to one another about a foot's length from the wall.

Seated Dumbbell Curls

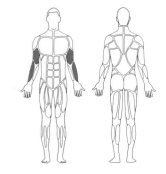

Main muscles involved:
This exercise trains the biceps *(m. biceps brachii)*, the brachial muscles *(m. brachialis)* and the brachioradial muscles *(m. brachioradialis)*.

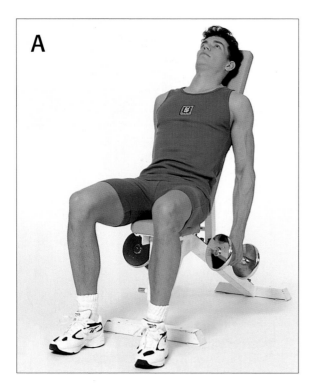

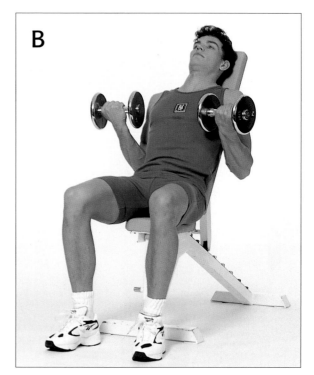

Starting position: Sit on an incline bench with the upper part of your body and your head supported by a back rest tilted back at about 30°. Hold two dumbbells of equal weight, one in each hand, with your palms facing one another. Because of the slant of the backrest, your slightly bent arms should be behind the axis of your body.

▷ Performing the exercise: Lift the dumbbells in an even, parallel motion close to your body. The upper arm should remain more or less vertical to the floor, while the forearm, turned at the elbow joint, moves upwards. In the course of the upward movement, the elbow should rotate 45° outwards. At the end of the movement, the backs of your hands should face forward. When lowering the weights, the palms again turn to face one another.

Variant: For variety you can also perform the exercise by alternating sides: in other words, when lifting one arm, lower the other and vice versa.

❗ Tip: To make the turning outwards or supination of the forearm more difficult, you can make the inner side of the dumbbell heavier than the outer. This, of course, only works with dumbbells where you can put the discs (weights) on yourself. This trick exercises the biceps *(m.biceps brachii)*, which has among its functions the supination of the forearm, even more intensively.

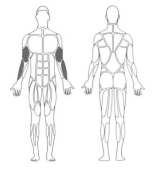

Main muscles involved:
This exercise also trains the biceps *(m. biceps brachii)*, brachial muscle *(m. brachialis)* and the brachioradial muscle *(m. brachioradial)*.

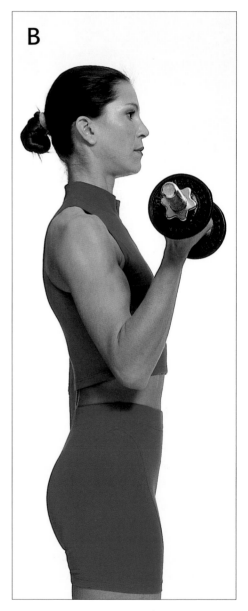

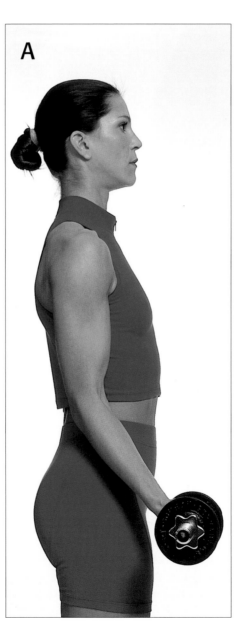

Starting position: Stand in the basic posture, feet in line with your shoulders, your arms slightly bent at your sides. Hold the dumbbells shoulder-width apart with your palms facing inwards. Make sure that your wrists are straight and that your head position is correct.

▶ Performing the exercise: Lift the dumbbells in an even, parallel motion. The upper arms should remain resting at your sides with the elbow joints acting as an axis, while the forearm, turned at the elbow joint, is drawn upwards. In the end position, the back of your hands should face forwards.

Variant: For variety you can perform the standing dumbbell curls while alternating sides. The effect is also different if you turn your forearm outwards during the upward movement.

❗ Tip: If you tend to involve your body in the exercise, try standing with one foot forward or lean the upper part of your body against a wall, placing your feet parallel to one another about a foot away from it.

Scottcurls

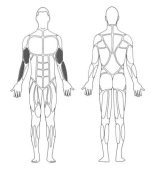

Main muscles involved: This exercise trains the same groups of muscles as in S20.

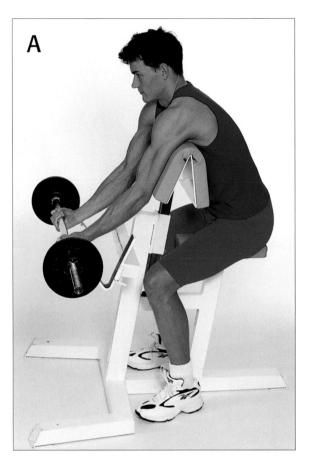

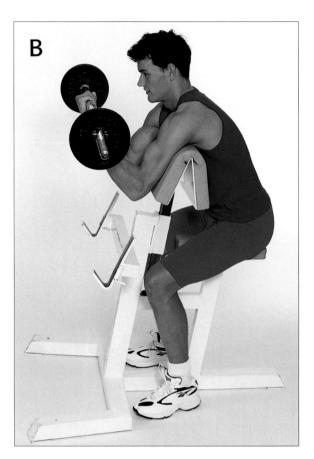

Starting position: For the Scottcurl the backs of your upper arms should be completely supported by the cushion on the special Scottbench. Your back and head should be kept straight, and your shoulders should rest directly on the edge of the cushion on the Scottbench. Grasp a barbell with your hands shoulder-width apart, palms facing upwards, keeping your arms slightly bent. Keep your wrists in a straight line with your forearms.

▶ Performing the exercise: Lift the barbell in a semicircular movement to a height where you can still feel the tension in the group of muscles bending the arm. Then lower the

barbell smoothly back into the starting position with slightly bent arms.

Variant: You can also perform the Scottcurl one arm at a time with a dumbbell. The advantage is that you can support the movement, if necessary, with your free hand.

❗ Tip: If there is no barbell support rack on the Scottbench, it is recommended that you have a training partner hand you the barbell.

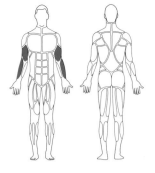

Main muscles involved:
This exercise trains the same groups of muscles as in S21.

Starting position: Sit lengthwise on the edge of a training bench. Place your left hand on your left leg, bend the upper part of your body slightly forwards and to the left. Hold a dumbbell in your right hand with the palm facing left and your arm slightly bent. Your right elbow should hang loosely close to your inner right thigh.

▷ Performing the exercise: Bend your right arm at the elbow joint, at the same time moving your upper right arm a few inches to the left. In the end position your right elbow should have moved some four to eight inches away from your right thigh, and your forearm should be bent as far as possible towards your upper arm. After maintaining this position for one or two seconds, lower the dumbbell with exactly the opposite movement. After you have done a set with your right arm, train the left arm in the same way.

Variant: For a somewhat different effect, start as in the basic exercise, but hold the dumbbell with your palm facing backwards. While lifting turn the forearm 45° outwards. This makes greater demands on the biceps *(m. biceps brachii)* in their function of turning the forearm outwards, thus intensifying the effect of the exercise on them.

❗ Tip: To get the right feeling for the movement, it helps to imagine that you want to show someone the condition of your upper arm by tensing up your bicep in front of your body. This is exactly the feeling you should have when doing concentration curls. Because it is a very isolated movement, you need much less weight for this exercise than for the other exercises which train the biceps.

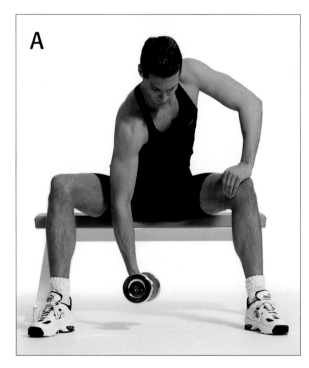

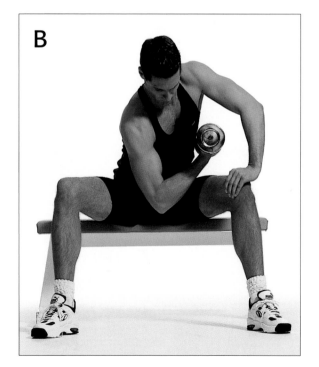

Preacher Curls

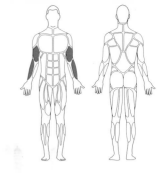

Main muscles involved:
This exercise trains the same groups of muscles as in S20.

Starting position: Sit upright on the seat with your spine straight. Adjust the height of the seat so that the back of your upper arm is completely supported on the pad of the machine. Make absolutely sure that your elbow joints are at exactly the same height as the axis of the machine, and that your arms are not straight but slightly bent at the start. Hold the grips with the palms facing upwards.

▷ Performing the exercise: Pull the grip or grips evenly up towards you, then lower them just as evenly. Make sure that your upper arms remain on the pad throughout the entire movement.

Variant: Different machines require the hands to be held varying distances apart. Some bicep machines allow you to hold the grips with the palms facing one another or downwards, which puts the emphasis on different arm-bending muscles.

❶ Tip: If you cannot adjust the machine so that your elbows are in line with the axis of the machine, it is better not to train on it – use a dumbbell instead.

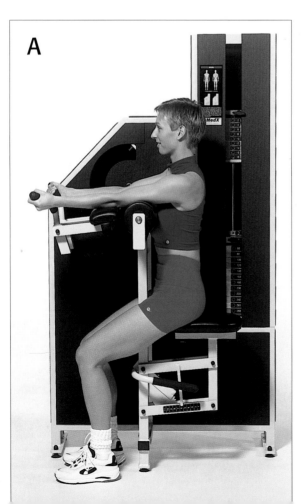

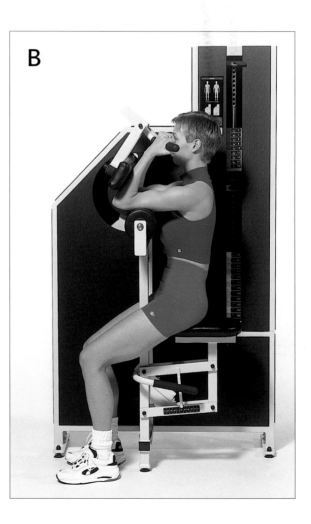

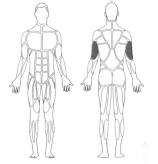

Main muscles involved:

Pulley pushdowns exercise the triceps *(m. triceps brachii)*, especially the side and middle part of the head of the muscle.

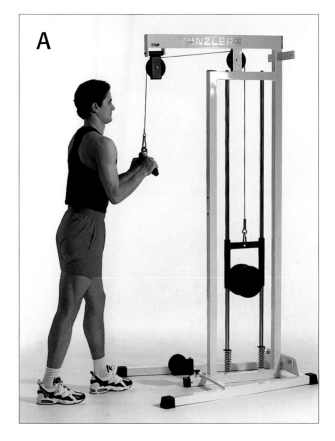

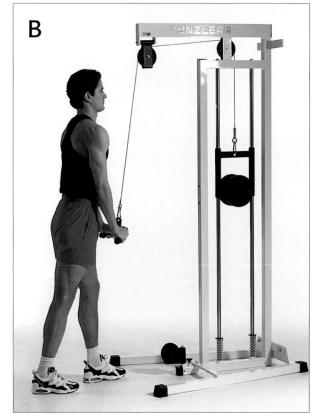

Starting position: Stand in the basic position, with feet either parallel or with one foot forward. Your upper arms should rest at your sides, while your forearms are bent at an angle of approximately 45° and your hands hold the bent, swiveling bar with the palms facing downwards.

▷ Performing the exercise: Straighten your arms in an even, semicircular movement until almost fully extended. While performing the exercise, your elbows should remain close to your body without moving. Then bring the bar back to the starting position with exactly the opposite movement. Make sure your wrists are straight and extended.

Variant: This exercise can also be performed with other sorts of bars or grip, for example a straight or single bar. In both cases the exercise can be successfully performed with the palms facing upwards, which means that the triceps *(m. triceps brachii)* can be tensed more.

❗ Tip: If it is difficult for you not to involve the upper part of your body, stand with one foot forward. When using this posture, make sure that your pelvis does not move backwards, but stays parallel to your shoulders.

One-Arm Dumbbell Tricep Extensions

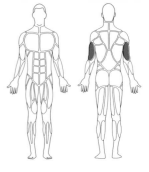

Main muscles involved:
This exercise trains all three parts of the triceps *(m. triceps brachii).*

Starting postion: Stand in the basic position with your feet parallel. One hand rests on your hip; the other arm, slightly bent, should be raised as vertically as possible. Hold a dumbbell in your hand with the wrist in a straight line with your forearm. The palm should face forwards.

▶ Performing the exercise: Keeping the upper arm vertical, lower your forearm by bending at the elbow until the upper arm and forearm form an angle of about 45°. Then lift your arm smoothly back to the starting position. After you have done the exercise on one side, perform it on the other side in the same way.

Variant: If you are advanced and can stabilize the middle part of your body well, you could perform the exercise with a dumbbell in each hand, simultaneously.

🛈 Tip: Use a Scottbench or a preacher curl machine and sit on it the wrong way around. Your back is supported approximately up to the bottom edge of your shoulder blades, so that you cannot come into contact with the back rest while lowering the dumbbell, as would be the case with a normal adjustable exercise bench.

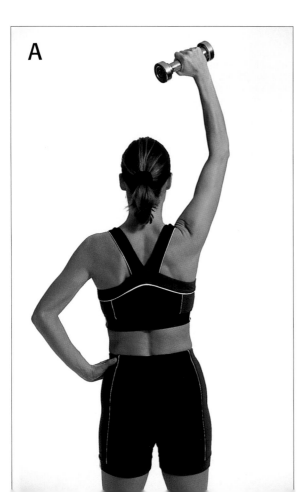

A

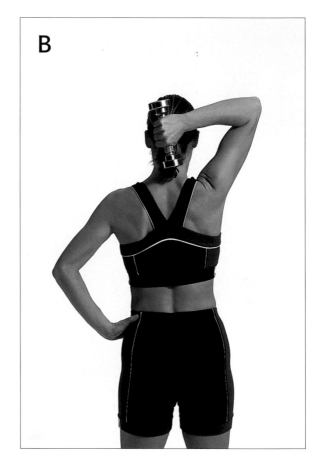

B

Main muscles involved:
In this exercise the same group of muscles is trained as in S25.

Starting position: Rest your left knee and lower leg on one end of an exercise bench and place your left hand on the other end. The upper part of your body should be parallel to the floor or slanted slightly upwards; in other words, your shoulders should be somewhat higher than your hips. Your right leg should be slightly bent and act as a support for the right side of your body. Hold a dumbbell in your right hand with the palm of your hand facing inwards. Your upper right arm should be parallel to the floor or, if possible, slanting upwards, and your forearm and upper arm should be at right angles to one another.

▷ Performing the exercise: Straighten your right arm slowly until it is almost fully extended. While doing so, keep your upper arm still and your elbow at a constant height. Then lower the forearm back to the starting position. After doing the exercise with the right arm, repeat it for the left side.

Variant: Perform the exercise with both arms simultaneously while lying on your stomach on an adjustable exercise bench with the back rest tilted at about 45°.

❶ Tip: If an adjustable bench is available, tilt the back rest at an angle of about 45°. Your knee then rests on the seat and the forearm of your bent arm on the tilted back rest. In this way the body is kept more stable.

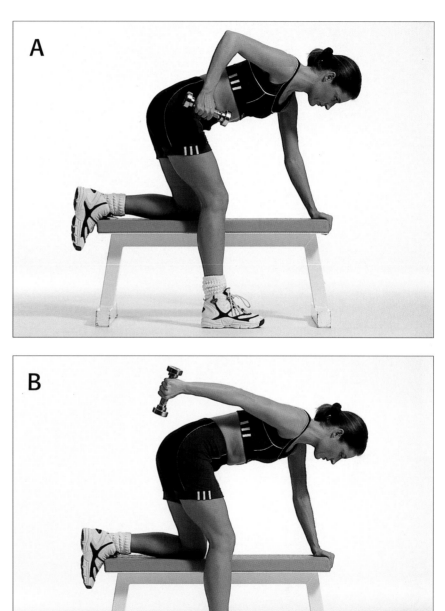

Close-Grip Bench Press

Main muscles involved:
Close-grip bench presses exercise both the greater pectoral muscles *(m. pectoralis major)* and the triceps *(m. triceps brachii).*

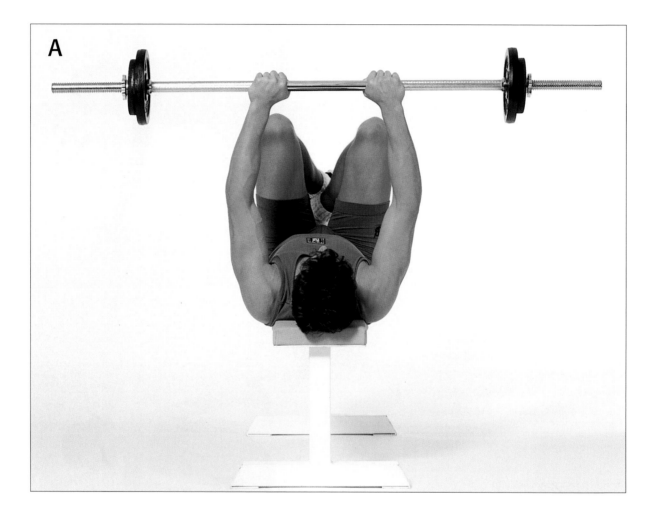

A

Starting position: Lie on your back on a level bench, looking upwards. Draw your legs up towards you and cross them at the ankles. Your eyes should be under the bar of the barbell with your hands at shoulder-width. The supports for the barbell should both be positioned at the same height, low enough for your arms to be slightly bent at the start. Your wrists should remain firm and in line with your forearms, and your palms should face downwards.

▶ Performing the exercise: Lift the barbell smoothly from its support and lock it with slightly bent arms above your chest. Now lower the weights smoothly down to chest level. The barbell should make gentle contact with your chest at approximately the lower end of your breastbone, and then lifted up again without jerking; in the end position the arms are again slightly bent. When performing the exercise, the elbows should be kept relatively close to the body.

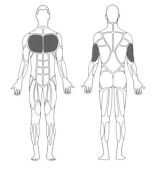

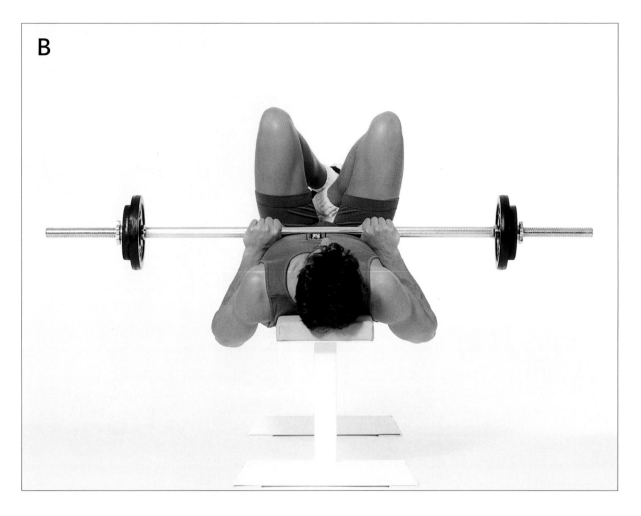

B

Variant: Hold the barbell with your palms facing towards you, not away from you. Otherwise, perform the exercise exactly as described. In this way, the long part of the triceps *(m. triceps brachii)* can be contracted slightly more fully and intensively. You can also perform the bench press with an EZ-curl bar. Here the weight is taken by the muscles in the same way, but some strain is removed from the wrists. The wrists gain even more freedom of movement and relief from strain, if you perform the

exercise with dumbbells. To do this, however, you need a good sense of balance to even out the weight of the dumbbells.

❗ Tip: Do not fall into the temptation of holding the barbell with your hands closer together than shoulder-width. This does not exercise the triceps any more effectively, since the angle of the elbow does not change, but just leads to more strain on the wrists.

Machine Dips

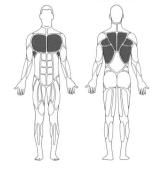

Main muscles involved:

Machine dips train a large number of muscles in the whole upper part of the body. In addition to the triceps *(m. triceps brachii)* and the greater pectoral muscles *(m. pectoralis major)*, the latissimus dorsi, the lower and middle part of the trapezius and the greater rhomboid muscles *(m. rhomboideus major)* are all involved.

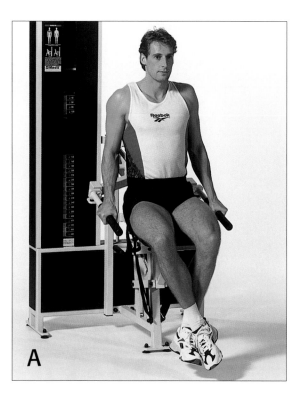

A

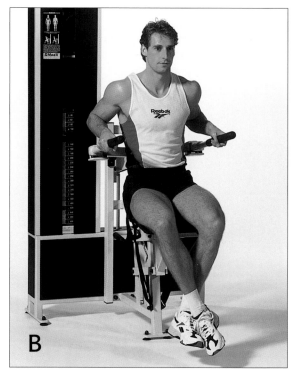

B

Starting position: Sit up straight with the upper part of your body against the back rest of the machine. If the machine has a start help, operate it with your legs to bring the weights into the starting position without taxing your arms. Hold your arms slightly bent and close to your body, and hold the levers about shoulder width apart with your palms facing inwards.

▶ Performing the exercise: Bend your elbows at a 45° angle. Keep your arms close to your body and leave the upper part of your body and your head supported by the backrest. Then extend your arms until they reach the starting position, where they should be slightly bent.

Variant: With some machines it is possible to hold the handles palm downwards. These machines are especially suited for doing a variant with the elbows extended outwards. This movement involves the latissimus dorsi more. Here the arms are not kept close to the body but deliberately angled away from it.

❗ Tip: In the case of weights approximately that of your body weight, you should fasten a belt around your waist so that your body is not lifted from the seat.

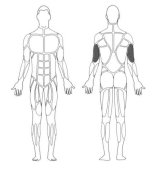

Lying Barbell Triceps Extensions

Main muscles involved:
All three parts of the triceps *(m. triceps brachii)* are trained with this exercise.

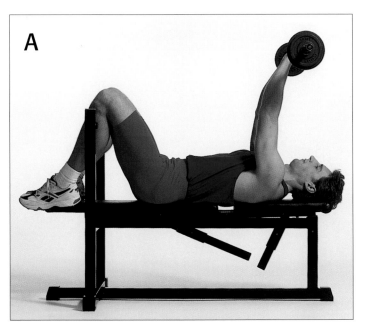

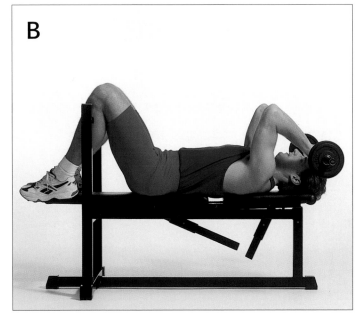

Starting position: Lie on your back on a level bench. Look straight upwards and place your feet on the end of the bench with your legs bent. This will ensure that you are in a stable position. Ask a training partner to give you an EZ-curl bar, and lock it above the upper part of your chest. Your wrists should be firm and form a straight line with your forearms and your palms should be facing your feet. Hold the EZ-curl bar behind the second bend from the middle.

▶ Performing the exercise: Lower the barbell in a semicircular movement down to your forehead by bending the forearm towards the upper arm at the elbow. While doing so, keep your upper arm where it was in the starting position; only the forearm should move. Shortly before reaching your forehead, stop the movement, change direction and raise the forearms

back to the starting position, where the arms should be slightly bent. Your wrists should remain in a straight line with your forearms.

Variant: You can change the effect considerably if you lower the barbell to a position just behind your head instead of towards your forehead. This means that your upper arms have to move a little towards your head, and then back to their original vertical position again.

❗ Tip: If you are training without a partner, do not place your head right at the end of the bench, so that you can set down the barbell there, if necessary, without having to let it fall. If the exercise bench is too short to allow this, put a second bench – if available – at its head end.

Lying Dumbbell Triceps Extension

Main muscles involved:
The same muscles as in S29 are exercised.

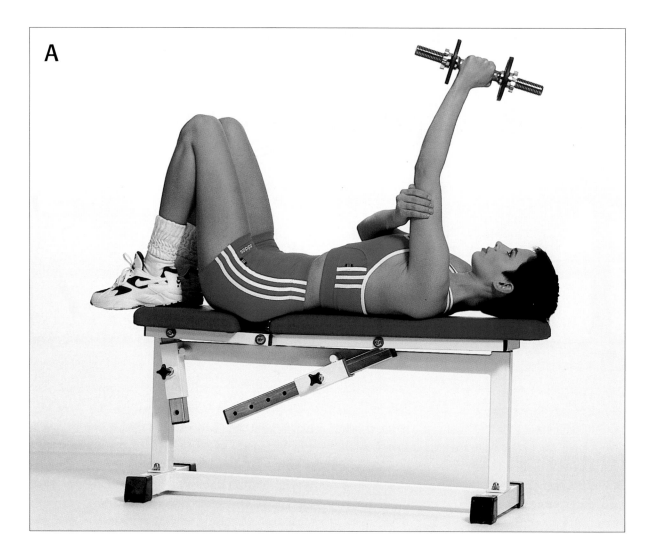

Starting position: Lie on your back on a flat exercise bench. Look straight upwards, your legs drawn up towards your body and your feet on the end of the bench to stabilize yourself throughout the exercise. Hold a dumbbell in one hand with the palm facing inwards. Your arm should be vertical and slightly bent. Lock the dumbbell above the upper part of your chest. Your wrist should be straight and form one line with your forearm. The other hand holds the upper arm of the arm being trained in a vertical position.

▶ Performing the exercise: Lower the dumbbell alongside your head in a semicircular motion by bending the forearm towards the upper arm at the elbow. The upper arm should remain immobile in the starting position; only the forearm should

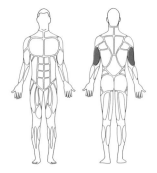

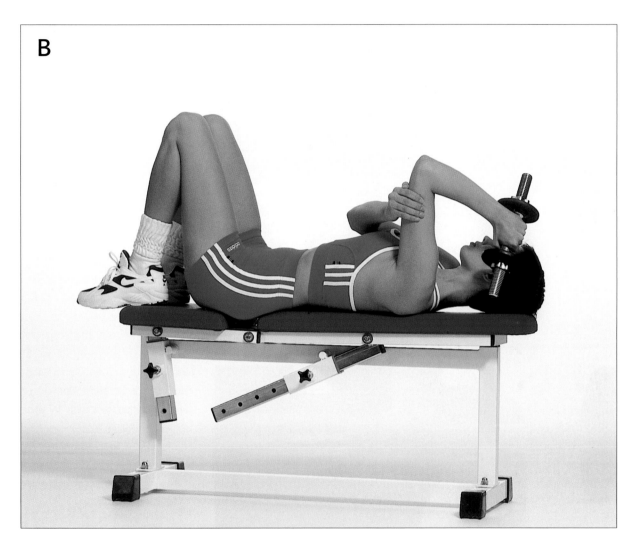

B

move. When the hand has reached the level of your forehead, stop the motion, change directions and lift the forearm back to the starting position with the arm slightly bent. During the whole exercise, make sure that your wrist does not bend, and always remains in a straight line with your forearm.

Variant: This exercise can also be performed using both arms. If you choose this variation, make sure that your upper arms always remain in one position while performing the exercise.

🛈 Tip: Experiment a little with the position of the palm at various angles between facing inwards and facing your feet, to find the most comfortable position for you.

Barbell Wrist Curls Palms Facing Up

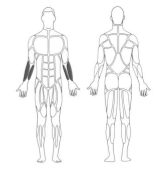

Main muscles involved:

Barbell wrist curls are primarily made possible by the ulnar flexors of the wrist (*Mm. flexores carpi ulnaris et radialis*).

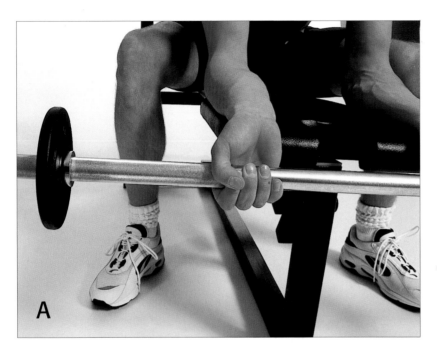

A

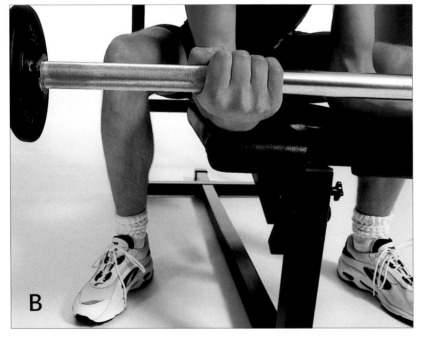

B

Starting position: Sit lengthways on an exercise bench. Bend your arms and rest your forearms on the exercise bench with your wrists and hands protruding over the edge. Hold a barbell with your hands shoulder-width apart, fingers underneath. In the starting position your hands should sink at the wrists; that is, your palms should face forwards and upwards. Your hands should be slightly open so that the barbell is held only by your fingers and not by the whole hand.

▷ Performing the exercise: First, close your hands by rolling the barbell upwards and then lift the barbell in a continuous movement without any hesitation. To do so, bend your hands at the wrist towards your forearm. Then lower the barbell smoothly back down until it is in the starting position, held only by your fingers.

VARIANT

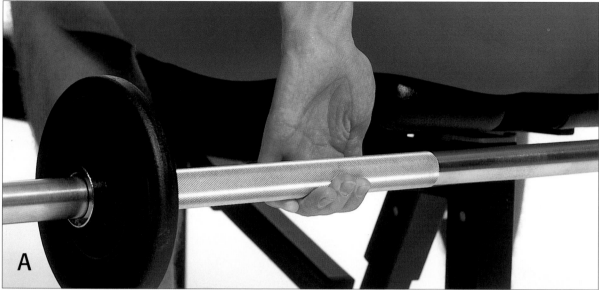

Variant: Hold the barbell behind your back while sitting backwards on the end of an exercise bench. The backs of your hands face your body and the barbell should be held only with the fingers. The barbell is rolled upwards by closing the hand and then lifted further in a semicircular motion by bending the closed hand at the wrist. The opposite movement is carried out to bring the barbell back to the starting position.

⚠ Tip: Work your way up to this exercise slowly. Use much less weight at first than what you could actually manage, so that the muscles, and above all the joints, can get used to the unusual strain.

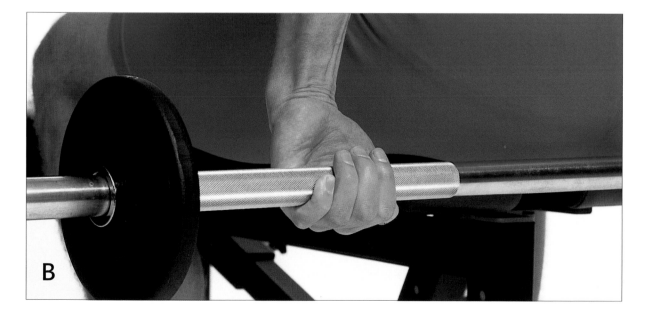

Dumbbell Wrist Curls Palms Facing Up

Main muscles involved:

The muscles mentioned in S31 are trained.

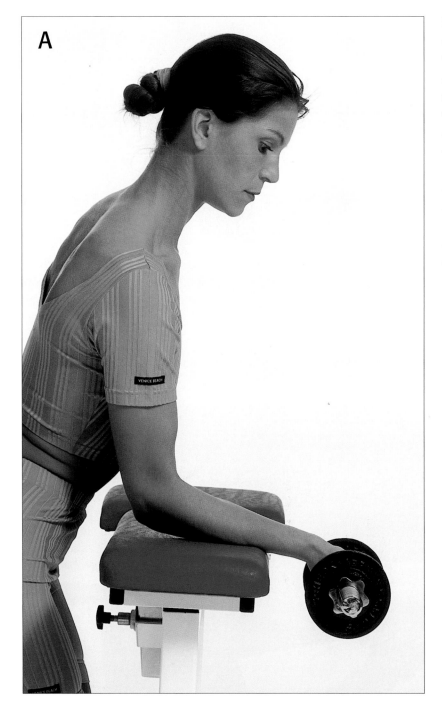

A

Starting position: Kneel on a mat in front of an exercise bench placed at right angles to your body. Your arm should be bent at about 90° and your forearm should be supported – along its entire length – with your wrist and hand protruding over the edge of the bench. Hold a dumbbell with your fingers underneath. In the starting position, your hand should be bent downwards at the wrist; that is, the palm of your hand should face forwards and upwards. Your hand should be slightly open so that the dumbbell is held just by the fingers and not the whole hand. The other hand should either hold the edge of the exercise bench or be placed on your hip.

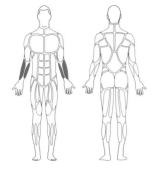

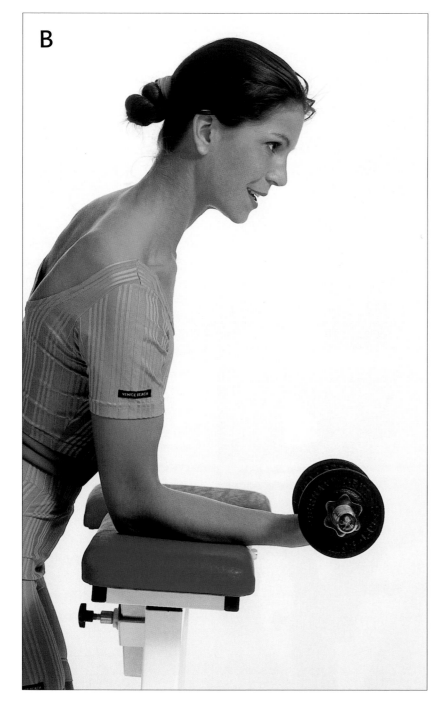

B

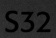 Performing the exercise: Close your hand by rolling the dumbbell upwards and then continue to raise it without hesitation in a continuous motion. Bend your hand towards your forearm at the wrist. Then lower the dumbbell in an even motion, until it is in the starting position again, held only by the fingers.

Variant: As a variation, this exercise can be performed using both hands simultaneously.

⚠ Tip: Do not open your hand too much in your first attempts at this exercise; otherwise, there is the danger for beginners that the dumbbell could slip from their fingers completely and fall on the floor.

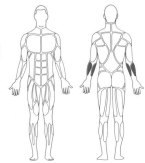

Main muscles involved:

Barbell wrist curls are mainly performed using the wrist extensors *(Mm. extensores carpi ulnaris et radialis).*

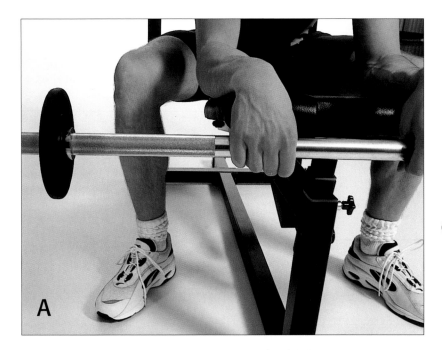

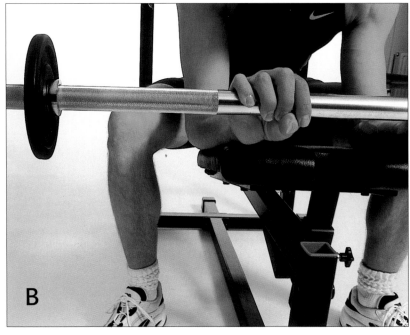

Starting position: Sit lengthwise on an exercise bench. Your arms should be sharply bent; your forearms should be supported along their entire length with your wrists and hands protruding over the edge of the bench. Hold a barbell with your hands shoulder-width apart, fingers on top. In the starting position, your hands should be bent at the wrists with the backs facing forwards and upwards.

▶ Performing the exercise: Raise both hands with the barbell in an even semicircular motion as high as possible until the backs of your hands are facing you. From here lower the barbell into the original position again. Make sure that you maintain tension even in the lowest position. Only the wrists should bend.

Variant: Perform the exercise using a pulley from below with a straight swivel grip. The transmission through the cable changes the way tension is built up in the muscles as compared to a barbell.

❗ Tip: If you are working with a barbell, you should have a partner take the weights from you after performing a set, if possible. Otherwise, there is a danger that fatigue in your wrist extensors could lead to your losing control over the weights and thus falling on the floor.

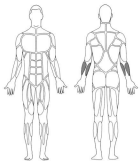

Main muscles involved:
The same muscles are involved as in S33.

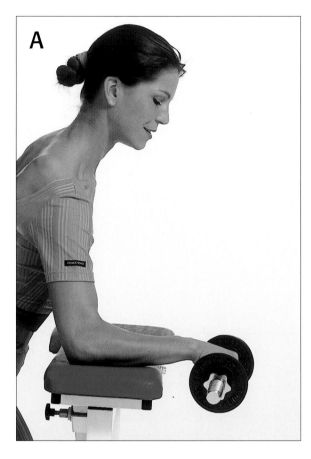

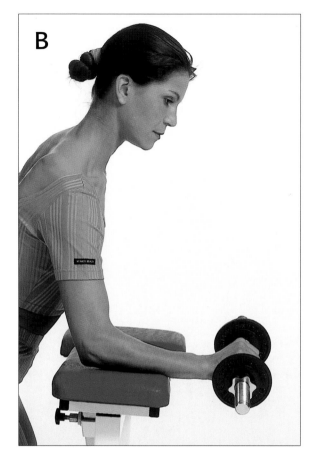

Starting position: Kneel on a mat in front of an exercise bench placed at right angles. Your arm should be bent at about 90° with your forearm supported along its entire length and your wrist and hand protruding over the edge. Hold a dumbbell with your fingers on top. In the starting position, your hand should be bent at the wrist and the back of your hand should face forwards and upwards.

▶ Performing the exercise: Raise the hand with the dumbbell as high as possible so that the back of your hand is facing you at the end of the movement. From here lower the dumbbell again slowly into the starting position. Make sure that you maintain some tension even in the lowest position. Only the wrist should bend during the whole movement.

Variant: As a variation you can do this exercise with both arms.

❗ Tip: Hold the bar of the dumbbell loosely in the lower position and strengthen your grip only during the upwards movement. This takes strain off the wrist.

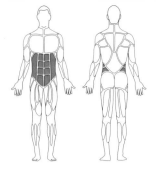

S35 Floor Crunches

Main muscles involved:

This exercise involves primarily the abdominal rectus *(m. rectus abdominis)*. The external and internal oblique muscles of the abdomen *(Mm. obliquus externus et internus abdominis)* and the abdominal tranversus muscle *(m. transversus abdominis)* play a subordinate role.

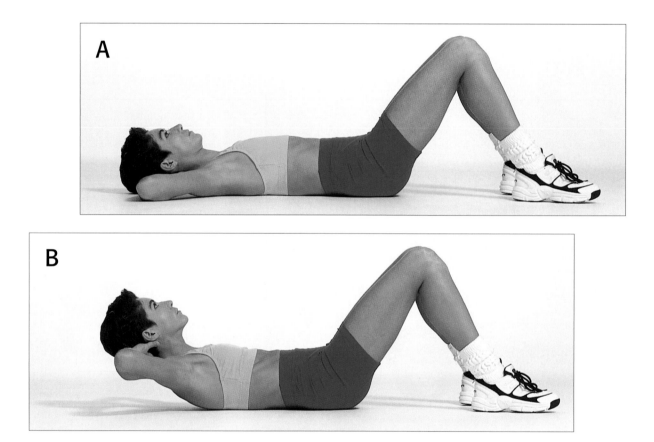

Starting position: Lie on your back with your legs bent and your feet placed on the floor as far apart as your hips. Bend your arms on each side of your head. Press your feet into the floor.

▶ Performing the exercise: Raise the upper part of your body a few inches forwards and upwards. Your hands should lie relaxed at the side of your head without pulling. The head should keep a constant distance from your body. Then lower your body just as slowly and evenly without letting it touch the ground completely.

Variant: To make the exercise easier, you can also cross your arms on your chest. It is made even easier if you slightly bend your arms in front of your body and slide them alongside your legs. This technique is to be recommended for beginners because the weight of the arms is not as noticeable and the danger of pulling on the head is eliminated.

❗ Tip: To obtain the best possible head position, the eyes should be directed at the ceiling for the whole exercise.

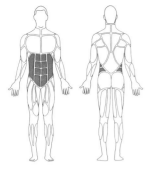

Main muscles involved:

Twisted crunches exercise the straight abdominal muscle *(m. rectus abdominis)*, the external and internal oblique muscles of the abdomen *(Mm. obliquus externus et internus abdominis)* and the transversus abdominal muscle of the respective side being trained.

Starting position: Lie on your back with your legs bent at right angles, your feet bent upwards and your heels pressed into the floor. Bend your arms on each side of your head with the fingers either touching your temples or supporting your neck without pulling on it. Your shoulders should already be slightly raised.

▶ Performing the exercise: Using your abdominal muscles, lift one shoulder towards the opposite hip. This makes the body roll a few inches diagonally upwards and forwards. Lower it again just as slowly and evenly and begin the exercise again.

Variant: A somewhat easier variation can be performed if you straighten your arm slightly and slide it along the leg on the opposite side instead of holding it angled at head level. You can also cross the leg – towards which the shoulder is moved – over the other one to stabilize your body.

❗ Tip: Do not try to reach the knee of the opposite leg with your bent elbow. That only twists the spine more without leading to better results.

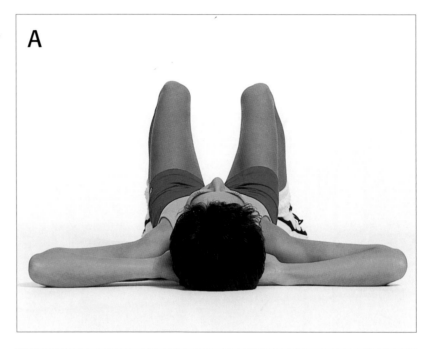

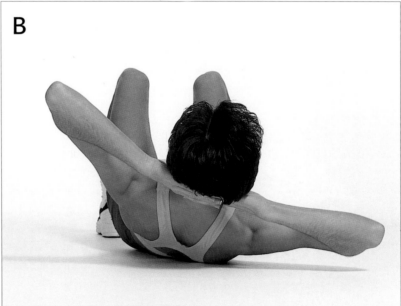

S37 Crunches Machine

Main muscles involved:

This exercise trains the same muscles as in S35.

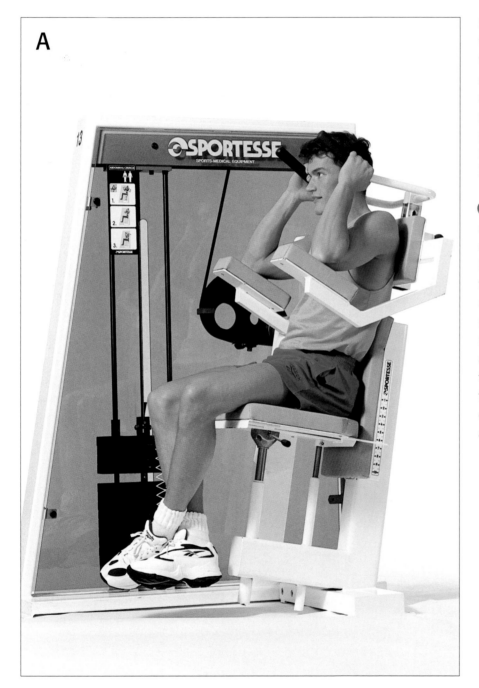

Starting position: Sit on the machine so that your pelvis is firmly supported and the pad of the machine is approximately at shoulder height. The height of the pad or seat can be adjusted to obtain this position. Bend your legs and, if possible, place your feet on the foot rest. If the machine has a belt to fasten the upper legs or the hips, put it on.

▶ Performing the exercise: Bend the upper part of your body forward slowly and evenly without moving the hips. The head should bend along with the rest of the spine. If the equipment has grips, make sure that you use the abdominal muscles and not the arms to perform the movement. At the lowest point, the abdominal muscles should have reached their maximum contraction. Now raise the upper part of the body again in an even motion until it is only slightly bent, and begin the exercise once more.

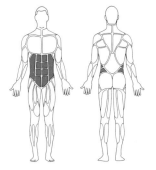

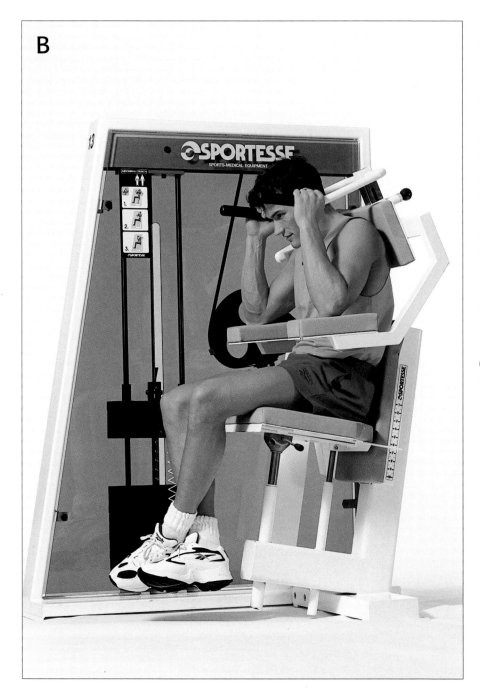

B

Variant: Depending on how the machine is built, there are different ways of keeping the body, and particularly the pelvis, still. The way in which the power of the upper body is transmitted to the machine also varies. Normally the pad is in front of the shoulders in the form of a cylinder, one long pad or two single pads, one for each shoulder. It is also possible that the elbows transmit the power. Here, the elbows are supported on two pads, the arms are sharply bent and the hands hold the two grips positioned above the elbow pads. The back is supported by the rest provided and the arms press the upper part of the body onto it, which then bends forward together with the pad.

⚠ Tip: To ensure that the spine bends evenly, it helps to imagine that you are watching an object falling to the ground. This makes the head sink smoothly downwards and come evenly back up again. If there is a footrest on the machine, you should push firmly against it. If not, cross your legs at the ankles and concentrate on pushing your pelvis back into the seat.

Main muscles involved:
This exercise trains the same muscles as in S36.

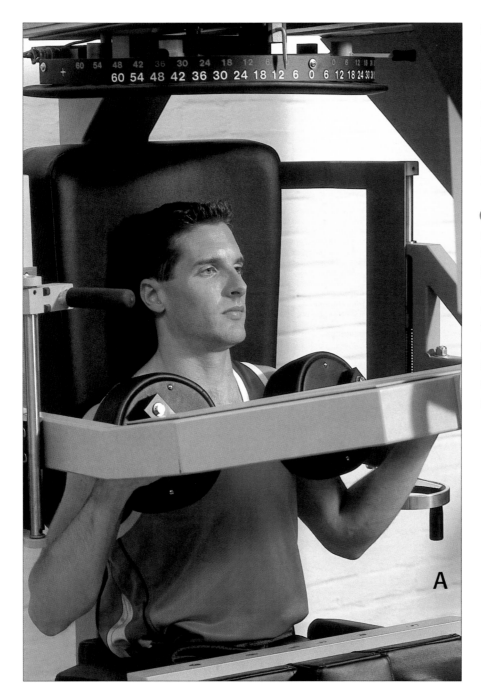

A

Starting position: Sit with your spine upright on the rotating seat of the twisting machine. Make sure that your spinal column is directly above the axis of rotation of the machine. Your head should form the natural extension of your spine and your hands stabilize the upper part of the body by holding the bars provided. Place your feet on the footrest.

▷ Performing the exercise: The maximum angle of rotation in this exercise is about twice 35°, i.e. altogether 70°. This means that the rotation to one side should not even be half of a right angle. Turn the upper part of your body slowly and evenly towards the side to be trained. While doing so, keep your shoulders in one line and as still as possible; your head follows the movement, remaining vertical to the shoulders for the entire exercise.

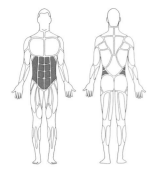

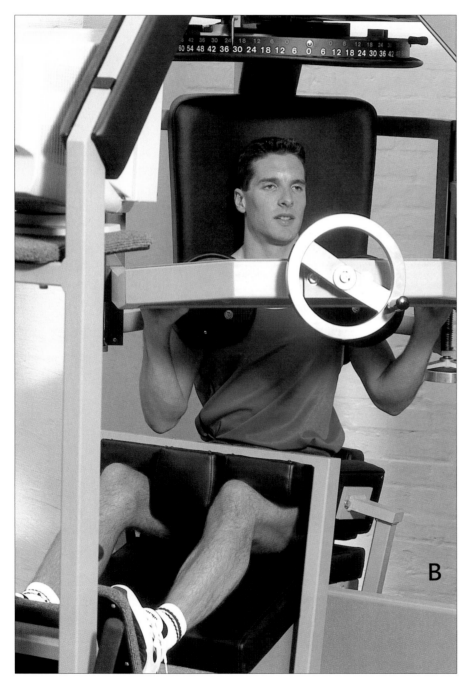

B

Variant: Many equipment firms make twisting machines that turn in two directions at once; that is, while the shoulders turn against resistance in one direction, the hips also turn against resistance in the other. These machines require better motor skills to avoid the body being contorted too much.

🛈 Tip: Have an observer tell you when the angle of turn is 70°, and perhaps note some reference points in the room to enable you to keep to this angle. Going beyond the recommended angle of rotation should be avoided; otherwise, the vertebral cartilage is put under unnecessary strain and the intervertebral discs are exposed to an unhealthy pull that can lead to premature wear and tear.

S39 Pelvis Raises

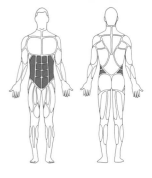

Main muscles involved:
This exercise trains the muscles described in S35.

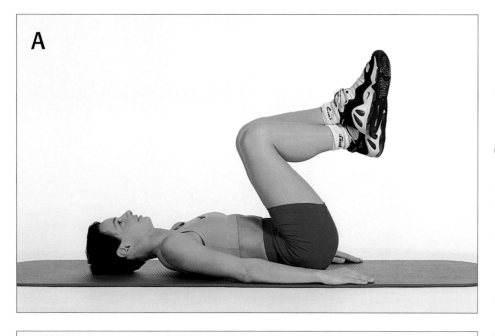

A

Starting position: Lie on your back on a gym mat with your head resting relaxed on the floor and your arms next to you, palms downward. Pull your legs up towards your abdomen and cross your legs at the ankles.

▶ Performing the exercise: Lift your hips several inches in a rolling movement towards your head. Then lower them again, without touching the ground.

Variant: Bend your legs slightly and stretch them upwards, thrusting your hips up as if someone were pulling them by the feet.

❗ Tip: To achieve greater stability of the upper body, place your gym mat at the end of a weight-lifting bench so that you can hold on to the legs of the bench with both hands to support yourself.

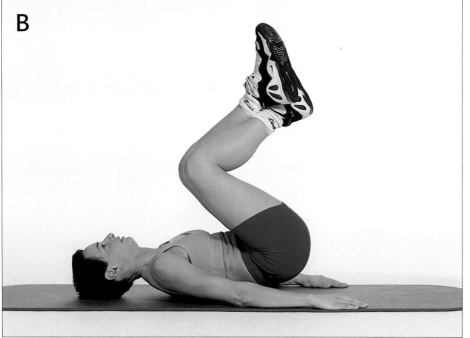

B

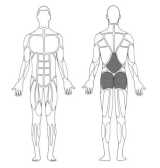

Main muscles involved:

Mainly the spinal erector *(m. erector spinae).* In addition, the greatest gluteal muscle *(m. gluteus maximus)* is trained.

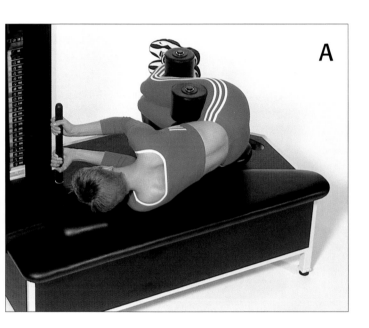

A

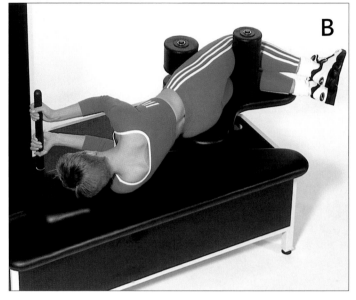

B

Starting position: Lie on the machine on your side and put your pelvis in front of the round hip cushion so that the hip joints are exactly above the axis of rotation the machine. The second cushion should be positioned just above the back of the knee. The upper part of your body is held in position by its own weight and by the handle, which you should hold with your palms facing you and your arms bent. Your legs should be drawn up so far that your lower back is somewhat rounded.

▶ Performing the exercise: Straighten out your body back-wards from the hips until your upper body is in line with your thighs. The upper part of your body should remain absolutely straight during the entire exercise with your head forming the extension of your spine. Bring your body forward again only to the point where the weight does not touch the ground and so that the tension in the lower back remains.

Variant: With another type of machine, you would not lie as described on your side, but instead sit on the machine. Your hip joints correspond to the axis of rotation of the machine. The back support that transmits the power of your muscles rests against your shoulder blades. Make sure that your hips move freely and that your spine is naturally curved in the end position.

🛈 Tip: Increase the weights very slowly because this exercise puts much strain on various passive structures such as ligaments, which take longer to recover than the active musculature.

Back Hyperextensions

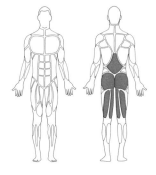

Main muscles involved:

In addition to the spinal erector *(m. erector spinae)* and the greatest gluteal muscle *(m. gluteus maximus)*, this exercise also trains the leg flexors. These are above all the biceps muscle of the thigh *(m. biceps femoris)*, the semitendinous *(m. semitendinosus)* and the semimembranous *(m. semimembranosus)* muscles.

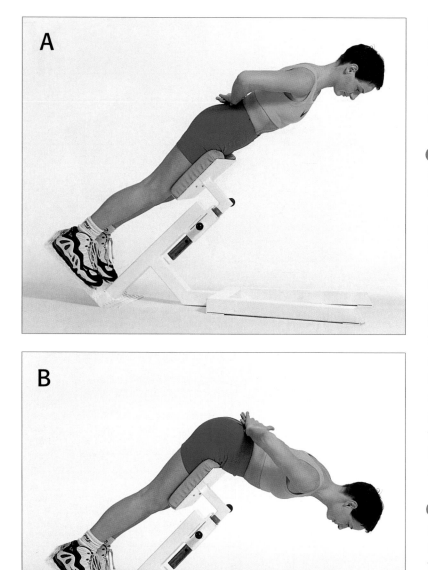

A

B

Starting position: Place your heels in the foot supports and adjust the leg pad so that your thighs are well supported, while your hips remain completely free above the edge of the pad. Your whole body should form a straight line with your head, as a natural extension of your spine.

▶ Performing the exercise: Lower the upper part of your body by bending at the hips. The whole trunk should remain completely straight and is lowered, depending on flexibility, only so far as it can remain straight in the lower part as well; the maximum angle between upper body and thighs should be 90°.

Variant: Bend at the hips as described in the basic exercise. This time however, bend your spinal column forwards one vertebra at a time from the bottom up. When the back is completely curved, begin the upwards movement by straightening up one vertebra at a time until the upper part of the body again forms a straight extension of the legs. This variation makes considerably more demands on the coordination than the technique with a straight back; however, it is possible to train the intervertebral muscles dynamically in this way, which is not the case with the other technique.

❗ Tip: You should not perform this exercise if your blood pressure is too high or low. This exercise is also not suitable if you have back problems of any sort, since the weight of the upper body cannot be controlled by you.

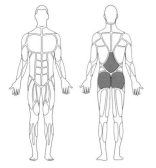

Hyperextensions Reversed

Main muscles involved:
Primarily the spinal erector *(m. erector spinae)*. The greatest gluteal muscle *(m. gluteus maximus)* is also trained.

Starting position: Lie on your stomach up to your hips on a raised surface. If you do not have a special bench, you can use a normal table. Hold the handles provided to keep the upper part of your body still. Bend your legs at right angles and let them hang over the edge; they should be parallel and as far apart as your hips.

▶ Performing the exercise: Extend your body in a smooth motion by simultaneously straightening at the hips and the knees. Your feet should remain drawn up towards the body. In the end postion the thighs and upper body should form a straight line.

Variant: If, after some training, this exercise becomes too easy with only the weight of the legs, you can fasten weights to your ankles. Another possibility is to do the exercise on a special machine. Here, a pad that transmits the weight to the legs lies on the back of your thighs just above the hollow of the knee.

❗ Tip: If you have problems at first with this exercise, try using only one leg at a time.

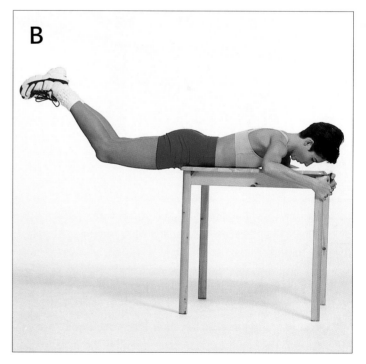

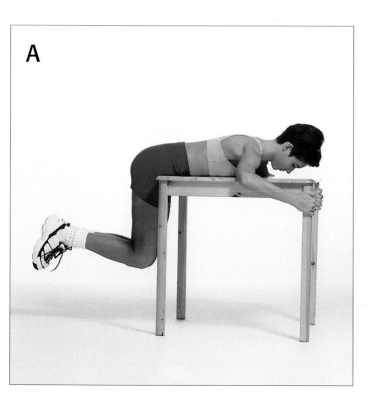

Main muscles involved:

The squat is one of the exercises that trains the greatest proportion of muscles in the body, either directly or indirectly. Especially exercised is the lower part of the body: the greatest gluteal muscle *(m. gluteus maximus)*, the quadriceps of the thigh *(m. quadriceps femoris)* and the soleus *(m. soleus)*. In addition, all the back muscles are exercised, especially the spinal erector *(m. erector spinae),...*

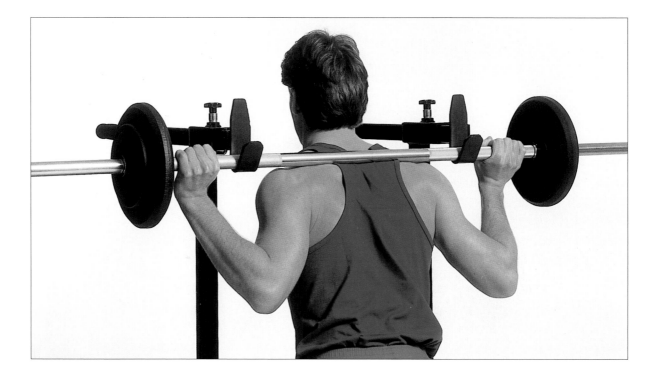

Starting position: Stand with your feet several inches apart and your feet pointing slightly outwards. Hold the barbell across your shoulders behind your head, resting on the upper part of the trapezius muscle. Your hands should be slightly further apart than shoulder-width. Distribute the weight of your body evenly onto both feet. Keep your knees and hips slightly bent.

▶ Performing the exercise: After lifting the barbell from the rack and taking up position two paces behind it, tense your back muscles and relax those of the knees, hips and ankles a little, then sink slowly into the knee-bend. The heels should not be raised from the ground and you should concentrate on lowering your hips. Your knees come slightly forward, your buttocks move a little backwards at first and then directly downwards, and the upper part of your body bends slightly forward (up to 45°). The spine remains in its normal, slightly curved state the whole time. The downwards movement should stop when the thighs form a right angle with the lower legs. At this point, change direction by straightening the body powerfully at the hips and knees. At the highest point the legs should again be slightly bent.

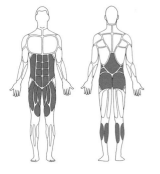

... and the abdominal muscles with the abdominal rectus *(m. rectus abdominis)*, the external and internal oblique muscles of the abdomen *(Mm. obliquus externus et internus abdominis)* and the abdominal transversus muscle *(m. transversus abdominis)* contribute to the necessary stability of the upper body.

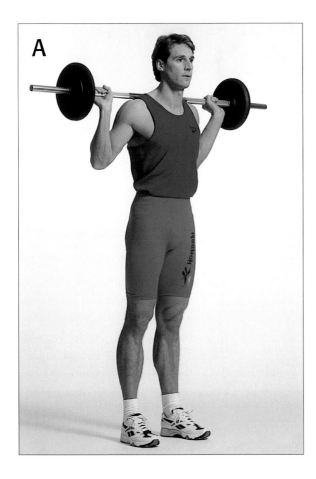

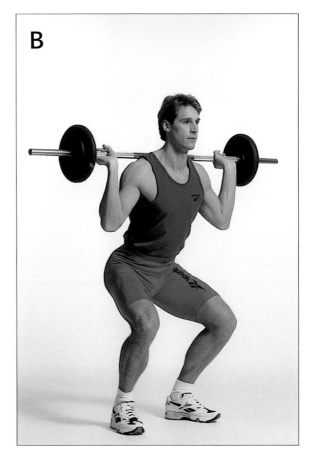

Variant: You can vary the distance between your feet from being a few inches apart to being at shoulder-width. Make absolutely sure that the tips of your toes are always in line with your knees and thighs even when standing with your feet further apart. With this stance you include the thigh adductors *(Mm. adductores)* as well.

❗ Tip: If you are not sure whether you are bending your legs too far or not far enough, ask a neutral observer to check on the 90° angle. If you use a mirror at the side to control the angle of bend, remember that your neck is no longer in its natural position when you look sideways. After checking briefly, rely on the motor sense of your body.

Main muscles involved:
More or less the same muscles are exercised as in S43.

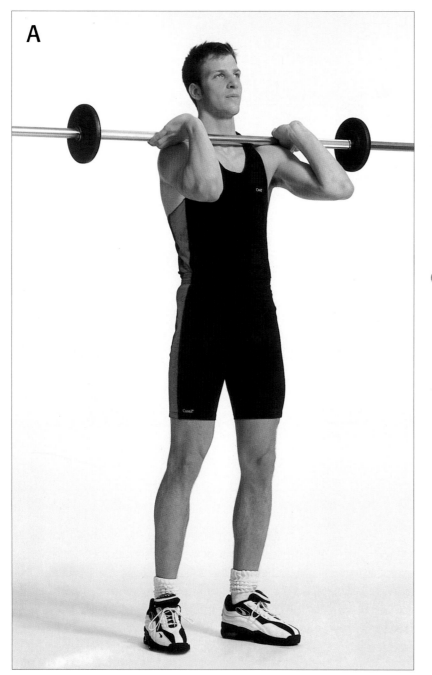

Starting position: Stand with your feet parallel. Hold the barbell with your hands slightly further apart than shoulder-width. Your hands should be under the barbell and your elbows raised as far as possible. The palms of your hands face the ceiling. While you are holding the barbell like this, the upper part of your back should remain straight. The wrists come under slightly more strain. Olympic weight lifters use this hold in training because it is possible to lift the barbell during the exercise.

▷ Performing the exercise: Tense your back extensors and relax your knee, hip and ankle muscles slightly before going down into the squat. Do not raise your heels from the floor and concentrate on lowering the hips. Your knees come forward a little, your buttocks move a little backwards at first and then straight downwards, and the upper part of your body remains nearly upright. The spine should remain in its normal, slightly curved state. Stop the downwards movement when your thighs are at right angles with your lower legs. Having reached the lowest position, change direction by straightening the body powerfully at the hips and knees until the legs are again only slightly bent.

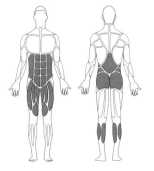

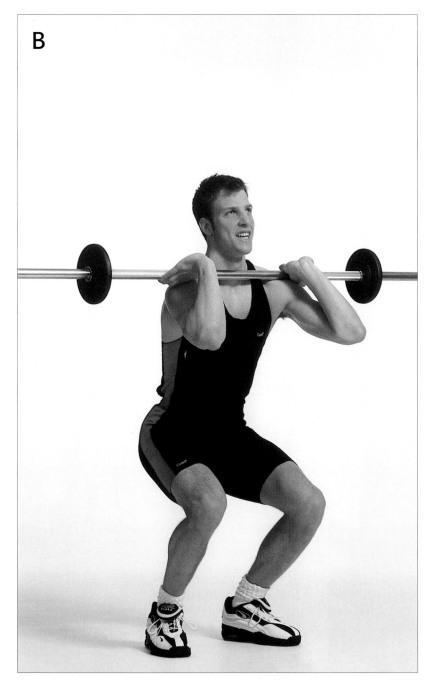

B

Variant: Stand with your feet parallel. Rest the barbell on the upper part of the chest and shoulder muscles. Raise your upper arms until they are almost horizontal and cross your forearms in front of you. Hold the barbell with your hands on top.

🛈 Tip: Because the muscles do not support the barbell as well in front of the body as they do in regular squats, it is better to wrap a towel around the middle of the barbell or use a special foam pad.

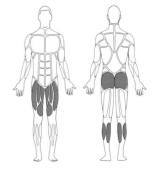

Main muscles involved:
The muscles of the lower part of the body described in S43 are trained. The upper body muscles are used far less.

Starting position: Lean the upper part of your body and your head completely against the backrest in whatever position the machine is used. Your feet should be placed as far apart as your hips on the footrest provided, the tips of your toes, your knees and your thighs should be in one line and your legs should be slightly bent at the knee. With a start help you can bring the weight into the raised position at the beginning, by using a lever so that the muscles involved can already build up the necessary preliminary tension in the first repetition while lowering the weights, and so that the joints are not put under unnecessary strain.

▷ Performing the exercise: Lower the foot rest slowly and evenly towards your body without moving your pelvis. Stop the movement when your legs form a right angle at the knee. Straighten the legs again until they are slightly bent in the starting position.

Variant: Place the feet higher or further apart on the foot rest if it is large enough so that the emphasis falls on different muscles. However, make sure that the tips of your toes, knees and thighs always remain in a one line.

❶ Tip: If the machine you are using does not have a start help, have a partner help you the first time you lift the weights. This considerably reduces the strain on the joints involved.

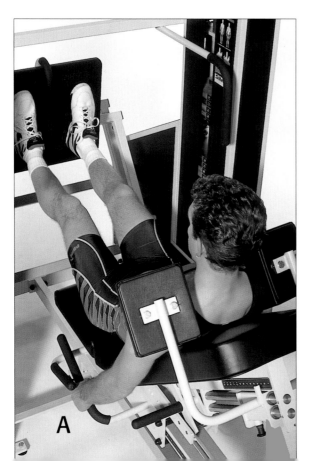

A

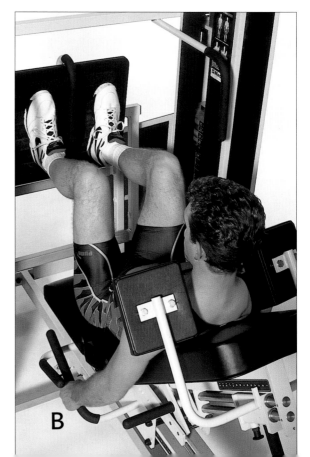

B

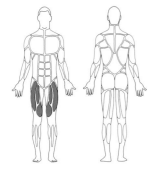

Main muscles involved:
This exercise primarily trains the quadriceps of the thigh *(m. quadriceps femoris).*

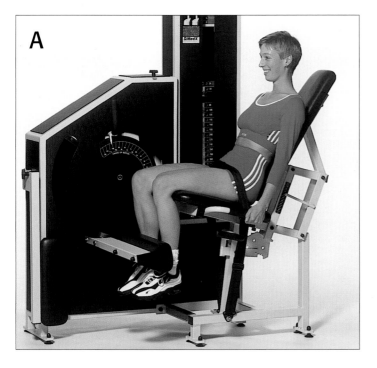

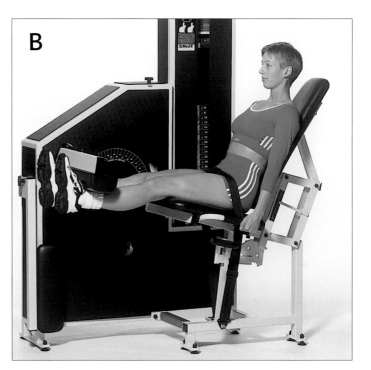

Starting position: Sit on the seat so that your knee joints correspond to the axis of rotation of the machine. Then adjust the backrest so that it makes close contact with your back and supports your pelvis. The foot pad should be adjusted to lie in the hollow between your feet and your lower legs. Bend your feet up towards your shins to stabilize your knee joints. Your hands should hold the body still by gripping the handles provided on the machine. In the starting position your legs should be bent at the knees to a maximum angle of 90°.

▷ Performing the exercise: Raise the legs slowly and evenly until they are almost straight. Lower your legs from this position just as evenly back into the starting position.

Variant: In this exercise you should not vary the way your feet are bent, since the knee joints come under unnecessary strain if the position is contorted in any way.

🛈 Tip: If you have access to a modern machine where the range of movement can be limited by determining the starting and end positions, you should fix the starting position at 90°, and the end position at the point where your legs are almost straightened. This prevents you from over-straightening your legs, thus also causing too much strain on your knees.

Lying Leg Curls

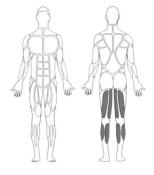

Main muscles involved:

This exercise mainly trains the biceps of the thigh *(m. biceps femoris)*, the semitendinous *(m. semitendinosus)* and the semimembranous *(m. semimembranosus)* muscles. If the feet are bent up towards the shin, the gastrocnemius *(m. gastrocnemius)* is also involved.

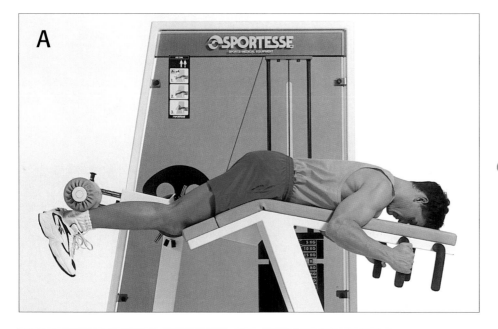

Starting position: Lie face down on the machine. Your knee joints should be in line with the axis of rotation of the machine. Position the cylindrical leg pad just underneath the calves. Draw the tips of your toes upwards towards the shins and bend your legs slightly.

▶ Performing the exercise: Lift the leg pad as high as possible in a slow, smooth and even motion. Make sure that you do not raise your pelvis from the bench. Lower the weight from the highest position just as slowly back into the starting position again, where your legs should be slightly bent.

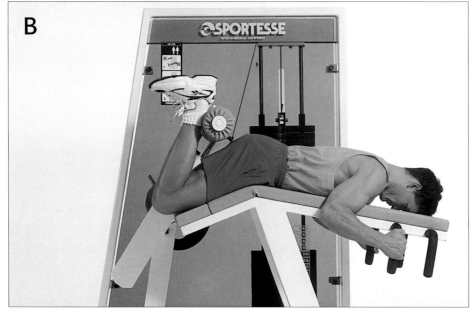

Variant: If this exercise is done with the tips of your toes drawn upwards, the gastrocnemius muscle *(m. gastrocnemius)* is actively involved and exercised. If you stretch your foot downwards at the ankle, however, this muscle cannot participate as much; instead, you exercise the thigh flexors more in isolation.

❗ Tip: If you place a rolled-up towel under your hips, it can help take strain off the lower back.

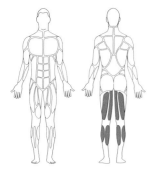

Main muscles involved:
The same muscles are exercised as in S47.

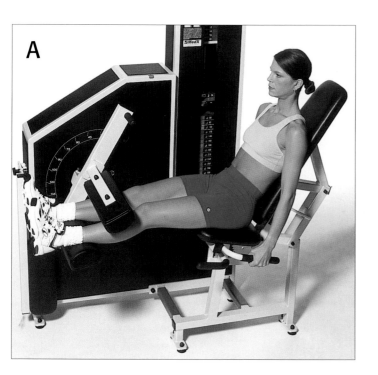

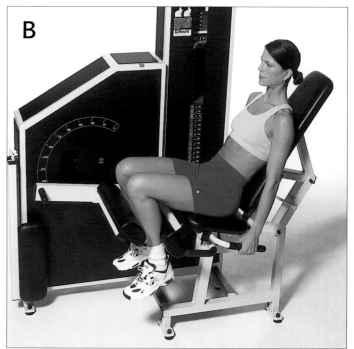

Starting position: Sit on the seat so that your knee joints correspond to the axis of rotation of the machine. Adjust the backrest so that it comes into contact with the back and supports the hips. Position the foot pad or the leg pad so that it is just below the calf at the back of the lower leg. Draw your feet up towards your shins. Hold your body still using the grips provided on the machine. In the starting position, your legs should be slightly bent at the knees. The machine you are using could have an additional pad to hold the thighs in position. Adjust it so that your thighs are held but not pressed unnecessarily.

▷ Performing the exercise: Pull the leg pad as far as possible downwards in a slow, smooth movement. Only your lower legs should move while doing the exercise. From the end position, where your legs are sharply bent, raise the weight just as slowly back into the starting position with your legs slightly bent.

Variant: If you bend your foot downwards at the ankle, the gastrocnemius muscle cannot participate as much; instead, you exercise the thigh flexors more in isolation.

❗ Tip: Check if the foot pad on your lower leg moves around. If so, you are not sitting correctly at the axis of rotation. Check and adjust your position until the pad does not move any more.

Leg Adduction Machine

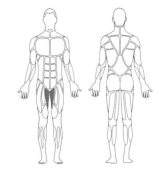

Main muscles involved:

Leg adductions are carried out by the the pectineal muscle *(m. pectineus)*, the long, short and greater adductor muscles *(Mm. adductores longus, brevis et magnus)* and the gracilis *(m. gracilis)* with help from the lower part of the gluteus maximus *(m. gluteus maximus)*.

Starting position: Sit on the seat provided with your whole back leaning against the backrest. Your head should form the natural extension of your spine. Place your legs, more or less bent according to machine type, against the outside of the leg pads. These are mostly positioned near the knee, just above or above and below the knee joint. Modern machines have a start help that enables you to get into the position with spread legs without strain. Your hands should support your body using the grips provided.

▷ Performing the execise: Draw your legs simultaneously and smoothly together into the middle until the leg pads touch. Move only from the hip joint. Move your legs just as evenly back into the starting position until you feel a slight stretch on the inner side of your thighs.

Variant: Depending on the type of machine, the muscles are exercised to slightly different degrees because the hip and knee joints are bent at differing angles.

❗ Tip: This exercise is very often mistaken as a "woman's exercise"; it is, however, just as suitable for men.

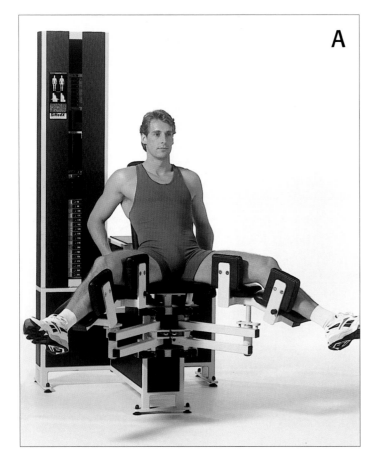

A

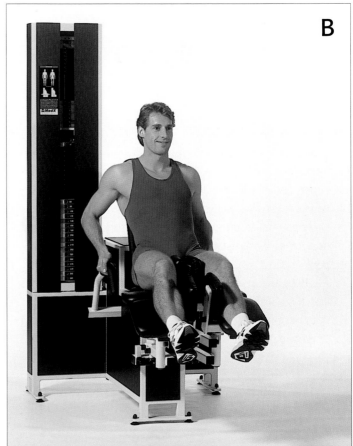

B

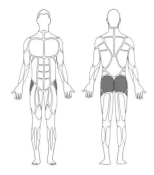

Leg Abduction Machine

Main muscles involved:
The main strength to carry out the abduction of the thighs comes from the medium and small gluteal muscles *(Mm. gluteus medius et minimus)* as well as the upper part of the greatest gluteal muscle *(m. gluteus maximus)*.

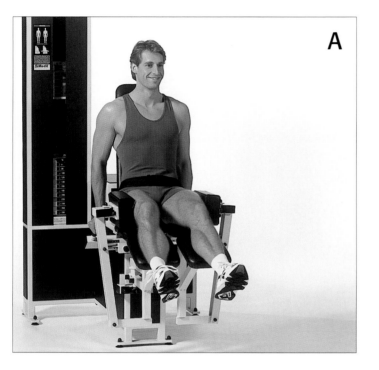

A

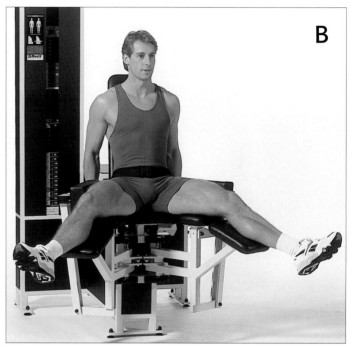

B

Starting position: Sit on the seat provided with your back fully supported by the backrest. Place your legs, more or less bent according to machine type, against the inside of the leg pads. These are normally positioned near the knee, just above or above and below the knee joint. Your hands should support your body using the grips provided on the machine. In the starting position the weight is already slightly raised, so the muscles to be exercised are already under some strain.

▶ Performing the exercise: Move your legs apart simultaneously and evenly as far as you can. The movement comes solely from the hip joints. Then bring your legs back into the starting position just as smoothly.

Variant: Depending on the type of machine, the knees are bent more or less and the angle of the hips also differs. This produces small differences in the way the muscles are exercised.

❗ Tip: Especially if you have only been training your pelvic muscles for a short time, the muscles being exercised are very susceptible to cramps, because such an isolated contraction of the pelvic muscles scarcely ever occurs in everyday life. If this is the case with you, you should stretch your pelvic muscles after every set. Remember to warm up well before training. If you still get a cramp, the only thing to do is stop and stretch the cramped muscle. Massaging the muscle gently also helps get rid of the cramp.

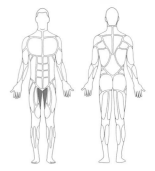

Main muscles involved:
This exercise trains the groups of muscles described in S49.

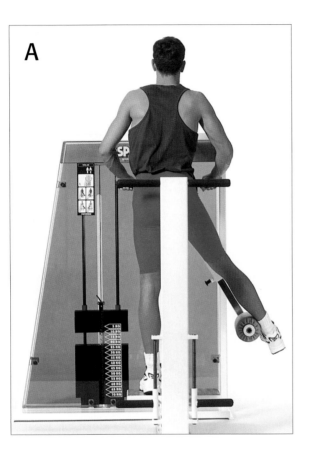

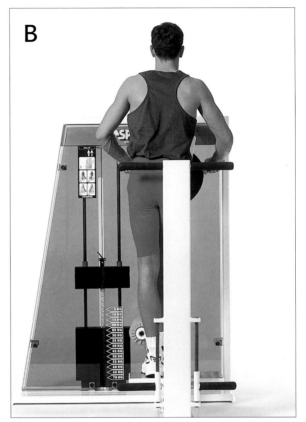

Starting position: Stand upright on the platform of the so-called multi-hip machine. Your body should be in the basic position with your muscles slightly tightened. Hold the grips provided to support and stabilize the body to avoid any undue strain. Make sure that the hip joint on the side to be exercised corresponds to the axis of rotation of the machine and that your hips are parallel with your shoulders. Normally it is possible for you to alter your position by adjusting the height of the platform as well as by standing at different places on it. Place the leg to be trained on the outside of the cylindrical foot pad. In the starting position you should feel a slight stretch on the inner side of the leg being trained.

▷ Performing the exercise: Bring your slightly bent leg with the foot pad evenly from the starting position into the middle. In the end position the leg being exercised should be exactly in front of the fixed leg without the hip being drawn forward. The rest of the body should remain as motionless as possible during the whole exercise and should maintain the basic tension.

Variant: Bend the upper body slightly forwards at the hip.

❶ Tip: Correct your posture, if possible, by checking in a mirror. Make sure above all that your hips do not move as result of the movement; keep them parallel to your shoulders.

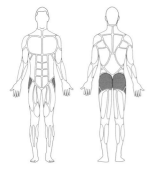

Main muscles involved:
This exercise trains the muscle groups described in S50.

Starting position: Stand in basic position on the platform of the multi-hip machine with the hip joint on the side to be trained in line with the axis of rotation of the machine. If possible, alter the height of the platform and your position to ensure that this is the case. Support your upright posture by holding the grips provided. Tighten your buttocks, abdominal muscles and the back extensor to build up basic tension in your body. You should make sure that the foot pad is adjusted to a height where your hips can still remain parallel to your shoulders. As in the multi-hip adduction, you should also feel a slight stretch on the inside of the leg to be trained while in the starting position. Cross your legs slightly for the starting position so that the pad is in a line with the fixed leg.

Performing the exercise: Push the foot pad with your leg slightly bent sideways and upwards from the starting position. Raise the leg only so far that your pelvis can remain parallel to your shoulders in the end position without one hip bending inwards. Keep the rest of your body as motionless as possible during the whole exercise.

Variant: Turn the leg to be exercised slightly in at the hip so that the foot is pointing somewhat inwards.

Tip: Do the exercise first with the weaker and then with the stronger leg and check your posture in the mirror.

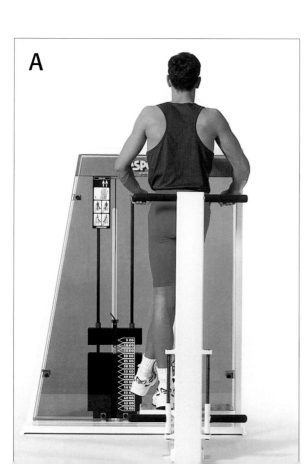

A

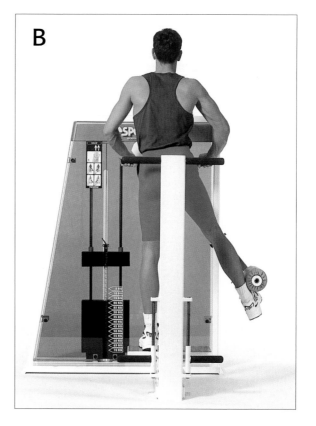

B

Multi-Hip Gluteal Exercise

Main muscles involved:
In this exercise the greatest gluteal muscle *(m. gluteus maximus)* is primarily trained.

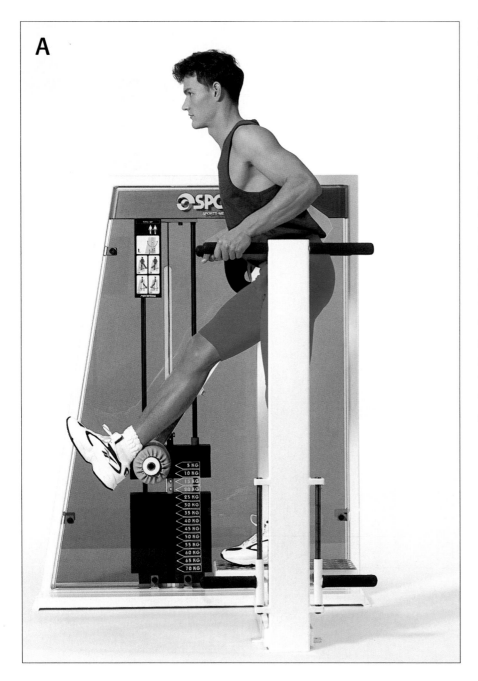

A

Starting position: Bend the upper part of your body slightly forwards at the hips. Build up tension in your whole body in this posture just like the tension in the basic position. Support your upper body using the grips provided to stabilize and support the bent posture. This exercise is carried out first with the weaker, then with the stronger leg. Your body should be parallel to the multi-hip machine. Make sure that your hip joints are in line with the axis of rotation of the equipment. You can alter your position both by adjusting the height of the platform and by standing at different places on it. The foot pad should be positioned behind your lower leg just below your calf. In the starting position the pad should be far enough in front of the hip to allow the leg flexors to move freely without creating tension in the lower back. Both legs should be slightly bent.

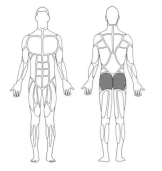

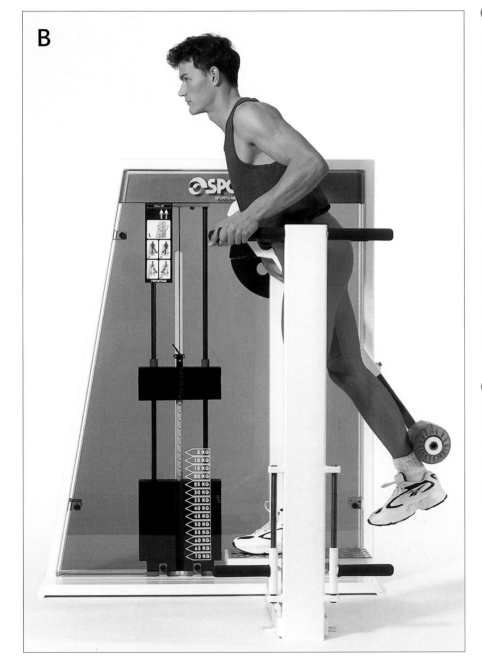

B

▷ Performing the exercise: Move your slightly bent leg with the foot pad evenly backwards and downwards from the starting position. In the end position your body should form a straight line. Your shoulders and hips should be parallel with one another. The rest of the body does not move during the whole exercise. From here bring the foot pad in a slow, smooth motion back into the starting position.

Variant: If you bend the upper part of your body further forwards at the hips, you can achieve a better preliminary stretching of the buttocks muscles and thus a more intensive contraction. This variant is only for the advanced, as the body is harder to stabilize.

⚠ Tip: Observe the front end of the foot belonging to the leg being trained. It should point forwards or downwards for the entire movement. If it points outwards, it is a sign that your hip has come out of line and is no longer parallel to your shoulders.

Standing Calf Machine Toe Raises

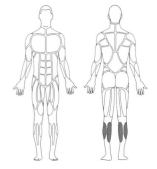

Main muscles involved:

This exercise trains primarily the gastrocnemius *(m gastrocnemius)* and the soleus *(m. soleus)* muscles. Other deeper lying muscles, which are not mentioned individually here, play a subordinate role.

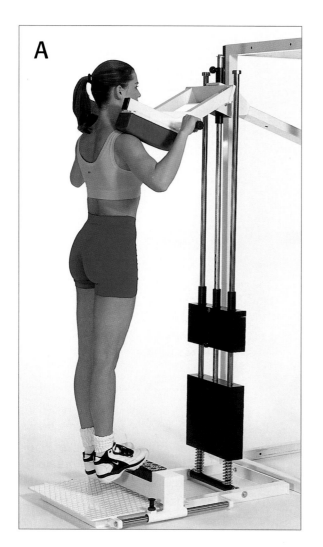

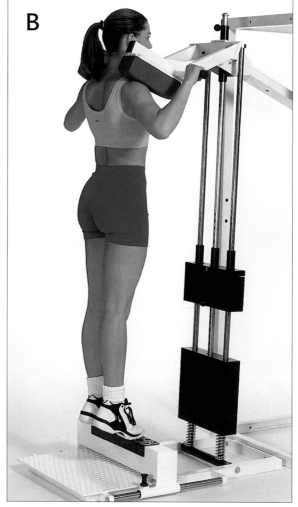

Starting position: Stand up on the step of the calf machine. The weight is transmitted to the shoulders via two pads. Your hands should support your body by holding the grips attached to the pads. Keep your legs slightly bent in the starting position, and place your feet a few inches apart on the edge of the step so that only the toes and the balls of your feet are on it. Bend your feet up towards your shins, causing your calves to stretch. Make sure that your gluteal, abdomen and back extensors build up basic tension that is maintained throughout the whole exercise.

▶ Performing the exercise: Raise your heels in a slow, smooth motion. This raising of the heels is the only movement that should take place in the whole body. Avoid trying to gain additional strength by straightening at the knee. In the end position your calf muscles are contracted and shortened as much as possible. From here, lower your body slowly back into the starting position.

Variant: You can also perform this exercise while sitting, if the right machine is available. Here, the weight is applied via pads resting on the thighs just above the knees. The machine has a lever as start help, with which you can raise the weight and the knee pads high enough to slide your thighs underneath them. While performing this exercise, be careful not to vary the position of the balls of your feet to avoid putting too much strain on your knee joints.

! Tip: Especially when starting calf training as a beginner, there is possibility of cramping, because such an isolated contraction in the calf muscles scarcely ever occurs in everyday life. If this is the case, you should always stretch your calf muscles before performing the exercise and also between the sets.

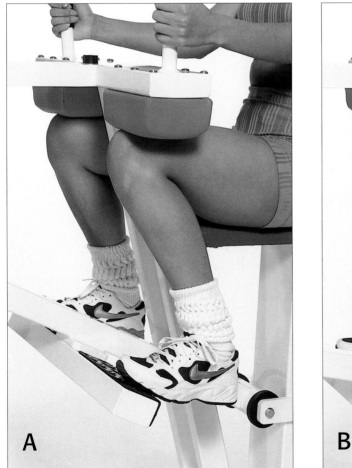

A

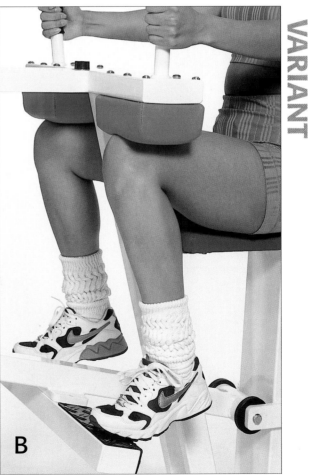

B

VARIANT

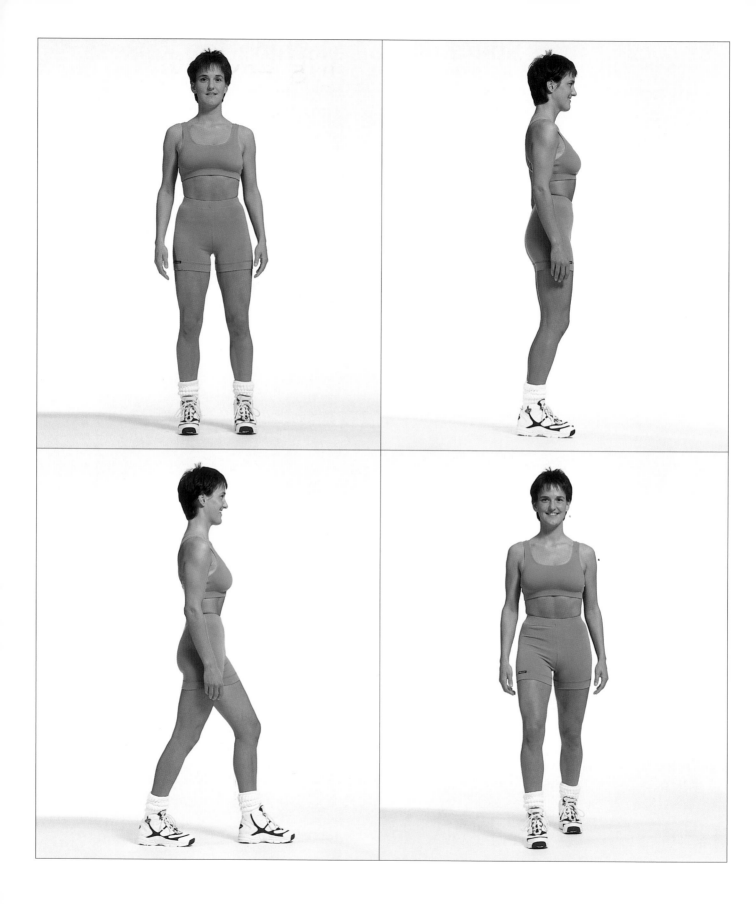

PHYSICAL STRENGTHENING

Physical Strengthening Exercises

In this chapter you will find a wide selection of exercises as well as many suggestions and tips which are intended to create an effective and motivating personal training program.

While weight training with the strength training machines and free weights (dumbbells and barbells) can be graded to a fine degree, this is not possible in the same way for strengthening exercises using body weight or training equipment to hold in the hand. Due to training with different bands to pull (*rubberband*, *tubes, Deuserband,* etc.), however, a special strength curve develops which is not spread as evenly on the motions as with a machine, but which increases continually from beginning to end of the exercise. Due to these differences there are some training restrictions for the physical strengthening exercises. By positioning the arms and legs in different ways a changed strain can be achieved in the exercises which are carried out with portions of body weight. If you use bands to pull, you can choose from different strengths. Despite these possibilities of differing degrees of training, the physical strengthening training is used first of all to improve the strength endurance. The same basic principles apply to the carrying out of an exercise as for the strength training with machines – namely the slow and controlled performing of an exercise.

In some physical strengthening exercises, small, mostly plastic-coated dumbbells are used. As already mentioned several times in the chapter on strength training, you should pay attention that the wrists form a straight extension of the forearms. If you use so-called "weight cuffs" to increase the resistance, please take care to fasten them tightly to your wrists and ankles with the velcro bands provided. The cuffs should be so tight that they do not slide back and forth during the exercises, yet they should not hurt. You should stand in the following basic positions for all exercises which are done standing up as long as a different position is not suggested explicitly:

Basic position with feet parallel: The legs are slightly bent and no wider apart than the hips. Gluteal and stomach muscles build up a basic tension for the middle of the body. The shoulders are slightly back and the head forms a line with the spine; it is thus pulled straight up (pictures on top row).

Basic step position: The feet are positioned as if you are taking a step forward so that there is about a foot's length between the front and the back foot. Build up a basic tension for the middle of the body, and hold your head in a straight line with the spine. Remember to keep the pelvis and the shoulders always parallel (pictures on bottom row).

Golden Rules

- Naturally you must also warm up adequately before performing these exercises.
- Always breathe out during the tension phase of the trained muscles, and breathe in during the relaxation phase.
- When you use bands to pull or a similar apparatus, use a resistance which enables you to repeat the exercises between 15 and 25 times.
- As a beginner repeat the exercise series twice per exercise, the more advanced three times per exercise.
- Always take care to strengthen both sides, one after the other with exercises which are performed to one side of your body or with one arm or leg.
- If performing exercises with one side of the body, always train your weaker side first.
- You should be able to perform even the last repetition of a repetition series with the right technique; otherwise use a smaller resistance or do an easier variation of the exercise.
- Stretch your trained muscles after training.

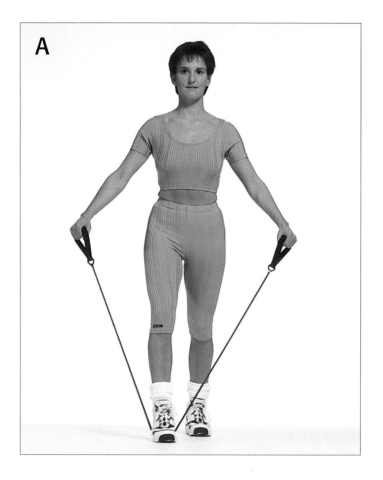

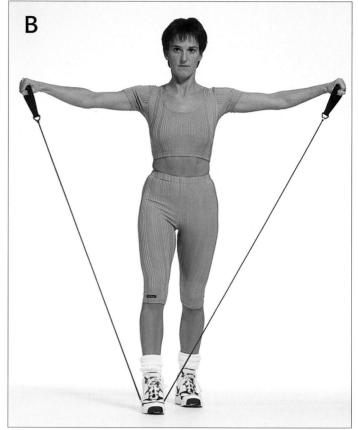

Starting position: Move from the basic position into a slight step position. The pelvis and shoulders should be in line. The front foot is standing on the middle of the tube, both handles are held sideways to the left and right of the body. The arms should be slightly bent.

▷ Performing the exercise: Pull your arms up to your shoulders sideways simultaneously and evenly in a semicircle. The arms stay in line with the body, i.e. they are not moved forwards but remain at the side while moving them upwards.

The wrists must remain firm and held in as an extension of the forearm. Keep your arms slightly bent from beginning to end of the movement and pull your elbows to the same height as your wrists. During this exercise it is important to keep the wrists firm, the spine straight, the pelvis and the shoulders parallel, and the arms slightly bent. Common mistakes during this exercise include bending the wrists downwards and twisting the spine, which means that the pelvis is not parallel to the shoulders. In addition to that, the arms could be lifted above shoulder level resulting in the upper part of the trapezius taking on the larger part of the strain. If you stretch your arms too much, strain is put on the elbow joints.

Variant: You can also lift the tube sideways by putting both feet on the tube. The legs are in the basic position with feet parallel. This variation provides a bigger strain as the loose ends of the tube are shorter and are thus stretched even more in the end position at shoulder level.

⚠ Tip: Tall athletes or athletes with long arms should consider the fact that they have to expend more strength on the tube than smaller athletes although they are using a tube or rubberband with the same degree of flexibility, as the tube stretches more and thus develops a larger tension.

VARIANT

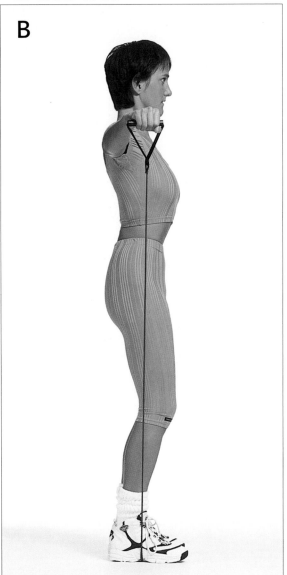

A

B

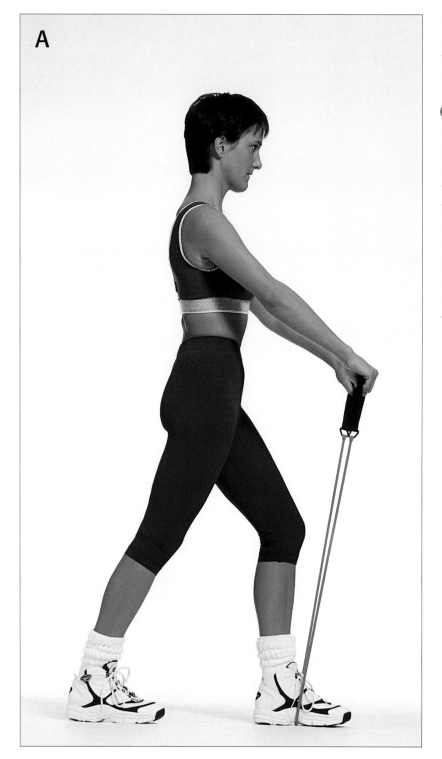

A

Starting position: Stand in the basic step position. The front foot fixes the tube in the middle of the floor. The back of the hands face forward.

▶ Performing the exercise: Pull both arms upwards evenly and parallel in front of your body. Take care that your arms are slightly bent and that the basic tension is maintained. The upper part of your body is bent forward a little. The backs of the hands point upwards in the end position. The arms are kept apart at about shoulder-width. Do not, on any account, lean the upper part of your body backward, and keep your wrists in line with your forearms.

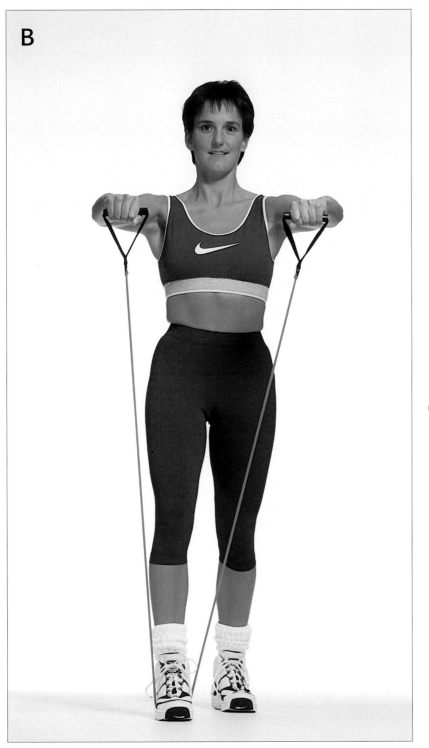

B

Variant: You can also lift the tube with only one arm. When using this technique, you have to be careful not to twist the upper part of your body during the movement of the arm, especially during the last, more difficult repetitions. Fixing the tube in the middle with the right front foot, you train the right front shoulder muscle – your left hand with the handle of the other end is on your left thigh. When you train the left front shoulder muscle, you perform this variation conversely. In another variation you raise your one arm while lowering the other, and vice versa. This means you are in a constant interchangeable rhythm. For this technique you should stand in the basic position with your feet parallel so that the tension in the free ends of the tube increases accordingly.

❗ Tip: Only lower your arms so far that you can still feel a noticeable tension in your shoulder muscles.

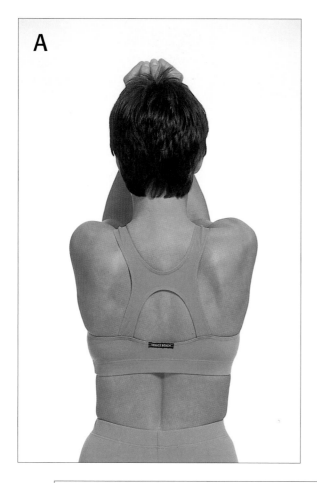

Starting position: Stand in the basic position and hold your arms bent at a right angle in front of your body. The elbows are on the same level as the shoulders, and the palms are facing one another. The hands are formed into fists. Hands and forearms touch lightly in the middle in front of your body.

▶ Performing the exercise: Move your arms as far back in a semicircle until the elbows are in line with the shoulders. In the end position the palms point forwards, the elbows are still on the same level as the shoulders, and the forearms are in a vertical position. The shoulder blades have been pushed together. Do not lower your elbows and keep the angle of the arms the same.

Variant: You can also do this exercise sitting cross-legged on the floor to integrate stretching the back muscles even more. It is now important to flex the back muscles so that the pelvis does not tip backwards.

❗ Tip: As you do not need any special equipment for this exercise, you can also do it in a sitting position, for instance at work or on vacation. Done regularly you can avoid drooping shoulders and tenseness.

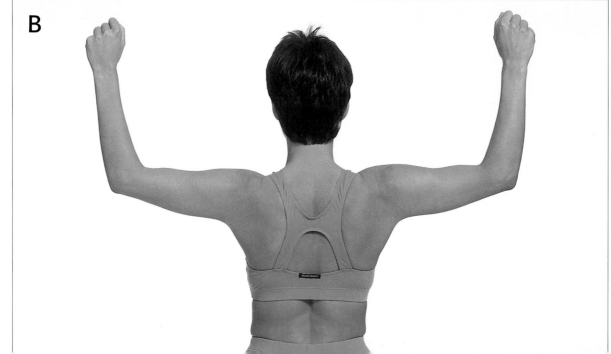

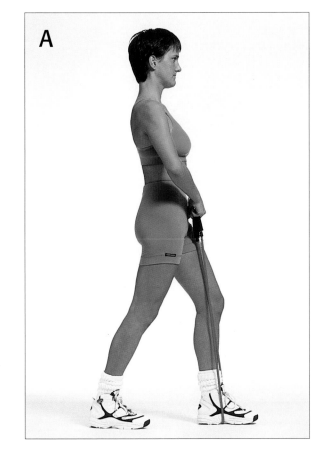

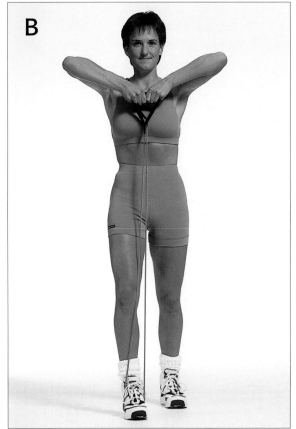

Starting position: Stand in the basic position. Remember that your pelvis and shoulders should be parallel. Both handles of the tube lie over one another and are held by both hands. In the starting position the arms are bent in the middle in front of your body.

▶ Performing the exercise: Pull both handles straight up in the middle of the body, as close to it as possible. The elbows move outwards and upwards while the shoulders remain lowered. In the end position, the elbows should be above shoulder level. The handles are often pulled up too far away from the body, resulting in unnecessary strain on the shoulder joint. In addition to that,

the head is often moved up which is an unnecessary strain on the cervical spine. Also, if there is not enough body tension in the basic position, the upper part of the body can bend backwards which strains the lumbar spine unnecessarily.

Variant: To make it more difficult, stand on the middle of the tube with both legs parallel.

🛈 Tip: If you prefer the step position but want to increase the tension in the tube, you can wind the middle of the tube once around your front foot. If you have tubes of different strengths at your disposal, you can differentiate even more finely.

Starting position: Take on the basic position with your legs parallel. Remember the basic tension. Take hold of both handles with one hand, and the middle of the tube with the other. That way the tube is double and the exercise thus more intensive. Hold your arms above your head a little wider apart than your shoulders so that the tube is stretched. Both palms should point forwards. The hands should form one line with the forearms.

▷ Performing the exercise: Pull both arms in even, slow movements out and downwards. Guide the tube just behind your head down to the back of your neck. Keep up the tension in the upper part of the body, pull back your shoulders slightly and do not move forwards. Do not push your head forwards.

Variant: In order to vary the exercise from easy to very difficult, do not hold the tube as usual at the handles but wind it one or more times – depending on the degree of advancement – around the backs of your hands.

❗ Tip: Feel how your shoulder blades push inwards and turn to one another.

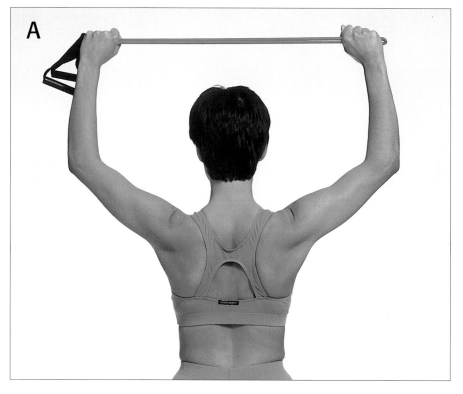

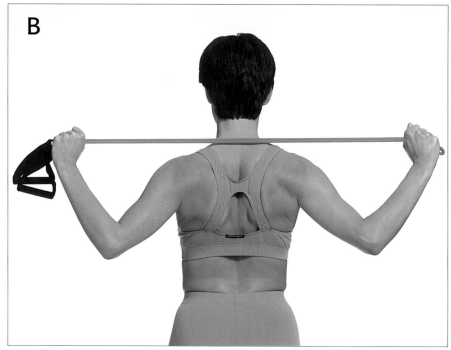

Starting position: Sit with noticeably bent legs and a straight, perpendicular back. Put your heels on the floor in front of your body, your legs together. As in the basic standing position, your head is in line with your spine. Place the middle of the tube under your feet, which are slightly parted. Then wind each loose end once around the respective mid-foot so that the tube ends are on the outside and can be pulled beside each leg. The palms should point inwards.

▶ Performing the exercise: Pull the handles in equal distance from the legs. Throughout the movement your hands remain in the neutral grip position. The palms are thus pointing inwards. In the end position the hands are close to the body, halfway between the chest and the navel. Although the upper part of the body should remain completely motionless, the shoulders should be pulled back. Do not move the upper part of your body forwards or backwards.

Variant: You can also move the elbows outwards. The palms then point downwards and are moved up and back towards to the chest. When using this position, you should take care not to move the shoulders up with the arms but to keep them down in their usual position.

❗ Tip: Take care to wind the middle of the tube around your feet so that the loose ends are the same length and the tension is the same. If you find it difficult keeping your back completely straight, then bend your legs a little more. In order to relieve the back in day-to-day life, you should stretch the biceps of your thigh.

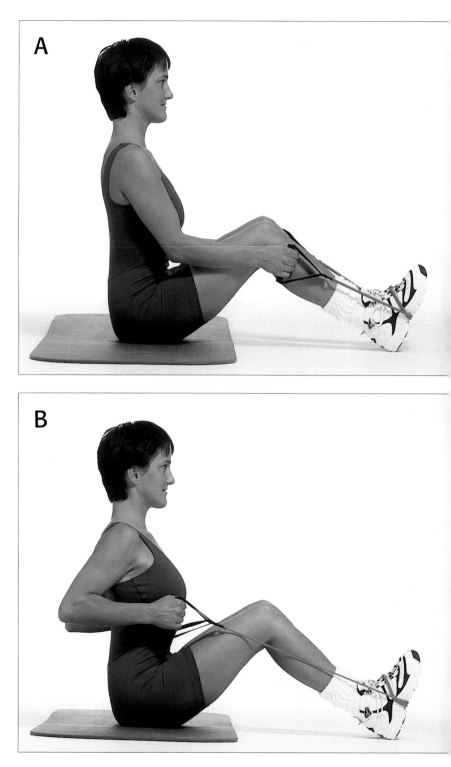

A

B

Bench Presses on Step with Tube

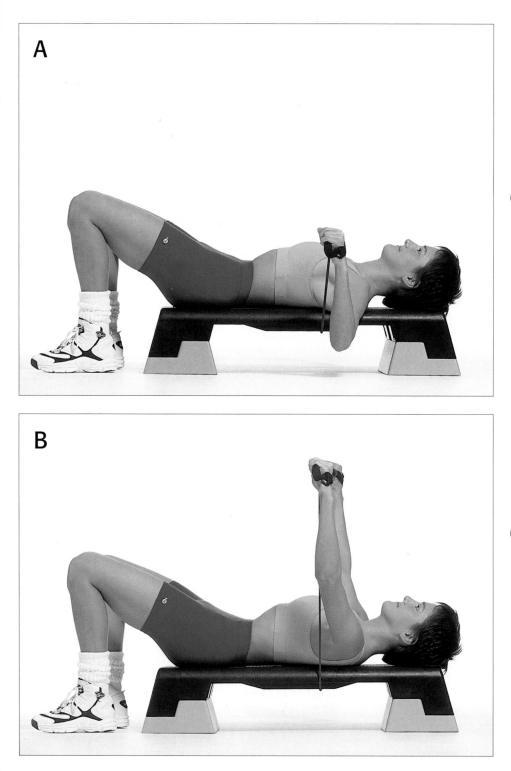

A

B

Starting position: Lie on your back on the step. Your legs should be bent and your feet flat on the floor at the bottom end of the step. Place the tube under the step near the breast bone. Then hold the tube slightly more than shoulder-width apart with your palms pointing towards your feet.

▶ Performing the exercise: Move your hands upwards in a semicircle. In the end position the hands should be shoulder-width apart and the arms slightly bent. Avoid a hollow back (do no forget your body tension), and do not straighten your arms completely.

Variant: If you do not have a step available, you can also do this exercise sitting down or standing. Then the middle part of the tube is placed behind the upper part of your back. The loose ends are moved forwards directly under your armpits, the backs of the hands point upwards throughout the movement. Again pay attention to a correct posture.

❶ Tip: In order to increase the effect of the exercise, you can wind the tube once around your hand. To prevent the tube from cutting into the inside of your hand, grasp the plastic part of the handle as far on the outside as possible. The inside thus juts out. Now lay the tube across the protruding plastic part.

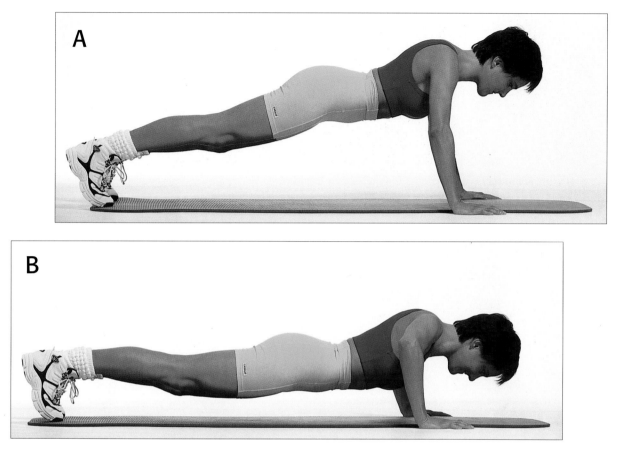

A

B

Starting position: Your whole body should be completely straight and stretched. Only the tips of your toes and the palms should be resting on the ground. The hands are just under the shoulder axis, flat on the ground, just a little wider apart than the shoulders. Bend your arms slightly.

▶ Performing the exercise: Lower your body evenly. In the end position the arms are bent at about a right angle. The tips of your feet provide the pivot of the movement. The body remains stretched and tense. The whole push-up is only advisable for the more advanced trainer. Do not let your body sag, do not straighten your arms completely and hold your head in line with your spine.

Variant: If you are a beginner or untrained,or if you find the complete push-up too difficult and you cannot keep the correct position, then change your starting position to kneeling on all fours. The knees should be padded with a gym mat. While lowering your body, the hip joint stretches a little and while raising, it bends again.

❶ Tip: With the usual push-up a certain strain is put on the wrists. In order to avoid this, you can also rest your weight on your fists, but pressure will build up on the knuckles. Therefore, in various combative sports, people like to use this technique to harden their knuckles. If the pressure makes you feel uncomfortable, place your knuckles on a mat or towel.

P9 Bicep Curls with Tube

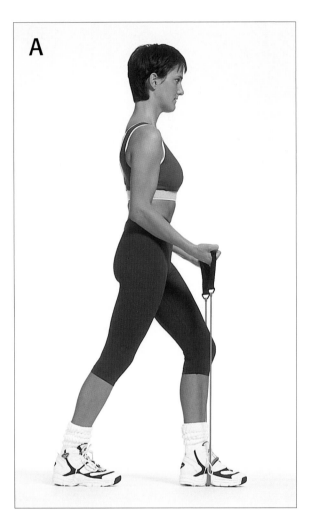

Starting position: Stand in the basic step position. The front foot fixes the middle of the tube on the floor. The arms are at the sides of your body, and bent so far that the tube is a little taut. Your hands form a straight line with your forearms.

▷ Performing the exercise: Move both ends of the tube simultaneously upwards in an even movement. Only the forearm is moved, the upper arm rests on your body. Do not lean the upper part of your body back and keep the elbows close to your body.

Variant: Move your forearms upwards in turn. To intensify the effect, you can also stand with both feet on the tube in the basic position with your feet parallel.

🛈 Tip: To isolate the muscles on the inside of your elbows, just imagine that both your elbows were joined by an axis. The elbows form the pivot joints, whereas the axis itself remains unmoved.

Starting position: Put your feet one step apart. Bend the front foot noticeably and lean the upper part of your body forward so that it is in line with your back leg. The tube is fixed under the front foot. The arm which will not be trained holds the one end of the tube, while resting on the front leg. The other arm is lifted so far into the upper arm that the elbow is clearly behind the back. It is stretched so far that you already feel a slight pulling in the arm extensor muscle. The palm of the arm being trained points forwards and slightly inwards.

▶ Performing the exercise: Stretch the trained arm completely without over-stretching it in the elbow. The only thing being moved is the forearm of the trained arm. The swinging movement here is relatively small as you are only supposed to move your forearm back so far that you can still feel the tension in the back of your upper arm. Do not move the upper part of your body and remember to keep your head in line with your spine.

Variant: The shorter you keep the end of the tube on the side to be trained, the bigger the strain on the muscles. You can also perform this exercise well by fixing the tube around a tree, a door handle or something else which is tightly fixed. You can then work on both arms at once. You can increase the effect of the exercise by placing yourself a bit further away from the tube's fixing point.

❶ Tip: Turn the back of your hand slightly outwards when moving it up so that, in the end position, it points up and the palms are then pointing down and not inwards. By doing this, a part of the arm extensor muscle is trained more intensely.

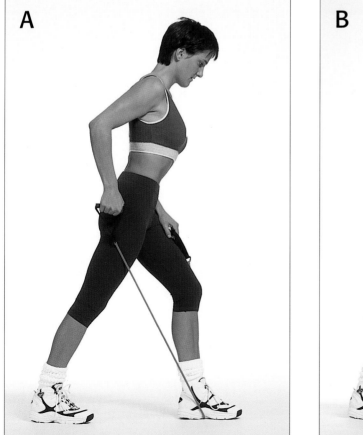

A

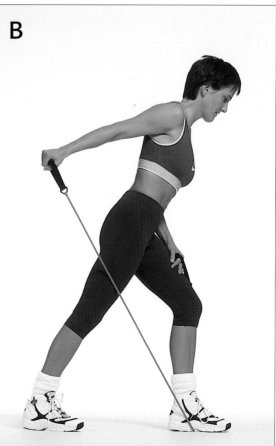

B

Starting position: You need a stable platform like a chair, a wall or something similar for this exercise. This platform should be at least 13 inches high, ideally it should be about as high as your knees. Place your hands from the top on the edge of the platform at shoulder-width. The arms should be slightly bent, and the legs at an angle of about 90° to your body. Hold your body upright.

▶ Performing the exercise: Slowly lower your body by bending your arms. In the end position the arms should be at an angle of around 90°. It is important to pay attention that your back remains straight throughout the exercise and that it is in line with your spine.

Variant: If you have another platform or something similar available, you can also place your feet on the second platform. The legs are then only slightly bent. This technique is advisable for the more advanced athlete as the arms can be bent even more which makes the exercise more difficult.

❗ Tip: Make sure that your support is clearly fixed. This exercise can also be done on vacation when your usual training equipment is not available.

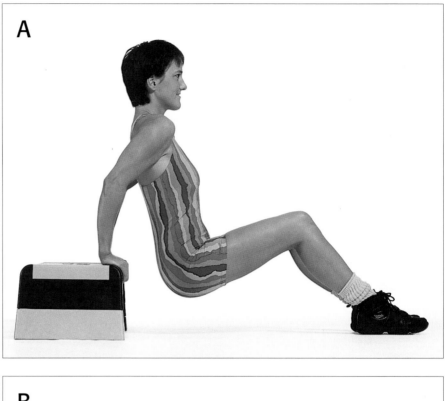

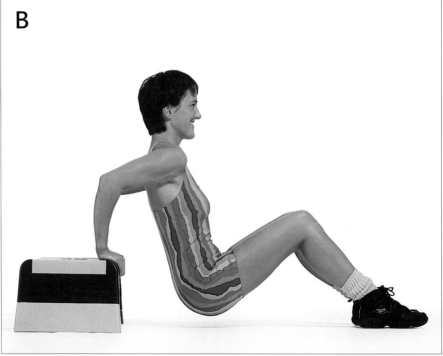

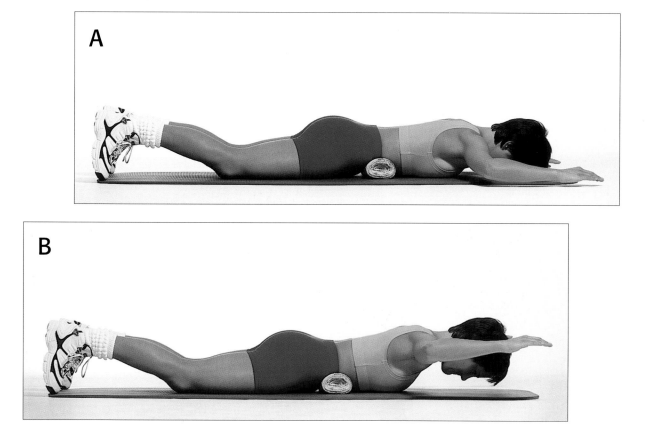

Starting position: Lie flat on your stomach on the floor. The tips of your feet should press onto the ground. Push your heels to the back. The whole body – especially the gluteal muscles – should be tensed and tightened. Your arms form a "U", the upper arms form an extension of the shoulder axis, and the forearms are bent at a right angle.

Performing the exercise: Lift your arms and shoulders up only a few inches. Watch that your lower back is not over-stretched in the end position and that your head is in line with the spine. The forehead is pointing down. The elbows remain in the raised position on the same level as the shoulders. As this exercise entails static strengthening, hold this position a few seconds before lowering the upper part of the body completely to the ground.

Variant: In order to be able to count the repetitions in this exercise, which primarily puts static strain on the muscles, do the following: With your shoulders raised, move your arms forward in line with your body and bring them back into the starting position again. Keep the upper part of your body in static tension while moving the arms back and forth in a flowing rhythm.

Tip: If you tend to over-stretch your lumbar vertebra by doing this exercise, place a rolled-up towel or a folded, soft mat under your stomach.

P13 Backward Bench

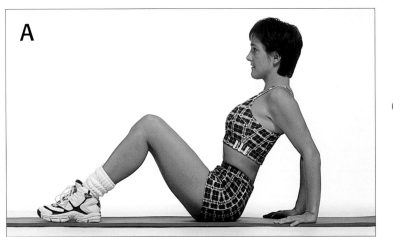

Starting position: Sit on a mat with your legs at a right angle in front of you. Place your hands on the ground just behind your buttocks, the fingers pointing to the front and a little outwards.

▷ Performing the exercise: Raise the pelvis until the thighs and upper part of the body form a straight line. By looking at the ceiling, your head would be in line with your spine. This exercise can be performed either static or dynamic. You can either keep the tension in the end position for some seconds before lowering your body completely, or you can raise and lower the pelvis in a regular movement, not quite touching the floor with your buttocks.

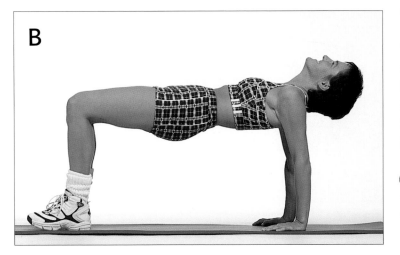

Variant: In the static variation you can take turns in lifting each lower leg and bringing it in line with the rest of the body, and with your stretched leg pull the tip of your foot back towards your body, pushing the heel forward. By doing this, not only the muscles are being trained but also the feeling for body and balance.

❗ Tip: Find out the difference of effect in the shoulders when you point your fingers to the back instead of to the front. Choose the position you prefer.

VARIANT

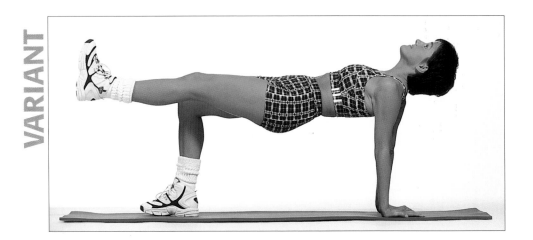

Raising Arm and Leg Diagonally Lying on Stomach

Starting position: Lie on your stomach and build up the basic tension by pressing down the tips of your feet, pushing the heels back and tensing the gluteal stomach muscles. Your arms should be stretched out in front of you, your forehead touching the floor. The hands are stretched, palms down.

▷ Performing the exercise: Raise the right arm and the left leg simultaneously a few inches. Take care to keep the hip from twisting. Keep your forehead on the floor as well. Stretch the raised arm and leg as far as possible. If you want to do this exercise statically, then hold the described end position for a few seconds. The dynamic exercise would be raising and lowering one arm and the opposite leg in a regular movement, again not touching the floor.

Variant: Do the dynamic exercise by taking turns in lifting the right leg/left arm and putting them down. Then do the same with left leg/right arm and repeat.

❗ Tip: Pay attention to your breathing especially in the static variation. You should always breathe freely. Concentrate on your breathing and count each breath. Put a rolled-up towel under your stomach in order to avoid over-stretching of the lumber vertebra region.

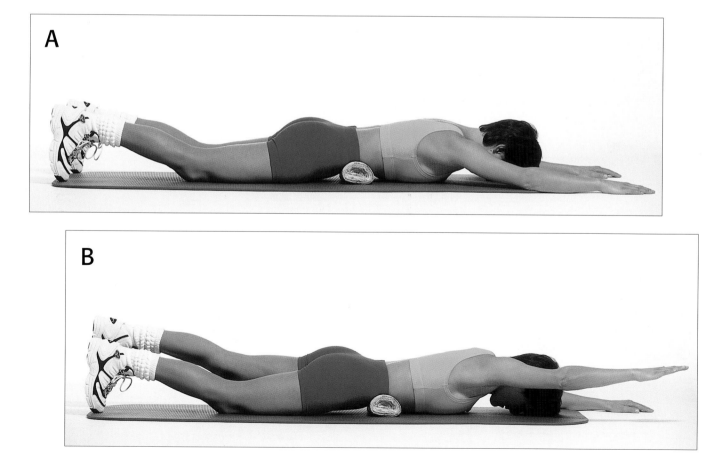

A

B

Leg Extensions with Rubberband

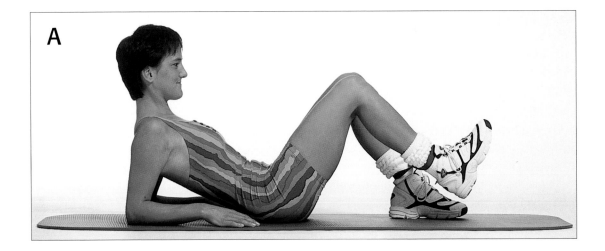

Starting position: Sit on the floor, the upper part of your body leaning back, propped up on the arms which are bent at a right angle. The rubberband should be wrapped around both ankles from the outside. Place one foot on the ground in front of the body, lift the other slightly to draw the rubberband tight. The legs are bent at a right angle and the tip of the second foot is drawn towards the shin.

▷ Performing the exercise: Now stretch the lifted leg completely without over-stretching it. Then move the leg just as far back so that the foot is not on the ground and tension remains in the rubberband. The rest of your body does not move throughout the exercise.

Variant: You can also perform this exercise sitting on a chair, a step or on the ground.

❗ Tip: If you do this exercise sitting on a chair or a step, you can hold and support the trained leg with both hands. This way you can concentrate more on the extensor muscle.

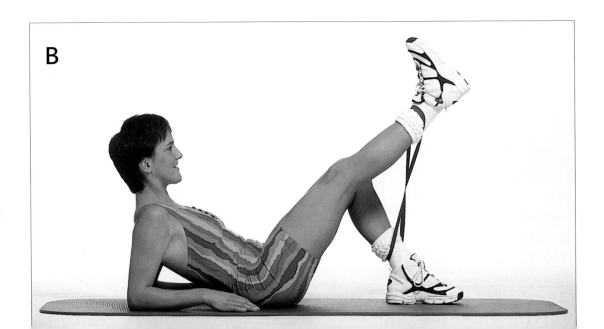

Starting position: Lie on your stomach with basic tension in the body. Wrap the rubberband around both ankles from the outside and cross it once in the middle. The tip of one foot is pressed firmly to the ground, the other is lifted a little.

▶ Performing the exercise: Bend the lifted leg and move it evenly in a semicircle towards your buttocks. The angle of the end position is between 90° and touching your buttocks. Take care to move only the leg being trained and to keep the basic tension throughout.

Variant: To intensify this exercise, you can place the rubberband around the heel of the resting leg. This way the rubberband will stretch even more and cannot slide up the leg in the end position.

❗ Tip: In order to relieve your back, place a rolled-up mat or towel under your hips.

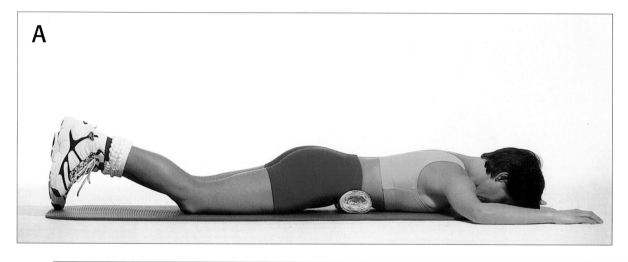

A

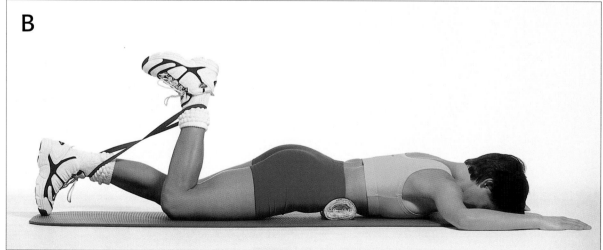

B

Starting position: Stand in the basic position with your feet parallel, legs slightly bent and the feet not wider apart than your hips. The tips of your feet should be pointing outwards a little, stomach and buttocks tense, slightly back, and the head in line with your spine. Look straight ahead. Place your hands on your hips or your thighs.

▷ Performing the exercise: Bend your knees and lower your body. In the course of this exercise the upper part of your body leans forward a little. In the end position, the legs are at an angle of about 90°. It is very important to breathe correctly, i.e. breathe in during the downward movement and breathe out evenly during the upward movement. After stretching your legs, you should be back in the exact starting position. Seen from the front, your knees, thighs and tips of your feet should be in line throughout the whole movement.

Variant: Place your feet wider apart in order to involve the adductors more. Remember to keep your knees, thighs and tips of feet in line again.

❗ Tip: If you do not have a mirror to check the 90° angle of the end position, take care not to push your knees further forward than the tips of your feet, i.e. you should be able to see the tips of your feet in front of your knees even in the end position. If this is not possible from the beginning, you are probably pushing your pelvis too far forward and not bending the upper part of your body enough. Simply bend your hips a little more.

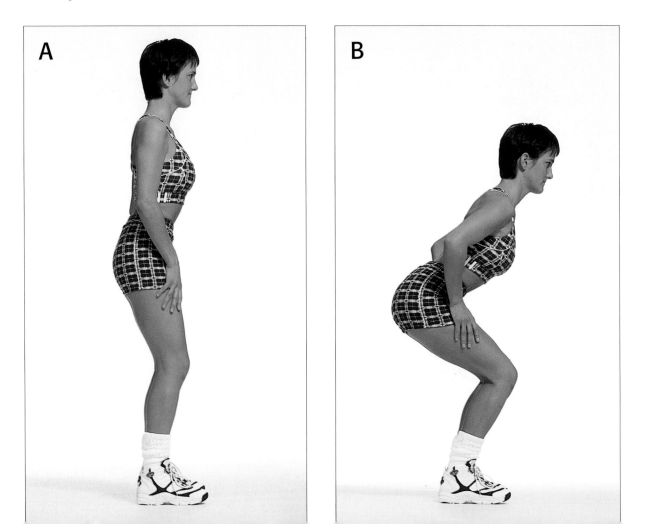

A

B

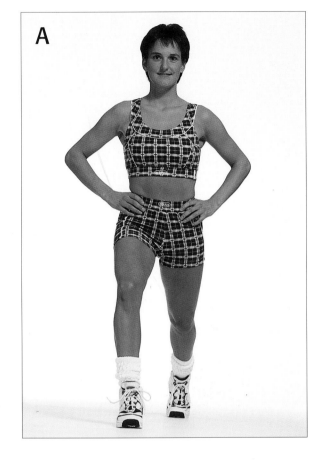

A

B

Starting position: Stand in a wide step position. Pelvis and shoulders should be parallel. Both legs should be slightly bent and the whole body has some basic tension. The upper part of the body is upright, hands placed on hips.

▷ Performing the exercise: Bend both your legs and lower your body. Keep the upper part of your body upright, this way equal weight is on both legs. The heel of the back leg lifts off the floor; in the end position only the tip of the foot remains on the floor. In the lowest position, the front leg is bent no more than at a 90° angle. The knee stays behind the tip of the foot. Do not stretch your legs completely when moving upwards.

Variant: In order to increase the training effect, you can hold light weights in your hands. Try this variation only once you have mastered the basic exercise as your hands can no longer support your body as before.

🛈 Tip: Experiment a little by placing the center of gravity more to the front or the back. This way you can not only train the muscles involved in various degrees, but you will also develop a proper feeling for how to take care of your joints the best way in this exercise.

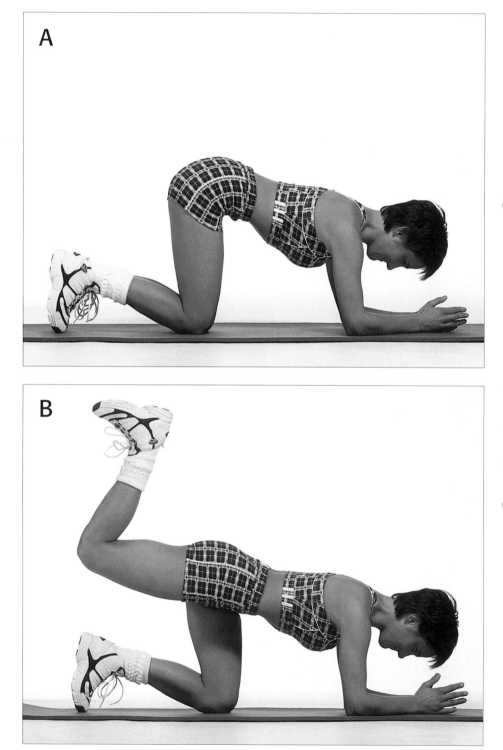

A

B

Starting position: Stand on all fours, i.e. the body is resting on the forearms and the lower legs (knees and tips of your feet), while you look down. Your hips are bent at a right angle. Your spine should be long, and your head in line with your spine. One leg is slightly raised and bent. Place your weight evenly on your forearms and the supporting leg.

▶ Performing the exercise: Lift the bent leg evenly. In the end position your thigh should be in line with your spine, while the lower leg stays the same throughout the whole exercise. Move the leg back into the starting position without letting your knee touch the floor. Your pelvis should be parallel to your shoulders during the movement. You should take care to only move the active leg. Keep your head in proper position.

Variant: If you are advanced enough, you can place a small dumbbell at the back of your knee to increase the effect.

❗ Tip: Do not forget to breathe evenly.

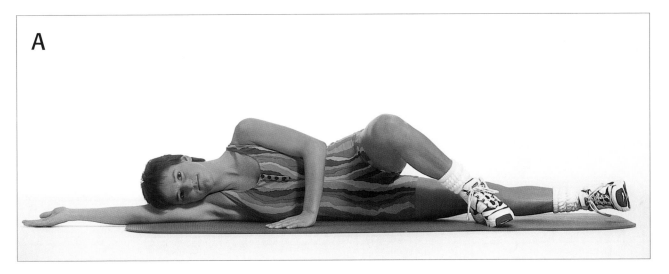

A

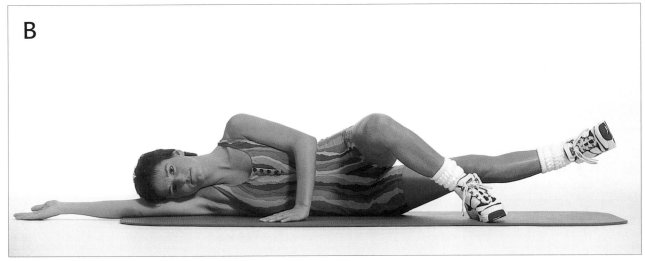

B

Starting position: Lie on your side with your head resting on your outstretched arm. The top leg should be bent at a right angle in front of your body with your foot touching the floor to stabilize the side position. The other leg is slightly bent and slightly raised in line with the upper part of the body just above the ground. The top arm also stabilizes the body at the front.

Performing the exercise: Raise the bottom leg as far as possible before lowering it again without it touching the ground. Take care to keep the upper part of the body in place.

Variant: Place your front leg on a step bent at a right angle. This way your body is even more stable and you can concentrate even better on the effect of the exercise.

! Tip: Place the body's center of gravity slightly to the front. The thigh can thus turn a little inwards in your hip joint, which makes the exercise more effective.

Leg Abduction in Side Position

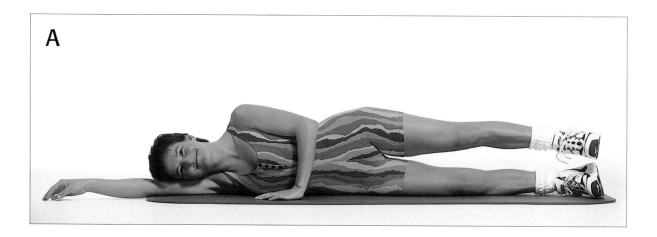

Starting position: Lie in the side position with your head resting on your outstretched arm, the top arm stabilizing the body at the front. The legs are slightly bent and parallel, keeping in line with the upper part of the body. Pull the tips of your feet towards your body.

▷ Performing the exercise: Lift the top leg 12–16 inches from the bottom leg, keeping the knees parallel. The hips should remain in the same position. Stomach and gluteal muscles are tense. Raise and lower the top leg repeatedly without the legs touching one another.

Variant: The more advanced trainer can intensify the exercise by placing a rubberband around his ankles. When using the rubberband, you can also do this exercise standing in the basic position with feet parallel.

❗ Tip: In order to train the muscles in different ways, alter the position of the moving thigh in the hip.

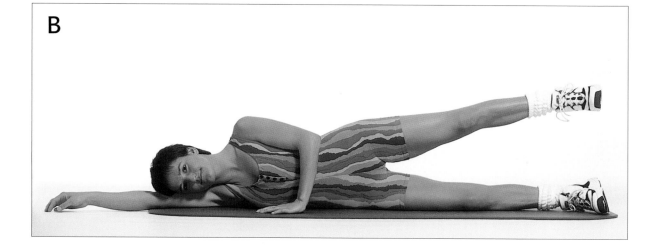

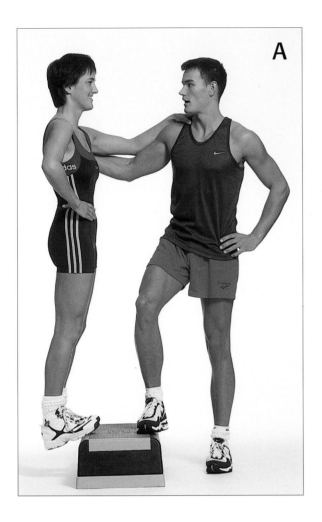

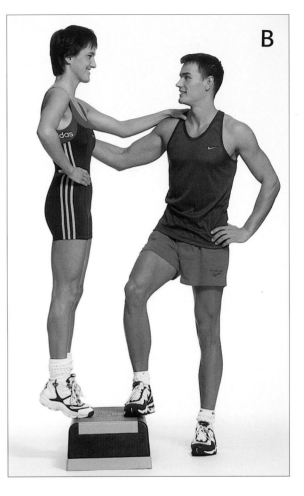

The body's center of gravity remains above your feet so that there is no movement forwards and backwards.

Starting position: Place the balls of your feet on the edge of a step in the basic position with your feet parallel and the rest of the foot jutting out. Remember the basic tension in your stomach and buttocks. You need to hold on to something to keep your balance, for instance a wall, a pillar, a partner or even a broomstick.

Variant: The more advanced athlete can also perform this exercise by using only one leg. The other leg is slightly bent and raised.

▶ Performing the exercise: Lower your body down as far as possible in your ankles and then stand on your tip-toes as high as possible. The only movement is in your ankle joints.

⚠ Tip: When performing this exercise, imagine that you are taking a box of chocolates from the top of a high cupboard. That way you will probably find it easier to stretch your ankles completely.

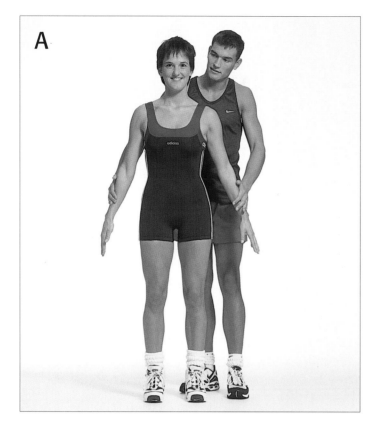

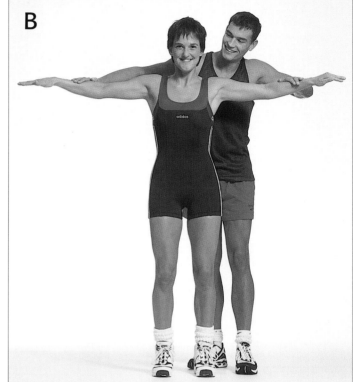

Starting position: If you are the person doing the exercise stand in front of your partner with your back towards him/her. In the basic position with feet parallel, keep your arms at the side of your body, bend them slightly. Your partner is also standing in this basic position and is holding your forearms from the outside just above your wrists. Both partners stand closely together without their bodies touching.

▷ Performing the exercise: As the person doing this exercise move your slightly bent arms upwards in one axis with the body against the resistance of your partner, until the arms are in the horizontal position. Then slowly let your partner push

your arms back down into the starting position. It should always be a flowing movement, the helper only using so much strength that the other can still move up his/her arms evenly. In the downward move, the helper only presses against the arms so much that they can be brought back into the starting position at a slow, controlled pace.

Variant: In order to level out the two persons' different strengths, the grip on the lower arm can be varied. The nearer to the elbow, the more difficult for the helper and the nearer your partner gets to the hand, the easier for him/her.

⚠ Tip: If the helper is much smaller than the other person standing on a step makes the exercise easier.

Starting position: Your are sitting cross-legged, while your partner is standing behind you with his/her legs wide apart and slightly bent. Hold your arms above your head bent a little to form a "U". The palms are pointing to the front, the hands loosely formed into fists. Without pressure the standing helper grips your wrists from the outside.

▷ Performing the exercise: Pull your arms down evenly against the resistance of your partner. Halfway down the upper arm should be parallel to the floor and at a right angle to the forearm. Your head is in line with the spine. In the end position, your head and arms form – as seen from the front – a "W". Then the arms are raised back into the starting position in a slow, flowing, movement. The helper takes care to keep a straight back, even when he/she leans the upper part of the body forward a little. The helper bends the knees to the same degree as you pull your arms down in order to follow the movement.

Variant: You can vary this partner exercise by holding your arms about 4 inches further apart or closer together, putting different strains on the muscles.

❗Tip: In order to avoid unnecessary bruises on your wrists, the helper should concentrate on using strength against the movement instead of on the grip. The grip should be as loose as possible. You may want to wrap a cloth or something similar around your wrists before doing the exercise.

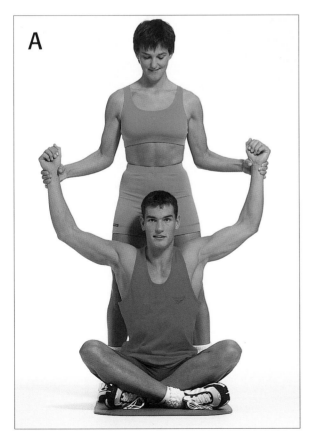

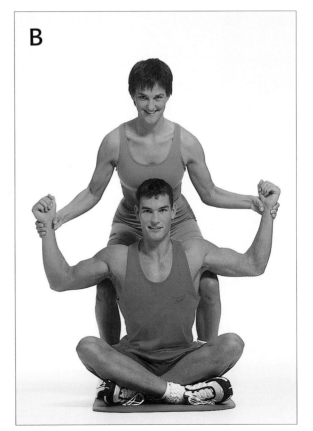

Partner Exercise for Back and Chest

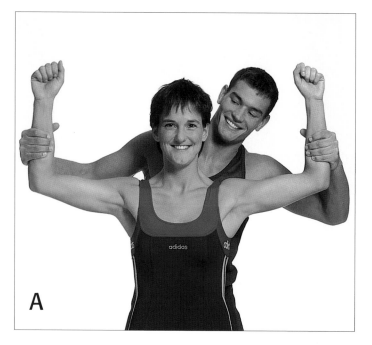

A

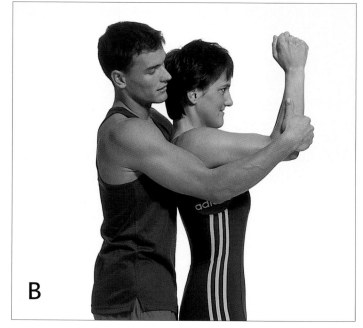

B

Starting position: Both partners stand in the basic position with feet parallel. As the person at the front, lean slightly against the chest of your partner behind you. Hold your arms bent at a right angle, the forearms pointing straight up and the palms pointing forwards (forming a "U"). The hands are loosely formed into fists. Your partner grips your forearms from behind just above the elbows and holds your arms up.

▷ Performing the exercise: Move your arms forward evenly against the resistance of your partner. In doing so, keep your upper arms parallel to the floor and the arms bent at a right angle. In the end position, the forearms are in front of the middle of your body either touching or nearly touching. Your partner pulls his/her arms back into the starting position evenly while keeping his/her own arms raised throughout the whole movement and the upper part of the body straight. Your partner takes the strength for this movement mostly from the

back muscles, which are trained with the deltoid muscles. Both partners should take care not to lean on one another too much, but rather that each of you keeps his/her own balance.

Variant: If you are the person exercising your pectoral muscles, sit on a chair, especially if your partner is much smaller. He or she then crouches down and, if possible, supports themselves on a chair in order to develop strength more evenly.

❗ Tip: Even if partner exercises are a lot of fun, take care to do the exercises evenly and correctly. As in all other strengthening exercises avoid jerking movements in this exercise. You are not meant to find out who the stronger person is. Your partner should only use as much strength as needed to keep the movement flowing.

Starting position: You and your partner should stand in the basic position with your legs parallel. You can also choose the step position with both partners putting the same foot forward. Stand no further apart than the width of two forearms. Both partners take hold of a short rolled-up or folded towel or something similar with both hands, palms pointing inward. Hold the towel at the top with your arms slightly bent, while your partner's arms are nearly stretched. Both you and your partners' upper arms remain close to the body throughout the whole exercise.

▷ Performing the exercise: Your partner bends the arms evenly against the resistance of his/her partner, keeping the upper arms completely unmoved. After the triceps are fully contracted, change the direction of the movement and now you extend your arms against your partner's resistance. When performing this exercise, one partner trains biceps and the other triceps.

Variant: Vary the standing distance.

❶ Tip: The closer the grip, the better the result. The wider the grip, the smaller the movement and the training effect.

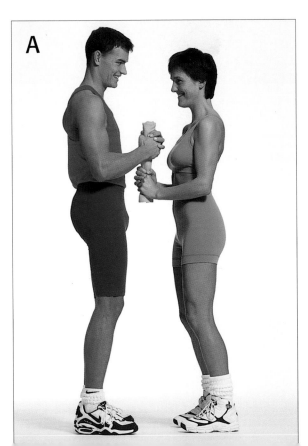

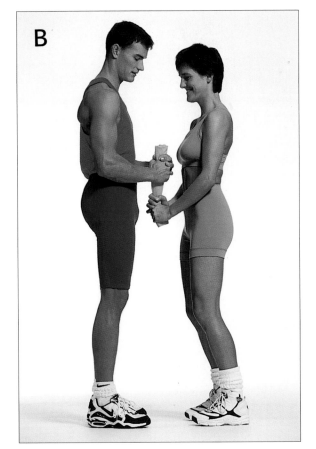

Partner Exercise for Biceps Muscle of Thigh,

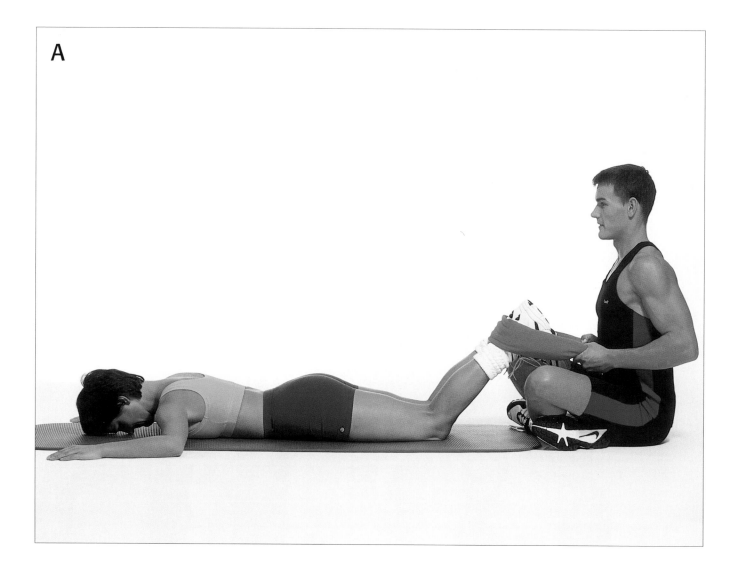

A

Starting position: Lie on a mat on your stomach with basic tension. Place your forehead on the mat with your arms on the floor, forming a "U" next to your head. Your lower legs are slightly raised and your partner is holding your heels back with a rolled-up or folded towel or something similar. Your partner sits behind you cross-legged, close enough so that he or she can hold the ends of the towel with nearly stretched arms. In the starting position, your legs are only bent a little while your

partner's arms are visibly bent. His shoulders are slightly drawn back and his head is in line with his straight back.

▶ Performing the exercise: Bend your legs against the resistance built up by your partner, who just about straightens the arms, moving his/her shoulders forward a little. In the end position, your heels are as near as possible to his/her buttocks, whereas your partner has the arms stretched out in front of

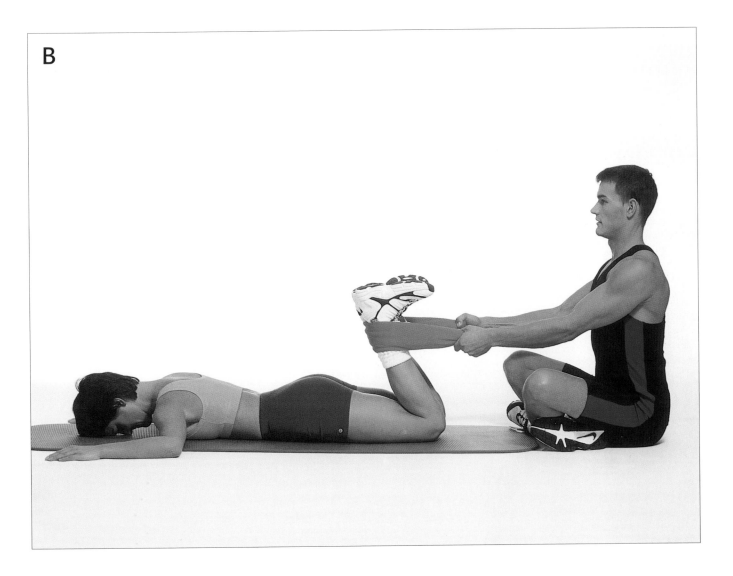

B

him/her with the upper part of the body upright. Your partner then pulls back his/her arms evenly, taking the shoulders back and pushing the shoulder blades together. Move slowly back into the starting position. This way you exercise the biceps muscle of your thigh and your partner trains all his/her back muscles and the biceps simultaneously.

Variant: You and your partner can also perform this exercise training only one leg at a time.

🛈 Tip: Putting a rolled-up towel or something similar under the pelvis relieves the strain on the lower back.

Partner Exercise for Leg Presses and Squats

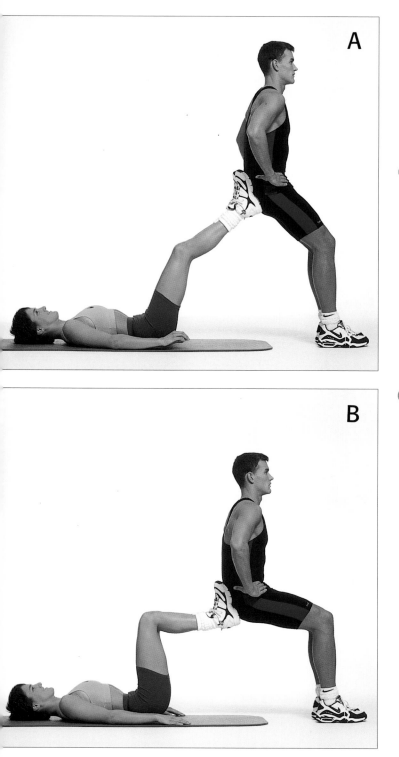

A

B

Starting position: Lie on your back with your legs slightly bent, your arms beside the hips. Your partner rests his/her buttocks against your raised feet with legs also slightly bent. Your partner places his/her hands on the hips and the head is in line with his/her straight back. To find the right distance between you and your partner, your heels should reach – in outstretched position on the floor – the tips of your partner 's toes.

▷ Performing the exercise: Bend your legs to an angle of about 90°, while your partner uses the strength of the biceps femoris muscle *(m. biceps femoris)* to press against it. Then you push your partner back up into the starting position. In the end position take care that your pelvis is kept on the ground.

Variant: If both partners have a good feeling for their body and a sense of balance, the standing person can keep his/her body as straight as a board by tensing all muscles. In this case you do not press against you partner's buttocks, but your feet are placed in the small of the back.

❗ Tip: When you try this exercise for the first time, the standing partner will find it difficult to keep his/her balance and to do the exercise evenly. So try changing the distance until you and your partner can do this exercise evenly without losing balance.

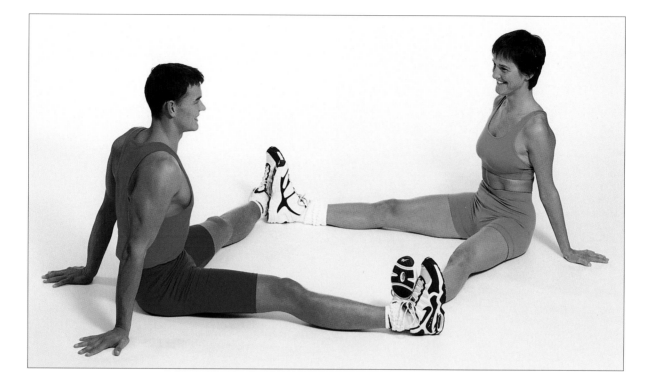

Starting position: You and your partner sit opposite one another with your backs straight. Your legs are slightly bent and form, as seen above, a "V", with the feet 8–12 inches wider apart than the shoulders. You sit so closely together that your inside ankles touch your partner's outside ankles. The arms support the upper part of the body, which is to be kept upright.

▶ Performing the exercise: You and your partner start pressing your legs outwards and respectively inwards at the same time. If both of you have about the same strength, the legs will hardly move in either direction. Nevertheless, a lot of tension is built up in the muscles involved. As there are no repetitions in this exercise, the best way to determine the duration is counting slowly or checking a clock. Ideally you should keep pushing for about 30–45 seconds. Breathe regularly during this static strain and only flex the muscles needed in legs and hips. Then exchange the positions of your legs, i.e. your partner pressing inwards should now press outwards, and vice versa.

Variant: If no partner is available or if he/she is of a different strength, the exercise can be done using a chair. Pad the legs of the chair with a towel to avoid uncomfortable pressure.

🛈 Tip: Leave off your shoes because hard soles cause unnecessary pressure on your partner's ankles.

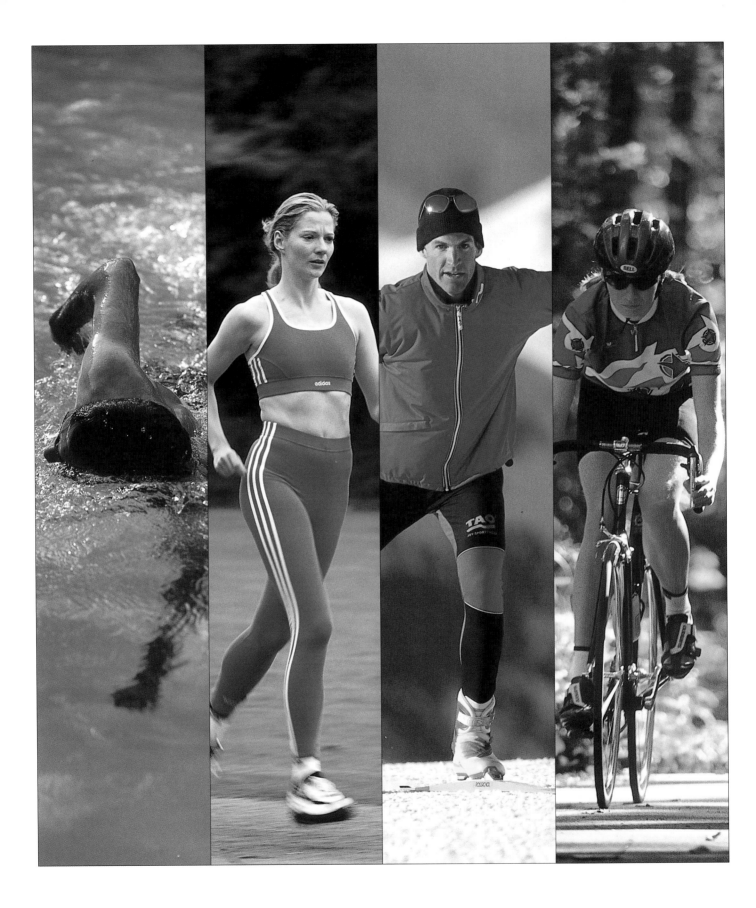

ENDURANCE TRAINING

Endurance Training – How Does It Work?

Of all the motor skills to be trained – power, endurance, mobility, speed and coordination – endurance appears at first glance to be the least spectacular. However, in terms of its contribution to health it actually comes first. In particular, there are numerous advantages in prevention. Regular endurance training tailored to the needs of individual performance has a wide-ranging positive impact on the cardiovascular system:

- greater heart efficiency
- reduced heartbeat through increased beat volume
- increased heart volume and weight
- increased oxygen intake capacity
- reduced oxygen consumption of heart musculature
- reduced blood pressure
- improved blood circulation and coagulation
- improved breaths per minute volume under exertion
- enhanced aerobic enzyme capacity
- enhanced coronary vascular system
- reduced heart risk by about 50%
- improved capillarization of body muscles
- enhanced glycogen content in body and heart musculature
- enhanced mitochondrion volume
- reduced levels of the "stress hormones" adrenalin and noradrenalin
- reduced LDL cholesterol level
- increased HDL cholesterol level

This list can be added to significantly. However, despite all these largely unchallenged advantages, endurance training is still the most important, especially among leisure-time sports practitioners who like to train with weights. A common reason why many people drop out of endurance training after a short trial period is that training intensity is increased too quickly. Very often exertion levels are not planned in advance. In practice, for example, people take up jogging, swimming, cycling or other sports with a view to trimming their figures. If they set out to cover a given distance, it often leads to excess demands on the body. Jogging, in percentage terms the most frequently practiced sport, can produce symptoms of excessive stress in joints and muscles if the initial stress is either too intense or too prolonged. The pains which indicate excessive exertion then lead to a long-term suspension of training.

As with weight training, you should tailor your endurance training to your current performance level. In the chapter *Training Guide* you will find two tests you can use to identify your own level. In addition, almost every fitness center today offers the opportunity to test endurance training capacity with an experienced trainer. Should your test result fall short of the average, it is particularly important that you lower duration and stress levels when you take up training. For this reason, in the subchapters on specific forms of endurance sports below, special programs are set out. As a rule of thumb your heart rate should be in the lower part of the tables presented here during the first few months. In this initial phase it is advisable to divide training into three or more short sections rather than carrying out a longer continuous training unit. In the breaks between these sections you should either rest (by, for example, swimming) or exercise with low intensity activities (for example, relaxed walking between the running stages in jogging). As your training experience and endurance capacity increase, you will be able to reduce the number of breaks step by step and steadily increase the duration of a training unit.

Anyone who has started a planned and regular program to improve their cardiovascular performance generally feels unbounded enthusiasm. A quotation by the well-known cardiovascular specialist Professor Wilfried Kindermann, graphically brings home the positive effects of this kind of training: "Endurance training effectively means saving on oxygen consumption, decreasing blood pressure, stabilizing the heart rate, stimulating metabolism and reducing coagulation and has no side effects whatsoever when properly carried out. What medicine is as effective or free of side effects as this?"

The Cardiovascular System

In order to understand just how endurance training works, certain basic points about the cardiovascular system need to be understood. The most important function performed by the heart, together with the vascular system and the lungs, is to provide oxygen for the whole organism. Ultimately, any positive accommodation in the cardiopulmonary system can be attributed directly or indirectly to an increase in the oxygen requirements of the organism or its individual cells. The heart is the pump for the vascular system and plays the role of a pressure and suction pump. Pumping is produced by a rhythmic contraction of the cardiac muscle. This involves a remarkably reliable endurance performance by the cardiac muscle since it cannot take a break for anything more than the time between one heartbeat and the next. The heart is protected by the sternum, two-thirds to the left and one-third to the right of the chest. It is a hollow muscle, about the size of a man's relaxed fist. Its size and weight, however, vary according to sex, age and use. Even if at first sight the heart resembles body muscles, there is a fundamental difference: whereas the body muscles may be contracted at will, the contraction of the heart is guided by a highly complex interaction of parts of the nervous and hormonal systems and its own system of stimulation.

The heart muscle consists basically of two individual pumps on either side which pump blood into the body's circulatory system and the lungs. In this way, every organ and indeed every individual living cell is provided with oxygen and nutrients by means of the vascular system. In addition to this irrigation system, used or metabolized substances can be removed. For example, oxygen from the lungs becomes carbon dioxide after metabolism in the cell has taken place and is then delivered back to the lung via the blood (see diagram opposite). Just how effective the cardiovascular system really is can be seen clearly by the fact that the entire blood volume of the body, about 8.8 pints to 10.65 pints liters, circulates throughout the entire organism in repose in about one minute. Blood also contributes to the protection of the body's immune system and keeps it warm. In sum, the heart can be seen as a pump, the vascular system as a transport network and the blood as the vehicle. If all the branches of the transport network were laid end to end, they would measure over hundreds of thousands of miles. Just as the heart is commonly compared to a pump, so too is the vascular system compared to a water irrigation system. However, this comparison is not entirely satisfactory since the copper pipes of a water system cannot actively dilate or contract as the vascular system can. A layer of muscle contained in each vessel makes this possible. This also explains why there are temporary alterations to blood pressure. Blood pressure is, after the heart rate, the second external yardstick which can be applied with relative ease in order to determine the current state of the cardiovascular system. Standard values for blood pressure were set out in the chapter *Training Guide*.

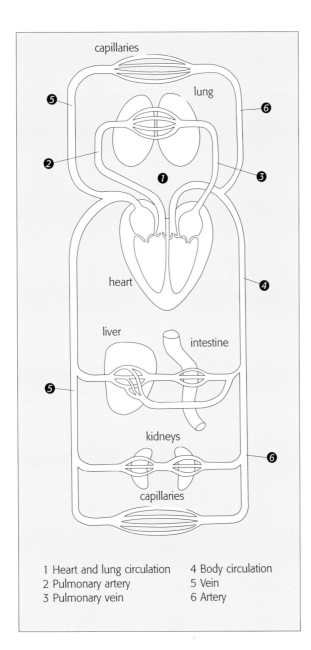

1 Heart and lung circulation
2 Pulmonary artery
3 Pulmonary vein
4 Body circulation
5 Vein
6 Artery

Presentation of Exercise Descriptions

The following descriptions of various endurance activities (cycling, walking, jogging, swimming, in-line skating, cross-country skiing, aerobics and cross training) follow a specific form of presentation. Firstly, practical clothing and the necessary equipment or sensible accessories are described for each activity. This is followed by detailed descriptions – as far as these are available – of the correct adjustment for the equipment and the relevant basic techniques. In addition, special tips for style improvement and a plan are provided which enable a clear improvement in endurance in the relevant discipline over a period of several weeks. Please note that irrespective of whether you are doing endurance training as part of a training unit for the improvement of overall fitness or as a separate training unit, a warm up and cool down followed by stretching of the muscles used must be done.

The main reason why people drop out of endurance training or do not take it up in the first place is perhaps because of insufficient motivation. Although the advantages set out above provide convincing arguments, endurance training is frequently considered monotonous and boring. One reason for this is without a doubt the fact that most endurance sports are essentially solitary. In order to avoid this negative motivation trap, or at least make a start, many people find it helpful to practice with others who are similarly motivated. In this case, it is essential to arrange to go swimming with a partner or a friend after, for example, an organized run. Once you have started and the first success experienced, motivation increases practically on its own.

Golden Rules of Endurance

- Always warm up at the start of training and never forget to cool down at the end.
- Keep to the times necessary for recovery between training days tailored to your own needs.
- Train at least twice and preferably three times a week.
- Observe the optimum training pulse rate for your age group and performance.
- Only increase the level of exertion when you are physically and psychologically fit to do so.
- Increase your exertion first in duration and then measured in heart rate intensity.
- Keep your training progress up to date by repeat tests.
- Train longer for sports which demand more and shorter where muscles are used less.
- Vary your training (see *Cross-Training*) to help prevent physical and psychological strain.
- Always take care to secure sufficient intake of liquid or prompt fluid replacement at the right time.
- Always use optimum clothing and equipment.
- Do not forget the fun and enjoyment of movement.

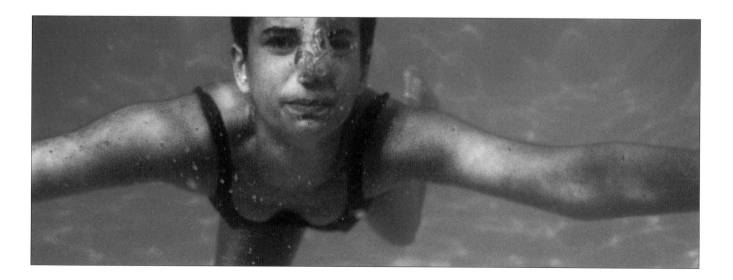

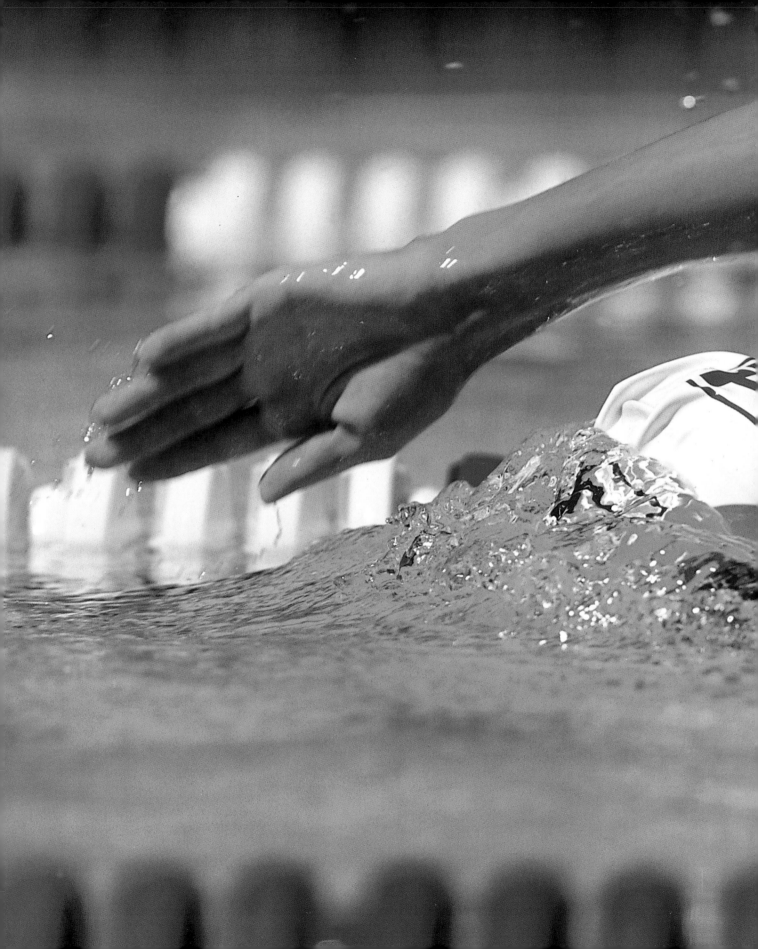

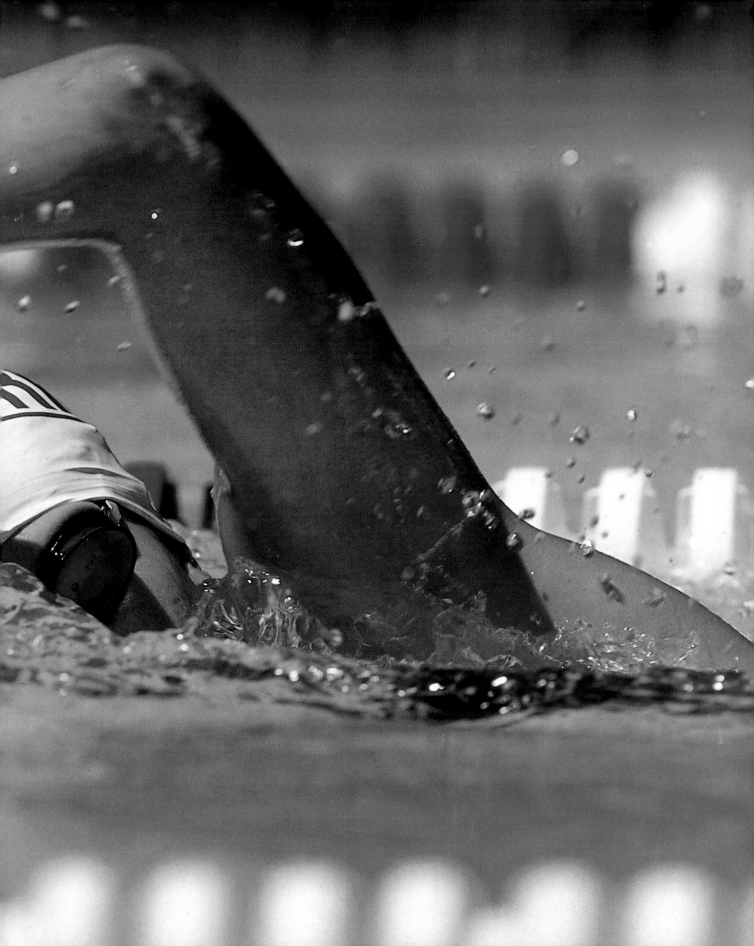

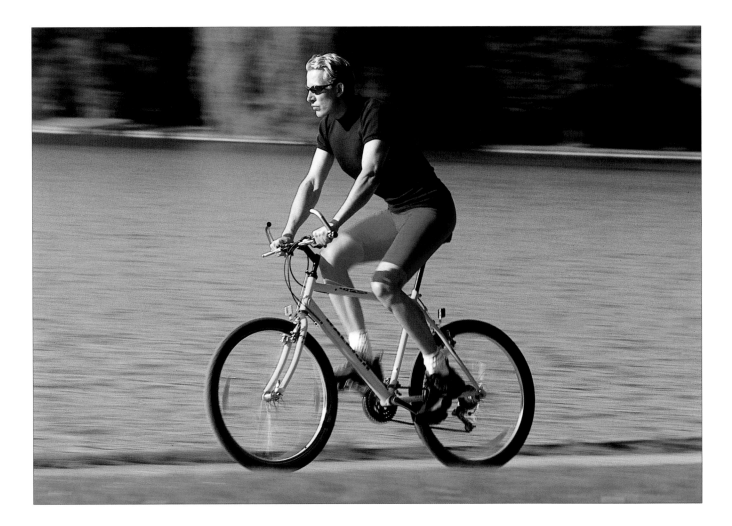

Cycling

Contrary to their nature, humans are increasingly developing into a sedentary being without any notable physical demands, only increasing psychological pressure. Lack of muscle movement and psychosocial stress are among the most dangerous risk factors for the emergence of diseases directly linked to our civilization. Coronary diseases can best be avoided by sports that train endurance. Cycling plays a major role here, since the weight of the cyclist is borne by the saddle. For this reason, cycling is a particularly appropriate sport for beginners with joint problems and excess weight. For people who have led inactive lives, cycling is also the ideal start-up sport because of the easy control of exertion. With his Tour de France win in 1997 Jan Ullrich also vividly demonstrated that cycling could also be practiced as a performance sport or competitive sport at international level. Whether cycling is practiced as a health activity or performance activity, the physical and spiritual well-being of the cyclist is enhanced with regular activity in the right amount.

Clothing

Even if you do not wish to dress as a professional cyclist, some clothing points should be taken into account. Because of higher speeds, headwinds are faster than in walking or running. On warm days, this can have a pleasant cooling effect but in cooler temperatures headwinds tend to make the body cold. For this reason, clothing should fit snugly against the body and provide adequate protection from the elements. You will therefore need short- or long-sleeved T-shirts as overwear. Ensure that the T-shirt does not flap too much and especially that it covers all of the lower back. In cool temperatures use two light pullovers over each other and wear a jacket made from breathable fabric over this in wind or rain.

Instead of buying expensive cycle shorts, beginners can use tights or tight-fitting jogging pants. However, as soon as you start regular training and cover longer distances in the saddle, you should add some further useful accessories.

Cycle shorts

The most important item of clothing for the cyclist is cycle shorts made of either wool or synthetic stretch fabric. These shorts come with a soft leather or synthetic lining and crotch support. Due to the special cut, they protect beginners and professionals from abrasions on hip bones, inner thighs and in the genital area. The legs of summer shorts should cover at least a third and preferably two-thirds of the upper leg and be crease-free. During cooler periods legs can be protected by a longer pair reaching to the ankles or by leggings used like tights over the

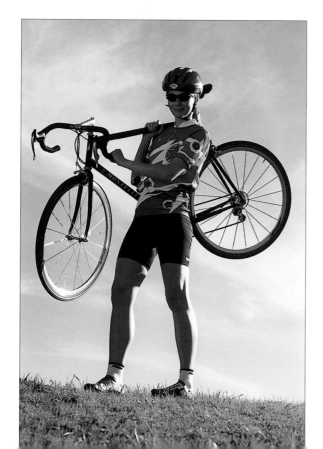

shorts. With longer pants it should also be ensured that they do not pressurize the knee joint and impede blood circulation in the process. Underwear should be made of a special mixed fabric that does not absorb sweat but transports to the outside.

Shoes

In the beginning, sports shoes with a firm sole are completely adequate. The shoes must provide a secure and firm grip on the pedals. However, in regular training it is worth investing in proper cycling shoes with clip pedals. Here, the foot is secured to the pedal so that pedal straps become unnecessary. Clip pedals guarantee a firm attachment between the feet and pedals and therefore facilitate optimum weight transmission and good rotation. When new, the shoes should offer a tight fit without cramping or pinching. An optimum weight transfer between the feet and the pedals can be guaranteed by a relatively stiff sole. Make sure that these shoes offer proper breathing for good foot comfort.

Vest

There are various vests with long or short sleeves, depending on the season. Vests make good sense because they protect the body from the sun and cold. A good vest will offer a tight fit, protect the kidney area and transport sweat as quickly as possible to the surface. For training outside daylight hours, bright vests with fluorescent and vivid colors should be used, since they can be better seen by other vehicles.

Useful Accessories

For safety reasons a helmet is absolutely indispensable. The helmets known as hard-shell helmets are especially advisable since they are built to offer effective shock absorption.

In the event of a fall, cycling gloves can protect the hands from serious grazes. Cycling goggles increase the pleasure of the cycling experience by blocking excessive UV rays, dust and irritating insects. A multi-function *tachometer* is also a useful aid in training. An anti-theft security chain is also a worthwhile investment for peace of mind during breaks.

Equipment

The cycle trade registers increasingly large numbers of bikes being sold each year. Rising sales figures show the upward trend. Ten to 15 years ago people bought bicycles almost exclusively according to color, features and size. Nowadays, choice for the non-professional cyclist is almost infinite: there are *trekking bikes, mountain bikes, racing bikes, city cruisers* and many others. In order to find your bearings in this constantly changing market, you require a good deal of specialized knowledge. You can find out about the pros and cons of the various new models and customized frames from specialty magazines and dealers.

In general, the intended use will determine the decision to buy a bicycle. A racing bike is only suitable for paved roads due to its very narrow tires. Even low curbs can crush wheel rims in everyday usage. Mountain bikes can be used in woods and difficult terrain. The thick tires and solid build naturally mean that they are heavier than racers.

Hybrid or trekking bikes offer a good compromise in terms of cycling comfort, sporting feel and intended usage. These "cross breeds" are perfectly suited to use on roads and in fields, wood and forests.

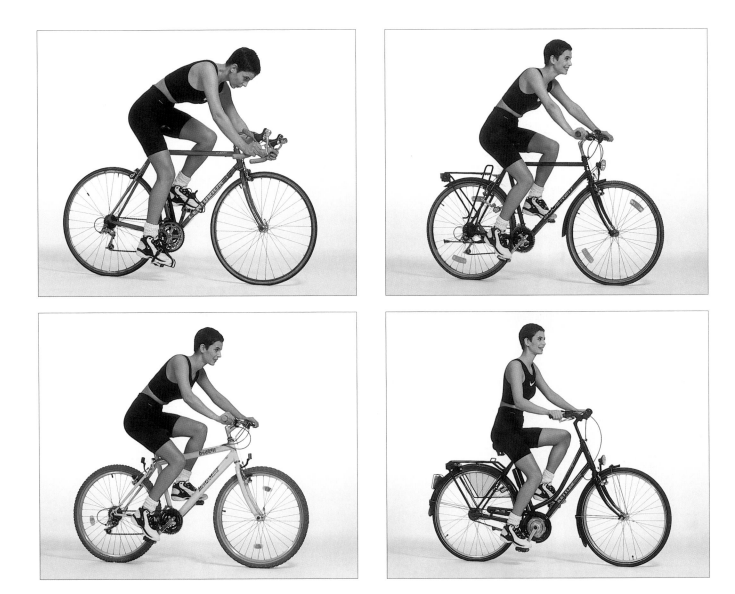

Adjusting Your Bike

Irrespective of the various models, you will need a bike that is suited to your build. It is only when cycle and body are in harmony with each other that optimum performance can be achieved. A good basis for this include the adjustment of the saddle position, good cycling style and a rounded pedalling action.

Correct seat position

If the dealer has set the frame measurements to the size of the user's body, fine-tuning of the individual seat position can be

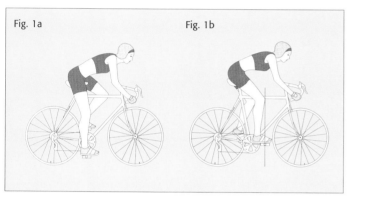

Fig. 1a   Fig. 1b

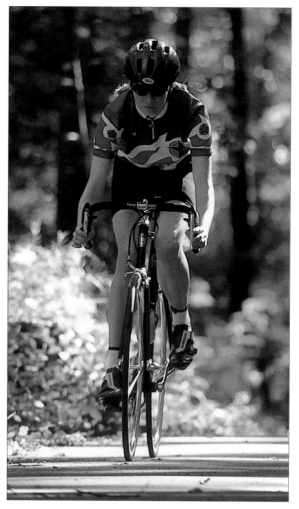

achieved by means of adjustments to the saddle and handlebars. An important principle when adjusting these are that all movements should be carried out with ease.

Adjusting the saddle height

To set the saddle to the correct height, sit on the saddle and place the pedal in the lowest position. When you put your heel on the pedal, the knee should be slightly bent (Fig. 1a). In addition, the tip of the foot should be able to reach below the pedal when the leg is fully stretched.

Setting the saddle position

Normally, the saddle should be set in a horizontal position, that is, parallel to the crossbar (if there is one) of the frame. It is best to adjust your saddle with a spirit level. Usually, the saddle support is to be found in the middle of the saddle. An optimum sitting position can be best achieved when the saddle is slightly adjusted to the rear or front after the correct height is set. This

position is known as saddle position. To ensure the correct saddle position sit on the saddle and bring both pedals into a horizontal position. Place the ball of the feet on the pedals. The correct saddle position is achieved when the knee is exactly vertical above the axle of the front pedal (Fig. 1b).

Adjusting handlebar height

Usually the correct handlebar height is the same height as the saddle. In all-purpose or touring bikes the handlebars are generally set higher than the saddle. Sports cycling involves reducing wind resistance by means of a hunched sitting position. According to training condition, handlebar size, intended use of the cycle and the physiognomy of the cyclist, the handlebars can be set slightly lower than usual in relation to the saddle setting.

Cycling Technique

Correct leg work and a round pedalling action are elementary techniques in cycling. Ideal leg movement entails leg movement parallel to the frame. The feet alternate, one forcing the pedals downwards, the other pulling upwards. In order to ensure such parallel pedalling and thereby also protecting the joints in this movement, the feet should be placed perfectly on the pedals. Here, the ball of the foot is exactly vertical above the pedal axle.

This rotational step, known as pedalling, is an art form which even trained professional cyclists need to refresh from time to time. Pedalling can only be learned when the feet are attached to the pedals by means of straps or other means. Many inexperienced cyclists content themselves with pushing the pedal up and down, thereby reducing the force of the foot on the pedal to a small arc. This means that they use only a part of the available pedal movement for forward motion. The style creates a cumbersome and chopped effect. Perfect pedalling increases the effective area of work by lifting and lowering the foot with downward pressure to the front and upward pull to the rear. Here, the tip of the foot alternates between pointing upwards and downwards in the pedalling process (Fig. 2b below). At very high speeds, however, it is almost impossible to lift the feet to the highest possible point. In

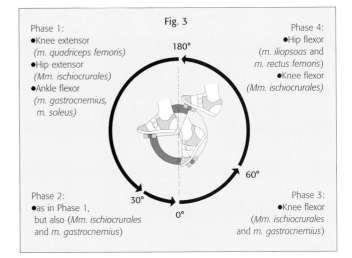

Fig. 3

Phase 1:
● Knee extensor
(*m. quadriceps femoris*)
● Hip extensor
(*Mm. ischiocrurales*)
● Ankle flexor
(*m. gastrocnemius, m. soleus*)

Phase 4:
● Hip flexor
(*m. iliopsoas and m. rectus femoris*)
● Knee flexor
(*Mm. ischiocrurales*)

Phase 2:
● as in Phase 1, but also (*Mm. ischiocrurales and m. gastrocnemius*)

Phase 3:
● Knee flexor
(*Mm. ischiocrurales and m. gastrocnemius*)

180° 60° 30° 0°

movement less effective, practice with the right foot. Exercise at the outset with a slow pedalling motion and low force. Then practise with both legs. While the right foot pushes the pedal downwards, the left foot pulls the pedal upwards. Remember that a good deal of pedal power as well as impulsion are lost if you do not actively lift your leg but let it passively rest on the upwardly moving pedal (Figs. 2a and 2b).

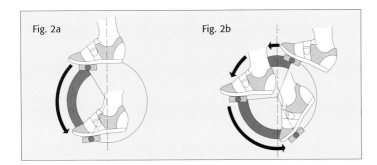

Fig. 2a   Fig. 2b

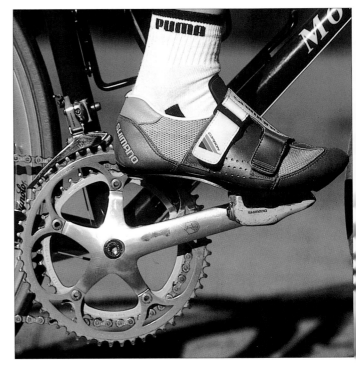

this case, the tip of the foot either remains horizontal or in a permanent downwards pointing position. Pedalling involves the harmonious interaction of three joints: hips, knees and ankles. Figure 3 illustrates the principal muscles used in the various stages of pedalling in a circular movement.

The circular pedalling action can be learned by training the movement firstly with one leg. Remove your right foot from the pedal strap and pedal with only the left foot. Try to pedal with equal force. As soon as your foot becomes tired and the

Good Cycling Style

The basic principle of a good cycling style is of course to maintain the body on the bicycle in such a position as to minimize wind resistance. A sports cyclist with a poor aerodynamic posture will have to deploy greater force than a cyclist with a good aerodynamic posture to achieve the same performance. You should, however, remember that health in sport is more important than aerodynamics. You should thus only adopt an aerodynamic

curves, pedalling should cease when taking a curve. As soon as you have left a curve, you should resume pedalling and accelerate.

Brakes are used during cycling in order to regulate and control speed. To slow down you should always use front and rear brakes simultaneously. In order to avoid falls when applying the brakes, ensure that they do not seize up. As a rule, the front brake is more effective than the rear, but it is also more likely to seize up. If you are forced to brake in a curve always apply the rear brake first. If

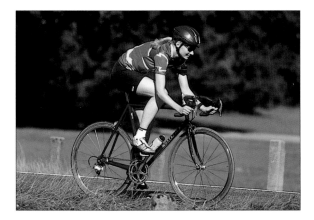

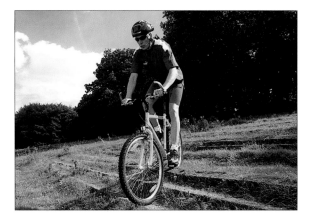

position if you are sure that no back, shoulder or wrist problems will result. For this reason, vary your grip and sitting position as often as possible during cycling to prevent muscle cramping and excessive strain on joints.

Body posture is to a large degree determined by the construction of the bicycle. Be sure to seek as much advice as possible when purchasing a bicycle and do not conceal any health problems. In riding the miles on a level road, the legs work in a parallel upward and downward movement like clockwork. The upper body should remain still throughout. Curves in the training course should be taken as quickly as necessary and as safely as possible. Make sure to keep the curve-side pedal in an upright position; in a right-hand curve the right pedal is therefore in the highest position, in a left-hand curve, it will be the left-side pedal. On account of centrifugal force, the cyclist should lean into the turn. Ideally, cyclist and cycle should adopt the same lean in the curve. In blind curves you must keep to the right for safety reasons. In the same way, left-hand curves should be negotiated in the middle of the road. With the exception of especially long

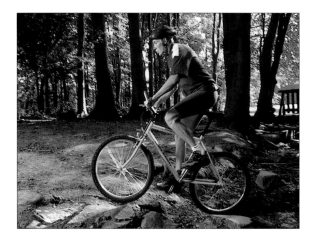

the front bake is applied too heavily, the front wheel will slide sideways in a curve.

Training Schedule

The endurance performance method can be used to improve aerobic performance in cycling. At the beginning of training, start with at least two training units of between 15 and 20 minutes. As soon as this can be achieved comfortably, increase the frequency to three times per week. Try now to increase the training distance while maintaining the same training heart rate. Over a long period of training the untrained cyclist achieves systematic progression up to the level of an advanced sports cyclist. The following basic principles should be observed, however: firstly, the frequency of training should be increased from week to week, then the increase of training distance and finally training intensity. The training unit can be graded in the following three areas:

1. Warm-up phase

The cyclist is best prepared for the real test by gradually running in. For this reason, the warm-up phase requires working at a lower heart rate than in the main phase. In order to monitor your heart rate in training distances derived from the Maximum Heart Rate (MHR), use a heart rate monitor.

Beginners

	Weeks 1–4	Weeks 5–8	Weeks 9–12
Training heart rate	60–70% of MHR	60–70% of MHR	60–70% of MHR
Training time per training unit	15–20 mins	20–30 mins	30–45 mins
Training units per week	2	2–3	3

Experienced

	Weeks 1–4	Weeks 5–8	Weeks 9–12
Training heart rate	60–75% of MHR	60–75% of MHR	60–75% of MHR
Training time per training unit	20–30 mins	30–45 mins	45–60 mins
Training units per week	2–3	3	3

Advanced

	Weeks 1–4	Weeks 5–8	Weeks 9–12
Training heart rate	70–85% of MHR	70–85% of MHR	70–85% of MHR
Training time per training unit	30–45 mins	40–60 mins	> 60 mins
Training units per week	3	3–4	3–4

2. Training phase

The content of the exertion phase depends on the performance and training objectives of the athlete. For this reason, training methods and exertion standards of the cyclist are established in accordance with the objectives.

3. Cool-down phase

The cool-down phase in cycling involves a long easing off period during which the heart rate remains clearly below the exertion level in the main part. Each training unit is ended with suitable stretching.

Indoor Cycling/Spinning® Program

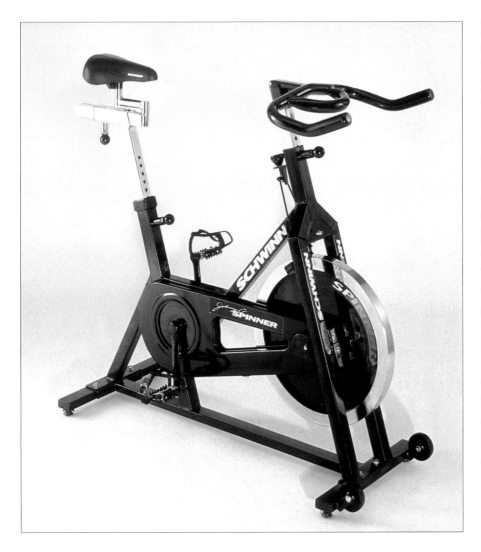

boring. During a course, the group is supervised by a specially trained trainer. He motivates the group and directs training intensity so that group members achieve their training objectives. With indoor cycling the heart rate should be monitored by use of a cardiograph. In practice, however, the participants frequently set resistance levels and step frequency according to their own subjective feeling. Insufficient or excess exertion can only be avoided by an objective control using a pulse monitor which also enables the individual adjustment of training programs. In this way, various performance and age levels can be individually supervised in one hour. Indoor cycling is therefore ideal for beginners in endurance training. Even cycling professionals can use indoor cycling as a substitute training unit or when bad weather persists. By virtue of its variety and motivation programs, indoor cycling is a commendable option to train endurance effectively while protecting your joints sufficiently.

Indoor cycling involves a varied form of endurance training on fixed bikes (indoor cycles). The indoor cycle was developed specifically for this purpose. A heavy flywheel is set in stationary motion by means of straps or chains. The resistance of the wheel can be varied by means of a carefully regulated control brake. In this way it is possible to tailor the exercise exactly to the performance ability of the cyclist and to bring the flywheel to a halt. The various indoor cycles are easily adjustable so that they may be set to the physical condition of the participants.

With regard to indoor cycling, the fitness center can also offer the Spinning® program. In the Spinning® program, cycling takes place in a group with musical accompaniment. It therefore offers a useful alternative to individual training, which is frequently

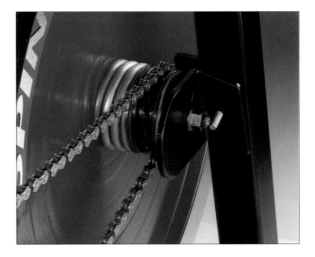

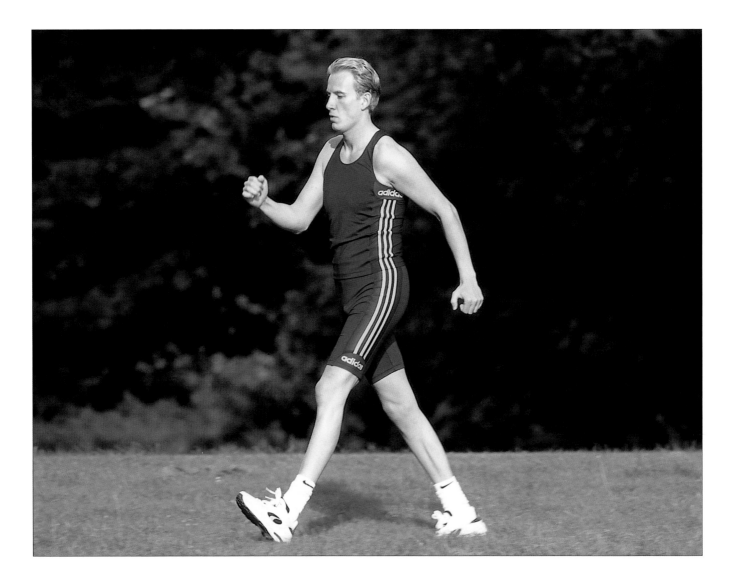

Walking

Despite its original meaning, walking is more than a simple variation on the stroll since it requires a specific technique. Walking has now become a mass sport in the USA – comparable to the jogging craze. Walking is a sport which is especially good for the promotion of health and protection of the joints because it places only minimal strain on the body in movement. For example, the reach and impact exercises in walking are about three times less than those in jogging. It is therefore better to take up walking before embarking on running. Because of its moderate technique,

walking is the perfect movement training for all people who show signs of wear and tear at the joints or the lower limbs and the spine and must therefore avoid impact strain on joints and on the back.

A further advantage of this moderate training form is that it involves a large number of body muscles (known as whole body training), thus enabling an effective and relatively low-risk capacity for endurance to be trained. Walking is not a performance sport, but a moderate form of sporting activity which can be practiced by everyone all year round. Experienced walkers and beginners, young and old, the healthy and less healthy – everybody – can easily learn walking and train regularly.

Choosing the Right Equipment

In the beginning, time-consuming and expensive equipment is not required. What is important is that your clothing is comfortable and that you feel good in it. Depending on weather conditions and temperature, you may opt for either airy or protective clothing. Should you wish to carry out walking all year round, you should invest in a protective cap and sunglasses for summer protection from UV rays. In winter you should use a warm cap, scarf and gloves to keep out the cold.

Although walking protects the joints you should ensure appropriate footwear for this sport. Some sports manufacturers already stock special walking shoes. However, in the beginning a good pair of general sports shoes is quite sufficient.

Before you buy your shoes, you should ask a doctor or specialist shop to measure your individual foot form first. When buying shoes, try on only those shoes which are appropriate to your feet (special shoes can work against deformation of the feet). An individually tailored footbed supports the arch of the foot and reduces the strain on foot movements. In addition, joints can also be relieved through special cushioning systems (air or gel-based). Additional insoles can act against the extremely rapid wear and tear of the soles and relieve the strain on your feet by means of additional cushioning.

In order to avoid pressure points, your walking shoe should normally be a full size or half size larger than your normal street shoes. The toes must be given sufficient room and should not be cramped or pinched. At the heel, the shoe should offer a firm heelpiece which covers the entire heel and offers stability and a close-hugging fit. In order to support the roll-off movement of the foot and the pressure movement of the toes during walking, the shoe should be supple and cushioned towards the front. Good circulation is guaranteed by a good ventilation system. On account of the special technique of walking and the accompanying individual strain on the shoe, you should use your new shoes solely for the purpose of walking.

As ability increases, people often wish for better equipment. Professional walkers can buy special walking shoes. Due to the special technique of walking, these shoes possess a low, cut-off heel. This wedged profile facilitates the roll-off movement of the foot. In this way, the toes do not "smack" the ground with the same force. Moreover, the front shin muscles are placed under less strain. In order to avoid blisters on the feet, great care should also be taken with the choice of socks. The best socks are made of polyester mixtures with low cotton content since they remove sweat from the skin and do not crease. Thin cotton socks store sweat in their fibers; in this way they can cause chafing and contribute to the formation of minor wounds.

Professional equipment also includes a cardiograph with which you can measure your heart rate during walking. This avoids either excess or insufficient exertion. There is an entire range of manufacturers on the market with various cardiographs. Ask advice from a specialty shop for your own individual purposes.

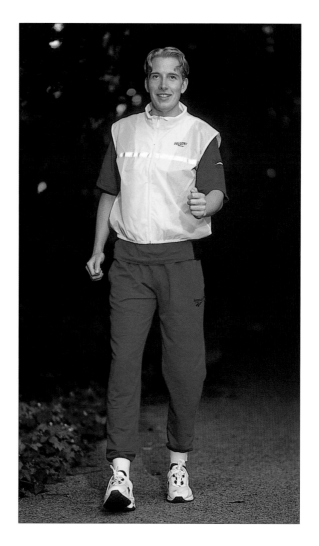

Techniques

Since the technique (see photograph) forms part of our everyday motor skills, it does not need to be acquired through protracted and intense training. However, the following principles should still be observed.

Posture

Straighten your upper body and keep it in a natural and upright position. The head should form the natural extension of the spinal column, the eyes should look straight ahead. Look at a point at a distance of approximately 12 to 15 feet in front of you. Your shoulders should be quite relaxed on the rib cage. When you push out your chest and keep your shoulders relaxed while doing so, the shoulder blades will automatically fall into the correct position. By maintaining an open chest posture, breathing can be considerably eased.

Arm technique/arm position

The arms should be kept close to the body and swing naturally parallel to the body in the normal walking rhythm. In the frontswing the arm should not go above chest height. In the backswing the hand should swing as high as the hipbone. At low speeds the arms are slightly less bent at the elbow. At high speeds the arm should be at right angles at the elbow joint. The hands are closed into a loose fist.

Stride/leg technique

Take quite normal steps. Stay relaxed in doing so, try not to influence your stride length. Long strides at this stage lead to premature fatigue. The conscious tread down and roll-off movement of the feet give the walking technique its ideal form. Ensure that the tips of the feet point in the direction of movement. The heel hits the ground first, then the rest of the whole foot up to the toes roll off. Make deliberate use of your foot and lower leg muscles and push off from the ground in order to introduce the next step. To relieve joint strain, the knee joint is bent slightly during the stepping phase.

Breathing

An upright posture gives the breathing organs room to work properly. Should you have breathing difficulties, first check your posture. In order to train the upright posture, open up your chest and raise your shoulders towards the ears. Relax and feel how the

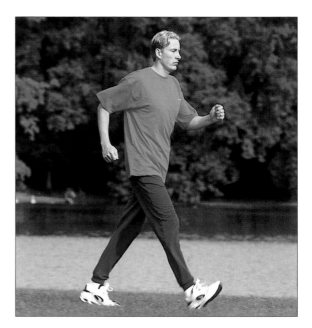

shoulders sink and how the shoulder blades sit in a relaxed position on the chest. Correct breathing means that you should breathe in deeply, but not at full capacity. Avoid shallow and rapid breaths (or "panting"). Each individual should find his own individual breathing rhythm. Try breathing in over the first three steps and then breathing out over the next three steps.

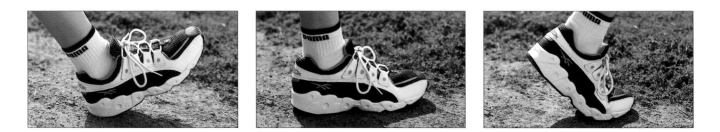

Walking Test

In this section you will learn a special walking test developed especially for fitness and health sports at the National Health Institute in Tampere, Finland. By building on these conclusions, the Institute for Sports Science in Frankfurt, Germany has further developed and evaluated the test. The outcome is an appropriate test with which you can monitor your current performance in endurance. On the basis of the test results, you can exactly determine your endurance capacity (or individual state of fitness) and take the appropriate steps for your future training.

If you are not ill, choose a 2000-meter stretch and walk along it in the technique described as fast as possible. The simplest way is to walk five times round a 400-

Average times (in minutes) and main variation

Age	Men			Women		
	below average	average	above average	below average	average	above average
from 20	>15:15	15:15–13:45	<13:45	>17:15	17:15–15:45	<15:45
25	>15:30	15:30–14:00	<14:00	>17:22	17:22–15:52	<15:52
30	>15:45	15:45–14:15	<14:15	>17:30	17:30–16:00	<16:00
35	>16:00	16:00–14:30	<14:30	>17:37	17:37–16:07	<16:07
40	>16:15	16:15–14:45	<14:45	>17:45	17:45–16:15	<16:15
45	>16:30	16:30–15:00	<15:00	>17:52	17:52–16:22	<16:22
50	>16:45	16:45–15:15	<15:15	>18:00	18:00–16:30	<16:30
55	>17:00	17:00–15:30	<15:30	>18:07	18:07–16:37	<16:37
60	>17:15	17:15–15:45	<15:45	>18:15	18:15–16:45	<16:45
65	>17:45	17:45–16:15	<16:15	>18:30	18:30–17:00	<17:00
70	>18:15	18:15–16:45	<16:45	>18:45	18:45–17:15	<17:15

	Test 1	Test 2
Test date		
Age		
Walking time for 2000 meter		
Heart rate (after test)		
Evaluation		

meter stadium running track. Immediately after the 2000-meter test, make a note of the test date, the time required and your heart beat in the table above.

In order to evaluate your time, use the table with the values for average times and standard deviations. Find the appropriate column for your age and sex. By comparing your time requirement with the reference data, you can calculate your current performance standard. Check from the table below if you have exercised appropriately. In order to interpret your personal test

pulse, find your age in the left hand column and then compare your pulse with the pulse values under maximum exertion in the second column. If, for example, your heart rate is over 220 minus your age, your exercise was too severe.

Age	Optimum test pulse (80–95% of maximum pulse)	Maximum pulse (220 minus age)
20	160–190	200
25	156–185	195
30	152–181	190
35	148–176	185
40	144–171	180
45	140–166	175
50	136–162	170
55	132–157	165
60	128–152	160
65	124–147	155
70	120–143	150

Training Plan

With the results of your walking test you can now select the appropriate training plan for your individual performance capacity. On the basis of your result you can obtain a general training recommendation for a period of several weeks. The results register the heart rate range derived as a percentage from the maximum pulse, known as the Maximum Heart Rate, your effective training time and the training units per week. After 12 weeks you should conduct a further test. It is highly likely that you will have improved on your first result.

Fundamentals of Walking Training

As soon as you have mastered the basic walking technique, you can start training. Find a training route you believe to be suitable to your current performance capacity. You should organize your training so as to avoid insufficient or excessive exertion. The basic principle is: the longer the selected test route, the slower your approach should be. As speed increases, so, too, does the heart rate. Always remain within the area for the training heart

Beginners	Weeks 1–4	Weeks 5–8	Weeks 9–12
Training heart rate	60–70% of MHR	60–70% of MHR	60–70% of MHR
Training time per training unit	15–20 mins	20–30 mins	30–45 mins
Training units per week	2	2–3	2–3

Experienced	Weeks 1–4	Weeks 5–8	Weeks 9–12
Training heart rate	60–75% of MHR	60–75% of MHR	60–85% of MHR
Training time per training unit	30–45 mins	45–60 mins	> 60 mins
Training units per week	3	3–4	3–4

	Weeks 1–4	Weeks 5–8	Weeks 9–12
Training heart rate	70–85% of MHR	70–85% of MHR	70–85% of MHR
Training time per training unit	20–30 mins	30–45 mins	45–60 mins
Training units per week	2–3	3	3

rate. In order to achieve an optimum training result, you should walk three to four times a week for 30 to 45 minutes. Training together with a friend or partner helps with motivation. Every training unit should be based on the following stages:

- warm-up phase (slow walking, gradual increase in speed, stretching)
- exertion phase (walking training in the stipulated heart rate range)
- cool-down phase (slow walking, stretching).

Variations

With the help of various walking techniques you can make your training varied and interesting. The selected variations act to increase intensity and should therefore only be carried out by walkers who have already mastered the basic technique. In view of recent and increased exertion incentives, the following styles can all be used when training success stagnates. The interval method can be recommended for the learning of the techniques. Alternate in training between the basic technique and specialized techniques.

small weight bands on the lower arms. With the additional weight the muscles of the upper body and arms are placed under greater strain. The weight bands can also be attached to the lower leg. The use of these weight bands increases the difficulty and training effect for the wogger.

Wogging

Wogging is an entirely normal basic technique of walking (as described). In order to increase intensity, the wogger carries small weights in his hands. It is, however, more comfortable to carry

Power Walking

Power walking is essentially walking at top speed. Ensure throughout that you are using the correct technique since high intensity exertion is particularly susceptible to small errors. Because of the endurance performance which is required, this variation is best suited to walkers who are used to walking at high speeds over long distances.

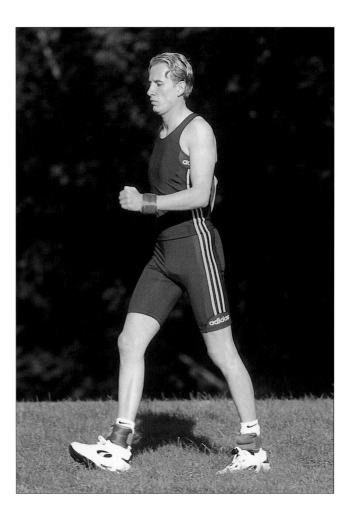

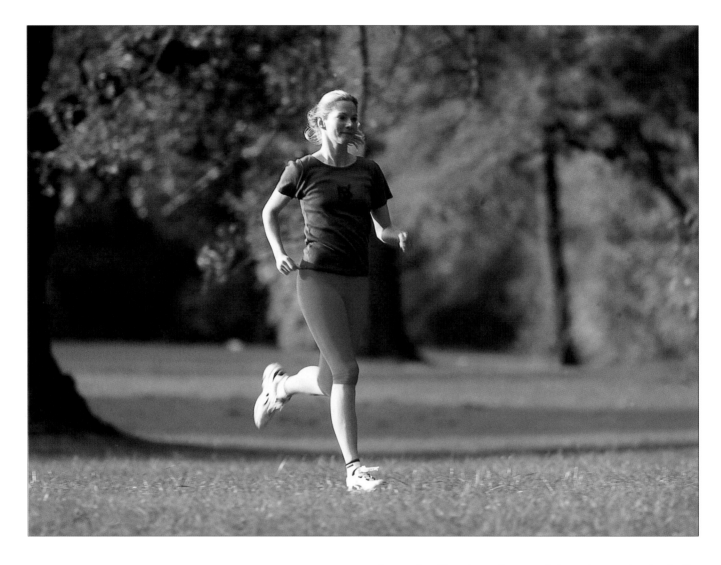

Jogging

Jogging is the most well-known and frequently practised endurance sport worldwide. About 30 million Americans jog on a regular basis. Many reasons account for the popularity and continued boom of jogging. Walking and running are movements which we tried out in our earliest childhood and have internalized. In comparison to skiing, for instance, they do not need to be learned from scratch. When a number of tips are followed, running can thus almost immediately be taken up. In addition, jogging is relatively independent of time and place. Jogging has particular recreational value in the open air and it reduces stress and calms the psyche. Since it requires very little equipment, jogging is, like walking, an extremely cost-effective sport.

Choosing the Right Equipment

The most important thing in running is good footwear. Beginners starting the sport should, since they do not possess a refined running style or frequently have insufficiently developed muscle support, take special care to buy good shoes. Practice is unfortunately rather different since often old sports shoes are dug out to make do for the start. Avoid these mistakes because poor footwear will quickly lead to running pains. Ideally before buying you should be examined by an orthopaedist and have your foot size measured. Two-thirds to three quarters of the population have some kind of incorrect foot posture such as clubfoot, collapsed arches, splayfoot, or hollow arches. When buying shoes these incorrect postures obviously need to be considered and corrected through adjustments to the shoe. If this does not take place the worst case result can be an aggravation of the incorrect posture through the shoe, thus also provoking problems in the joints. Do not be put off by high costs and remember that jogging and walking are some of the most cost-effective sports around. For the sake of your health, do not feel inclined to make savings on your shoes. Having said that, the most expensive footwear is not necessarily the best. The most expensive shoe is often little more than the latest fashion trend or high-tech material developed for competitive sport at the highest level. When purchasing we are often easily tempted into buying an especially lightweight shoe. Nevertheless, do bear in mind that a firm shoe provides better support.

Running shoes are only as good as their fit. Accordingly, you should observe the following tips when buying your shoes.

- From sports shops in your area, find the one which offers you the best advice.

- You are advised to buy your jogging shoes in the afternoon since in the morning your feet are still thin. However, they swell in the course of the day, meaning that your shoes can otherwise pinch in the evening.

- If you own old running shoes, take them with you to the shop and show the sales assistant. A good salesman will recognise your running technique from sole erosion. Tip: A good running style can be seen from the fact that the sole has been worn down most at the rear on the outstep and at the front on the instep.

- When buying, the weight of the jogger, running style and underfoot conditions of the running area must be taken into consideration. A cushioned sole will help to compensate the impact of the body in the landing phase. However, the heavier and faster the sportsman, the harder the sole must be. Therefore, when choosing your footwear be careful to see if the heel can easily be pressed in. If this is the case then the shoes are unlikely to be suitable.

- Good protection against the problem of foot twisting commonly seen in beginners is provided by a splayed sole. Provided the running route consists of straight paths with rooted soil you should consider whether to use ankle-high shoes, since they reduce the risk of twisting. The height, length and the material of the heel piece also provide support for the foot. The heel should therefore be made of synthetic material and covered with and protected by either synthetic material or leather. The heel of the shoe should be softly cushioned to avoid any damage to the Achilles tendon.

- Do not assume that the shoe needs to be broken in, because a good shoe will fit like a glove when first tried on. An appropriate shoe should not pinch or cramp anywhere. The foot should provide good support and at the front there should be about half an inch gap between the toes and the toe of the shoe.

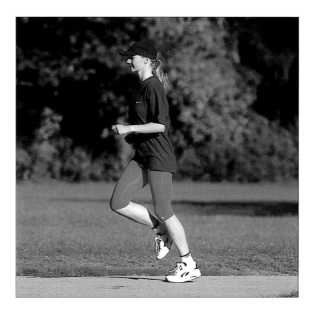

- If you are training daily, you should have several pairs of shoes to choose from. Not every shoe is equally appropriate for all seasons and underfoot conditions. Frequent use wears shoes down more quickly and they become unstable. After a training unit a shoe needs to be rested for 24 hours so that the material in the mid-sole area can regain its original form. Changing running shoes also helps prevent potential foot problems.

Clothing

There is no such thing as bad weather, only wrong clothes! For this reason, optimum clothing depends on weather conditions. Unfortunately, many people ignore this basic principle with the result that training becomes less pleasurable and the body can either become too hot or too cold. On the one hand, clothing should transport sweat and heat efficiently to the surface; on the other, it should provide ample protection from cold, wind and rain. When the weather is warm, a T-shirt or running vest plus a pair of shorts are sufficient. When the sun is strong, you are advised to use appropriate sports sunglasses and a protective cap. In autumn, when the days become cooler, you should also use a training jacket or sweatshirt. And to protect the legs from becoming cold, long and snug-fitting running pants known as tights or running pants are well regarded. For women runners several manufacturers offer special sports or running bras.

The material used is actually more important than the fashion aspects of sports clothing. Since natural fibres such as cotton absorb a lot of humidity and are considerably rougher than synthetic fibres, they tend to cause skin abrasions. A sweaty item of clothing sticks to the body and with the evaporation of accumulated moisture in low temperatures and strong winds quickly provoke chills. By contrast, synthetic fibers are smoother and cause less abrasion to the skin. In addition, they transport sweat from the skin to the outside. In this way, the skin remains comfortably dry and chills can be avoided. In the beginning, running beginners can safely use their own clothes. However, in time, you should invest in more suitable clothing in order to avoid potential health risks due to inappropriate clothing. To avoid health risks, high-tech fibers are an absolute must either in extreme weather conditions or long distance competitions.

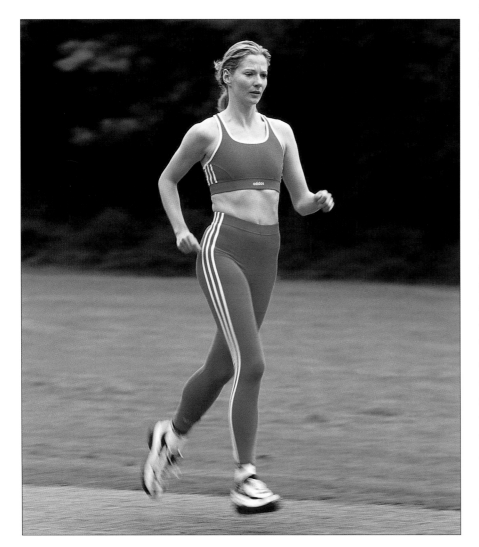

Clothing Tips

On cold training days you are best advised to dress according to the onion layer principle. That means using several layers of clothing. An undershirt, T-shirt and training jacket offer a higher number of isolating and thus heat-retaining layers of air between the pieces of clothing than a thick sweatshirt and a jacket.

When you are jogging in darkness or at dusk, which is likely to be a regular occurrence in the winter months, you should wear brightly colored clothing with a fluorescent top or fluorescent stripes on top for safety reasons. A small flashlight can also be extremely useful and a minor inconvenience. Bear in mind that most jogging accidents occur in the dark.

Techniques

The running technique involves a functional technique which must be followed by all runners. The terms running technique and running style are frequently used as if they were synonyms. However, the style refers to the individual form of running – e.g. light- or heavy-footed. In time, every runner will develop his own running style.

Body Posture

While running, the body posture should be relaxed. The upper body should be as upright as possible, possibly in a slight forward lean. The head is held in a continuous line with the spine so that

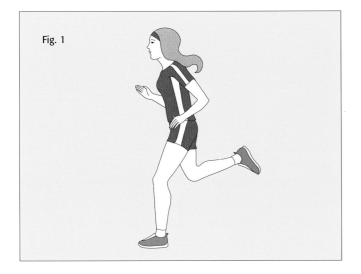

the view reaches the ground after a distance of 30 to 45 feet (Fig.1).

Arm Technique/Arm Posture

The arms are held at right angles at the elbow. They should be held close to the sides of the body and swing diagonally to the leg movement. This means that the right arm and the left leg or the left arm and the right leg move in the same direction at one time. This technique has usually become internalized through everyday walking and does not need to be acquired. The frontswing of the arms should reach up to about chest height, while in the

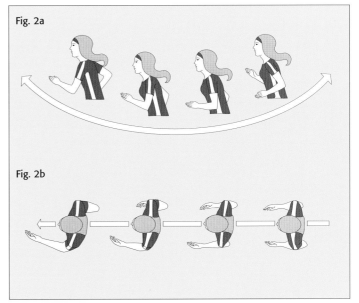

backswing the hand should swing back to waist height. During the swing of the arms the hands should be held half open or loosely closed. Avoid closing your hands into a tight fist (Figs. 2a and b).

Stride/Leg Technique

During the impact phase the foot first hits the ground at the heel and then rolls through the whole foot. The tip of the foot points in the running direction throughout. Also bear in mind that the leading foot should be slightly bent at the knee. This is because the impact waves are directly transferred to the running joints when the knee is overstretched. The bent knee joint also means that the foot hits the ground closer to the body's center of gravity. This technique is both economical and protects the runner's joints.

Experience shows that the running beginner has short strides and runs more slowly. Here, the roll-through movement as described is very difficult to achieve. Instead, the runner will inevitably hit the ground with the full sole. After a few training units the stride becomes longer and the speed higher. At this stage and with a little concentration the roll-through movement over the balls of the feet is possible. Good technique can be judged by the almost silent contact with the ground. If you hear a loud slapping sound, then your running style is closer to stamping and you should work on your technique.

One of the keys to running is economy of effort. An economical running stride depends on the length and form of the stride. So try not to force your body into a specific stride length. Instead, you should run as easily as possible; you will then find the optimum stride length. Always bear in mind that long strides demand greater energy. Shorter strides are therefore better at the outset because they economize energy and do not place the foot at too great a distance from the body's center of gravity.

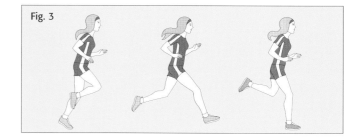

Fig. 3

Breathing

Many runners try to adjust their breathing rhythm to their running rhythm from the very start. Instead, you should first ensure that your breathing is even. Only after you have the correct running

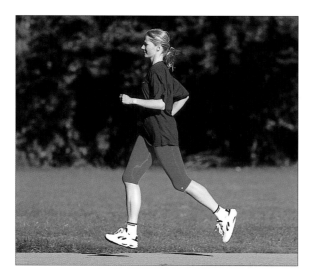

technique should breathing rhythm be adjusted to running rhythm. In the case of beginners and slow jogs the three-on-three rhythm is frequently used. This means that you breathe in over the first three steps and out over the following three. There are of course one-on-one, two-on-two and four-on-four rhythms – breathing in over one, two or four steps and out over one, two or four steps. Try to find your own individual rhythm. Breathing through the nose is preferable to breathing through the mouth since the nose humidifies, cleanses and warms the air more effectively. In this way, even in winter flu infections can be prevented. In order to guarantee optimum oxygen exchange, the emphasis of breathing should be on breathing out.

Running Phases

There are two phases in running (Fig. 3):
• the impact phase (characteristic: one foot has ground contact);
• the flight phase (characteristic: both feet are in the air).
Both phases are further subdivided in the following way:
The rear impact phase starts when the foot is slightly to the rear of the body's center of gravity and ends when the foot leaves the ground. The front impact phase starts with foot impact and ends when the body's center of gravity is either slightly ahead or exactly in line with the impact foot. Specialists still have not reached agreement on whether the runner should hit the ground first with the ball of the foot (pedal style) or the heel (stride style) (Fig. 4). It is, however, clear that there are good top-flight runners and record-holders in both styles. There is agreement that running on the ball of the foot is better suited to short runs, whereas middle-distance running is best performed by running on the middle of the foot. Leisure runners and long-distance runners are recommended to adopt the heel posture for biomechanical reasons.
The flight phase starts when the foot leaves the ground and ends when the other foot lands. During the flight phase the lower thigh swings, as the leg leaves the ground, towards the backside. This process takes place passively through the centrifugal force of the foot lift. When this movement is carried out actively, the running technique is uneconomical and wastes energy.

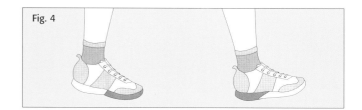

Fig. 4

Training Plan

The following section should help with the optimum build up of your running training so that you can achieve the objectives set. Experience shows that inexperienced runners have to stop after a few minutes of constant running due to breathlessness and muscle fatigue. It should always be remembered that although

beats per minute. When the heart rate falls below the necessary norm, you should increase walking speed or start with another running phase. The plan therefore acts only as a guide. If you feel that it is either too easy or too difficult, you should not hesitate to adjust it to your own exertion levels by adjusting the running or walking intervals to your needs.

Once you can run for 10 to 15 minutes without interruption, you can progress onto the minimal program. Experienced runners can start straight away with the optimum program.

Both programs help you to stabilize and extend your endurance. Remember that in weekly training four training units of 15 minutes are more effective than one training unit of 60 minutes. Increase gradually the route while remaining within the same training heart rate range.

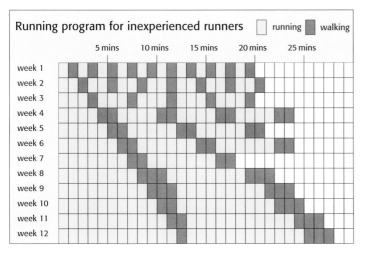

jogging is primarily an endurance sport, it is actually a form of whole body training with the full muscle application which that implies. The first training plan therefore aims to enable you to complete 2 x 12 minutes without difficulty within twelve weeks.

The training plan has been drawn up following the principle of interval training. This involves the alternation of exertion and relaxation phases. While the running intervals represent the exertion phases, the relaxation phases take the form of walking. In the first week you will run 1 x 10 minutes and walk 1 x 10 minutes per training unit. In order to observe the training plan the running intervals become longer from week to week and the walking intervals proportionately shorter. Training units are also systematically increased: in the beginning there are two to three units per week, in the following month three and in the last month three to four training units per week. The running speed will be set down by the individual heart beat range. Here, the use of a cardiograph makes good sense. You should always stay within the established range so that the heart and circulation system is neither under- nor over-exerted. In the walking phases you should select your pace so that the heart rate does not fall below 100

Training program

	Minimum	Optimum
Weekly exertion range	60 mins run ca. 5.6–7.5 m	3 hrs run ca. 21.7–24.9 m (at 7 mph)
Exertion intensity	50–60% of heart circulation performance (Vo_2 max.) HR = 160 – age	70–80% of heart circulation performance HR = 180 – age
Exertion duration	Minimum: 10–12 mins Maximum: 30 mins	Minimum: 30–35 mins Maximum: 60–70 mins
Training frequency	5 x 12 mins up to 2 x 30 mins per week	6 x 30 mins up to 3 x 60 mins per week
Effectively used in	Men: Vo_2 max. < 2.988 fl. oz./lb, or lower than 2 W	Men: Vo_2 max. < 3.361 fl. oz./lb, or 3–4 W
Caloric consumption	Women: Vo_2 max. < 2.39 fl. oz./lb, or lower than 1,5 W	Women: Vo_2 max. < 2.838 fl. oz./lb, or 2–3 W
	ca. 800–900 kcal	min. 3000 kcal

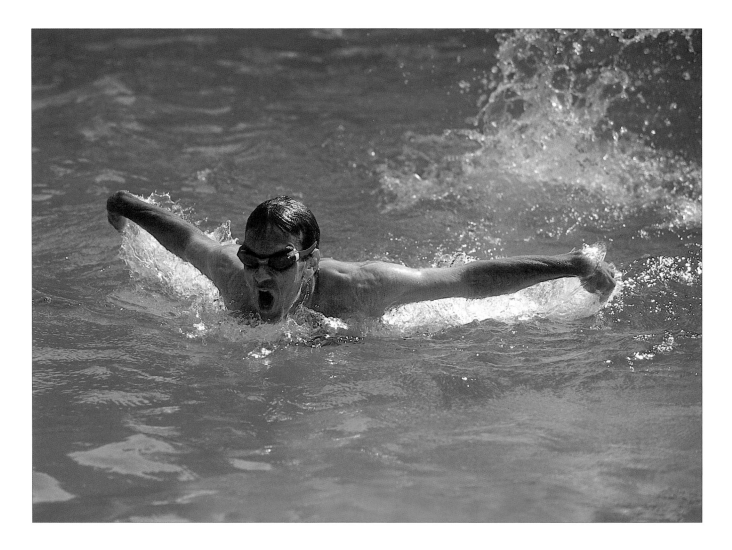

Swimming

Due to the changed perception of the forces acting on the body, movement in water is something special. On the one hand, each movement requires greater exertion because of the need to overcome water resistance, the movements are more difficult than on land (as you will quickly see if you try to jog through thigh-deep water). On the other hand, the buoyancy (lift) in water makes it possible for everyone, including heavy people, to float or glide peacefully almost without effort.

The impact of the cold and pressure of the water promotes blood circulation in the muscles. In this way the pulse is slowed and there is also a quicker recovery from exertion. In addition to the positive effects on the heart, circulation and breathing it is important to note the protection of the stroma. Since swimming does not involve any hard impact (as in running, for example), and buoyancy produces a significant reduction of body weight, the joints in particular are protected from excessive exertion. For this reason swimming is one of the most recommendable forms of endurance sport. There is a psycho-physical aspect, too: despite the exertion and exhaustion, water carries the body, lets you relax and soothes the organism. This leaves you with the sensation of pleasant tiredness. And that makes us feel good.

In addition to swimming there is now a range of other sporting activities which make use of the peculiarities of water already mentioned. Aqua-jogging takes place in shallow and deep water, in the latter case especially for therapeutic reasons after injuries. The same applies to "Aqua-Training", originally a form of gymnastic rehabilitation which focuses on strengthening and movement exercises. From the endurance angle, however, swimming in the classic sense remains the most appropriate water sport; it is also the easiest.

Mastering Water

All forms of swimming follow certain principles which should help you gain the confidence and courage to make it easier to acquire individual swimming techniques.

- Always keep your eyes open so as not to lose your sense of direction in the pool and drift from your lane.
- Learn to use *hydrostatic lift.* The more your body is under water, the more powerful the effect of buoyancy. Try playing "dead" (lie on your back with outstretched arms and legs), then lift your head and arms out of the water. Can you feel how you are really dragged down into the water? In other words, the more you use buoyancy, the less force you will need to keep your body floating on the surface. The muscles are more relaxed and you can use more energy for forward motion. In concrete terms, this means that in the crawl you should try to keep your head as far as possible under water and in the breaststroke you should immerse your head in order to glide evenly and easily.
- Always alternate between exertion and relaxation. There is, in any form of swimming, a constant alternation between impulsion and relaxation. This applies to arms and legs. Only if you give your limbs short periods of rest will they be able to move your body forwards in the water over an extended period of time. When your arms become "heavy" you should try deliberately to relax by pushing the arms in the crawl in a more relaxed fashion or extending the gliding phase in the breaststroke.
- Bear resistance in mind. Swimming depends on discovering and using "positive" resistance which pushes the body forward. You should always have the sensation that you wish to slide in the water using arms and legs along a large surface. On the other hand, it is necessary to overcome "negative" or "braking" resistance in water. Any surface of your body placed in the direction of your swimming brakes you. So try to keep yourself as small as possible.

Choosing the Right Equipment

You are bound to have a swimsuit and a towel and are unlikely to forget them if you go the pool. Frequent swimmers are strongly advised to buy a pair of swimming goggles since the chemicals used in pools can burn the eyes. And, of course, swimmers who keep their eyes open under water are less likely to be afraid of putting their heads under water. If possible, see if the goggles offer an air-tight fit around the eyes when you buy them.

There are several accessories for genuine swimming training, such as swimming boards, flippers, pull-buoys and paddles. Besides making you more experienced in water, they also help improve force and the technique of specific individual movements. These accessories can usually also be borrowed at the pool itself.

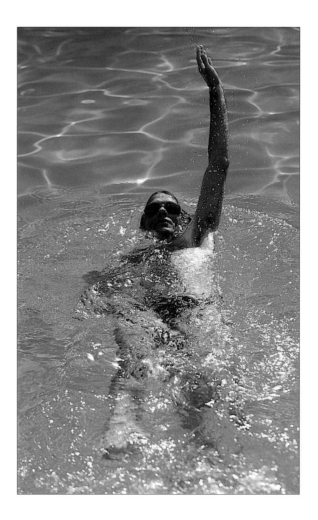

Basics of Swimming Training

This chapter should offer you incentives to make systematic use of your swimming and improve on it from a fitness angle in order to enhance your overall endurance capacity. The points below offer you guidelines. Remember that you are trying to do yourself some good – so do not spoil your enjoyment of the water.

Precede intensive swimming with a warm-up and stretching. Wait for a few minutes before leaving the pool after training until your pulse returns to a regular rate.

1. Short lengths well swum: the technique must be right.

The right technique is the key to economical and healthy swimming. To refresh your memory the following two pages re-acquaint you with the principal swimming techniques.

- Identify your technique through variations. More important than the precise repetition of specific movement forms is the development of a feeling for a movement which is economical and successful. To do this, you should vary individual movement elements as follows:
- In the front crawl, first perform a wide kick and then a narrow kick or firstly with high and then with low frequency; pull your arms into the water either at full stretch or bent; roll heavily or slightly from side to side; swim a length with as few arm movements as possible, that is to say, vary the length of the gliding phase, etc.
- Do you notice the changes? Find a style which allows you to make "fast and easy" progress. With the following program get slowly used to the idea that the quality of a movement is not reduced by fatigue:
- First swim a short distance, say one length (10–20 m) at a fast pace. Measure the time you required to do so (with the aid of a partner, a pool clock or a waterproof watch). The subsequent relaxation period at the pool-side should last five times the exertion phase. Repeat this five times. In the course of the training units increase the number of repetitions until you reach about 15 and reduce the duration of the breaks to a proportion of 1:1.
- In addition, practice the arm and leg movements in isolation in order to stabilize the technique – as shown under point 4.

2. Increasing the range: endurance swimming.

The next aim is to keep swimming over a longer distance. Here, you should start with a technique you master well.

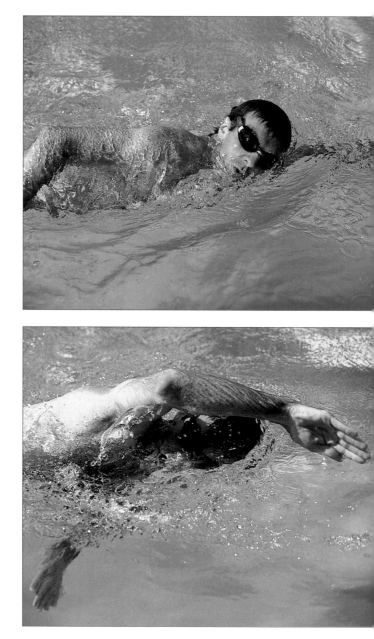

- Swim for at least five minutes, that is to say, distances of over 200 m, if possible without a break. Your pace should be moderate. You should swim so that the exertion does not make excessive demands on your body. In the course of the week, increase the range of swimming by swimming longer. You will discover how quickly you can increase your range. Within a few training weeks you will be able to swim between 800 and 1000 m.

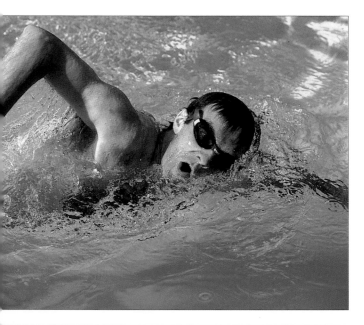

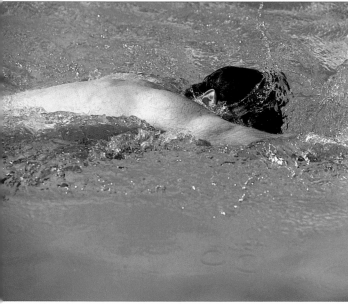

1. What time do you require for the total distance?
2. Reduce this time by 8 to 10%.
3. Subdivide this total distance in smaller units, say 10.
4. Divide the reduced time as calculated under number 2 by the number of smaller units. This is then the time in which you should swim these smaller units.
5. The breaks between the smaller units should each be one third of the time of the swimming time.
6. Make a note of when you should start again (after swimming and break times).

Example: You can swim 3000 feet in 25 minutes, that is 300 feet in 150 seconds. You should now try to swim ten times 300 feet in about 2:20 minutes. Take a break of about 40 seconds, that is to say, start every three minutes. Gradually, the breaks (30 seconds) and the smaller units (150 feet/75 feet) will become shorter and subsequently the swimming speed (-10%/-12%) will be increased.

4. Variation is the name of the game.

Alternate between continuous exertion and intervals, vary the length of the intervals and also the speed during endurance swimming. Vary also the swimming techniques and give yourself leisure periods in the water, by either playing or trying out new techniques. Practice arm and leg movements in isolation. For this purpose the equipment set out in the beginning will be of great use.

- Place the stretched lower arms on the swimming board and make only kicking movements (as in the crawl or breast stroke). For the back stroke secure the swimming board under your head with both hands.
- The use of flippers on the feet greatly facilitates forward motion in the techniques which require variation. They therefore promote motivation. In addition, through the stabilization of the body, they also help to concentrate attention on arm movements.
- By placing the pull-buoy between the legs, you can make specific improvements to arm movements.
- By using paddles in the hands, you can not only improve aspects of conditioning, but also improve awareness of the right kind of pull in the arm movement.
- Combine elements of various swimming techniques in order to improve coordination capacity. Try combining the butterfly arm movement with the leg movement of the breast stroke or vary the crawl between breast and back positions so that the body carries out a continuous rolling movement.

3. Increasing speed through intervals.

When you have become accustomed to swimming distances of over 1500 feet without interruption, you may start to increase systematically the speed of your distance. Subdivide the total distance into smaller units. Each unit, with its own break, is in turn swum at a faster pace than the total distance. Work out a plan at home for this approach by observing the following points:

Variation Techniques

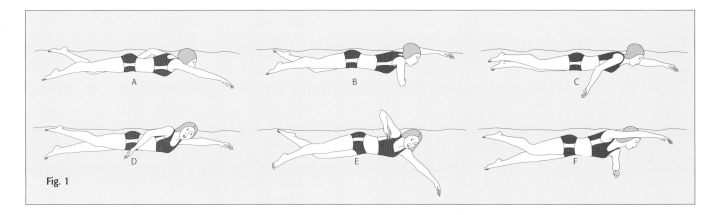

Fig. 1

Front Crawl

Those who swim the front crawl save energy. When carried out correctly, the classic crawl is the most effective use of energy deployed. The front crawl is thus suitable for the fastest possible completion of distances and also for long-distance swimming.

Technique

The body lies flat in the water and carries out a slight rolling movement along its length. The head on the water looks down to the front (see Figs. 1 and 2).

The arm stroke begins by pulling water by the hand. Catch a layer of water which you wish to hold onto and drag past. The second part of the stroke should build on the sense that you are trying to move forwards by means of the broadest possible contact surface (hand and lower arms) and automatically means that the elbow becomes bent and is held high. At shoulder height the hand should be under the body, the elbow joint is bent at a right angle. In the final pull phase the arm is extended under the chest and stomach to the rear. Always breathe out throughout the entire propulsion phase.

When the hand leaves the water, the arm relaxation phase begins. While the body rolls onto the other side, the elbow and lower arm leave the water. During this phase breathe in through the mouth. The head is tilted a little further but remains on the water surface. Breathing takes place on one side only. The upstretched elbow is now brought forward in relaxed way close to the body, bringing the relaxed hand and lower arm with it.

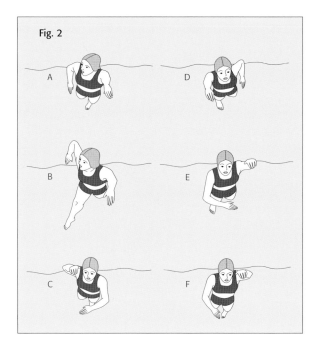

Fig. 2

Immerse your hand again in front of the shoulder. At the moment of immersion your other arm will be changing from the propulsion to the pressure phase. At this point the arm is outstretched and enters the water. With the simultaneous removal of the other arm, the body is rotated on the side of the immersed arm. The palm of the hand now begins to drag water again.

The alternate kicking movement serves primarily to stabilize the body position. The movement starts at the hip. Push the upper leg downwards. With water resistance this will produce a passive bend at the knee. The active elongation of the lower leg which follows now provokes a "kick" which propels the body forward.

The feet are stretched out and point inwards slightly. The upward movement takes place with extended legs and relaxed feet. A continuous six-beat leg movement produces three leg kicks for each leg of each arm cycle.

Back Crawl

The back crawl is the most sporting variant of the various back stroke techniques. These enable the swimmer to breathe with relative ease and relax the neck and spine. The alternate movements of the arms propel the body forward and the kicking and high, flat body position in the water correspond to the front crawl.

Technique

The body rolls along its length and lies with a high pelvis on its back flat in the water. The head remains still and is slightly tilted towards the chest (see Figs. 3 and 4).

The arm movement begins by immersing one arm behind your shoulder with the small finger side leading. Now push the arm forward and slightly downwards. Your body will now roll slightly to the side of this arm. By turning your hand downwards and then backwards you can begin pulling water. Once again the feeling that you are pulling yourself or rolling along the water should determine your movement here. Try to pull yourself along by using a broad surface of the hand followed by the lower and then the upper arm. In doing so, you will produce a bend at the

elbow which will also be held downward. At shoulder height your hand, elbow and shoulder should form a vertical triangle with the largest possible elbow bend in the direction of swimming. Now force your hand surface and the outstretched lower arm towards the upper leg. A clear downwards flip of the hand will support shoulder lift and also help lift the arm from the water.

The arm will be fed backwards in an outstretched position parallel to the body. Breathe in while the arm is being fed backwards and out when the arm is being fed forwards. The movement of the legs corresponds to the kick of an inverted front crawl. Similarly, one complete arm stroke will mean six complete leg strokes.

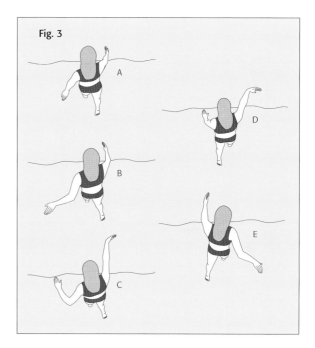
Fig. 3

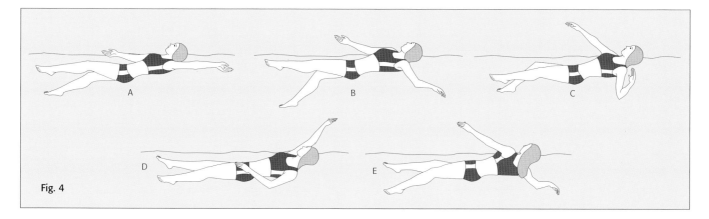
Fig. 4

Simultaneous Stroke Techniques

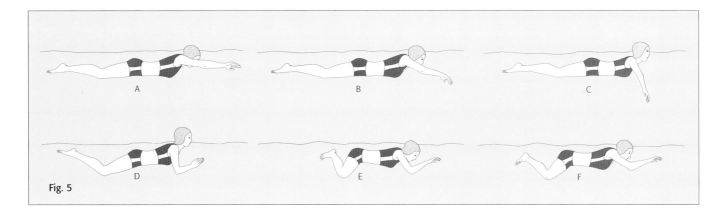

Fig. 5

The Classic Breast Stroke

The breast stroke is the most popular form of swimming since it allows a relatively "unhindered" form of breathing during swimming, an easy sense of direction and from time to time even a quick chat between lengths. On the other hand, frequently inappropriate techniques in breast stroke swimming place a particular strain on the neck and the small of the back, as, for example, "keeping the head out of the water."

Technique

The movement begins from the gliding phase. Here, the head lies in a relaxed way between outstretched arms. Your line of vision is towards the bottom of the pool. In order to drag water, turn your hands outwards in order to start the stroke phase (Figs. 5 and 6).

In the following outwards and downwards movement of the hands you should use the broadest possible hand and lower arm surface in order to pull yourself along the water surface. For this purpose it is important to bend the arms slightly at the elbows and to keep them high to the front. Once your hands have reached the line of the shoulders, pull your hands and lower arms quickly together. At this point, your head and shoulders will have reached their highest position and are above the waterline. This is the right time to breathe in. Stretch out your arms by pushing your hands forward and rest your head on the water surface again. Breathe out at the end of this stretching phase. The leg movement begins when the arms are being pulled together. The feet are pulled up in relaxed mode to the backside and bent. The outstretching of the

arms induces what is known as the straddle kick of the legs. To achieve this, turn your toes outwards and swing in a semicircular movement outwards, backwards and downwards. You then peel away from the water by using the insides of your feet and lower legs. Finally, the legs are quickly closed almost at full stretch. The soles of your feet should be pointing inwards at this stage.

The brief pause of the outstretched arms leads to a "relaxing" gliding phase whose length may be varied. Water catching should only ever begin just before you close your legs. There is therefore a brief overlapping of the arm and leg movements.

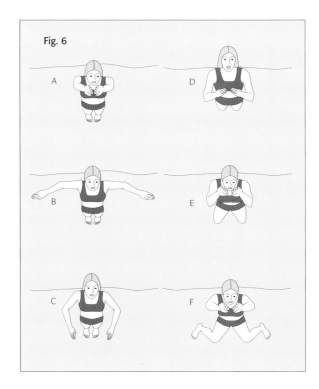

Fig. 6

Butterfly Stroke

The butterfly stroke creates the impression of beauty, power and speed. Although the impression of power is correct, the butterfly stroke does not allow the same speed as the front crawl. Particularly from the endurance angle, the butterfly stroke is recommended only for experienced swimmers since it places high demands on condition and coordination.

Technique

The most important characteristic of this kind of simultaneous stroke is the wave-shaped butterfly movement initiated by the head. This can only be achieved by good coordination of your arm and leg movements (see Figs. 7 and 8).

In the arm movement, the arms move at the same time and in the same way. The arm movement under water resembles the arm movement of the front crawl. The propulsion phase resembles a symmetrical, key-shaped stroke pattern. After the water catching phase, the stroke phase may begin. Your arm starts by pulling outwards and then downwards. As they bend, try to keep your elbows as high as possible and breathe out at the same time. The hands come together under the chest and finally push away towards the upper legs. This pushing phase must be given particular attention. It also involves lifting the head in order to start the return phase which brings the arms over the water. First, the arms and elbows are lifted from the water and quickly thrust forward as far as possible. The head, arms and shoulders achieve their highest position at this stage. Once again, the head reintroduces the next stroke. This involves bringing your head

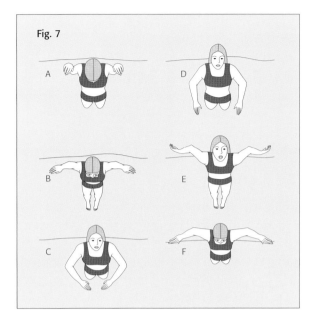

Fig. 7

forwards and downwards into the water. The hands then follow suit, turned slightly outwards at about shoulder width.

During an arm cycle you should kick twice. The first kick takes place when the arms enter the water and the second while the arms push backwards towards the upper legs prior to leaving the water again. The legs too follow a parallel movement. The kicks are similar to those used in the crawl. The movement is started from the hip. The downwards movement of the upper leg leads to a bend in the knee joint which is straightened by the whiplash upwards kick of the lower legs which follows. In this way the wave movement is produced which is so indispensable and characteristic of the butterfly stroke. The outstretched legs are brought upwards again. Keep your feet relaxed and turned inwards slightly during the downwards phase.

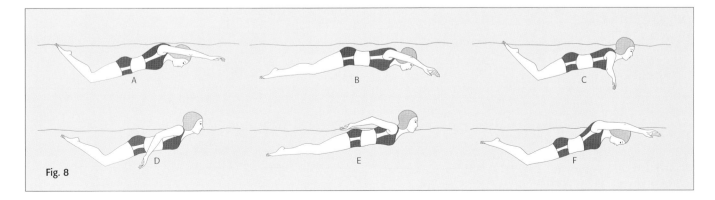

Fig. 8

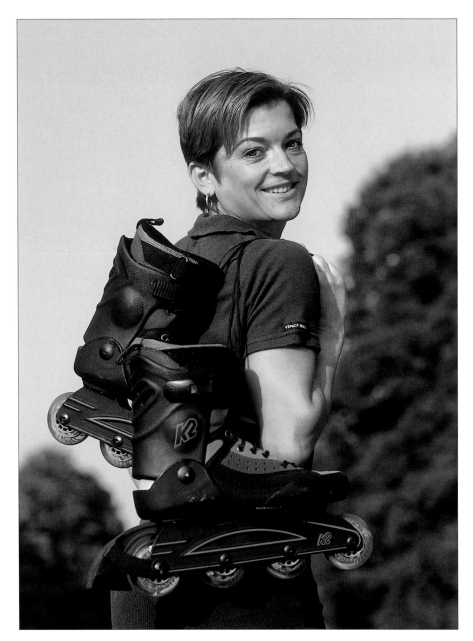

In-line skating is another form of skating. Its name comes from the special positioning of the wheels – in a line. They are therefore quite distinct from conventional skates in which the wheels are located side by side.

In-line skating combines training endurance, coordination and power and is therefore the ideal sports activity at a time when movement has become so scarce. However, because of the danger of falling, it is also a potentially dangerous sport which should be practiced with caution. Nevertheless, the dangers can be minimized by the appropriate protective equipment and firm mastery of the most important braking and running techniques. The basic techniques can be learnt in a relatively short time. Anyone capable of walking or running can do in-line skating. It is therefore a sport for all age groups. People who know now to ice skate are particularly in a position to learn the new techniques since ice skating technique is very similar to the in-line skating technique. But if you want to play it safe, sign up for an introductory course at an in-line training school.

Choosing the Right Equipment

The irresistible boom in in-line skating has been further strengthened by the development of new high-tech materials. Specialty traders sell the models appropriate for the various forms (street hockey, stunts, speed skating, fitness skates).

Although beginners are confronted with an almost impenetrable mass of materials and concepts before buying, a trained sales assistant or a specialist from among your friends, and reading the right specialty magazines can help in buying the right pair. Ask skating enthusiasts about their experience with skates.

In-line Skating

In-line skating is a sport which originated in the United States a few years ago. Almost no other sport has registered as much worldwide growth as in-line skating. In the USA there are already more than 19 million skaters – almost as many as jogging has attracted over decades.

You might even be able to try out a pair before buying. If this is not possible, you can take a trial run by borrowing or renting skates and protective equipment from your local sports store or in-line skating school in return for a deposit. Frequently, the deposit is then deducted from the subsequent sale.

The Skates

A basic distinction is made between soft boots and hard boots. The soft boots look like any other leisure shoe, only set on wheels. The inner and outer shoes are welded together. Due to the leather-like properties of its outer material, the soft boots are usually superior to the hard boots in terms of comfort and shape. Hard boots are made of an outer shoe shell and a removable inner shoe. The outer shells of top-of-the-line boots are made of polyurethane. They generally look very futuristic but provide a better foothold due to their shell design. Whether to recommend

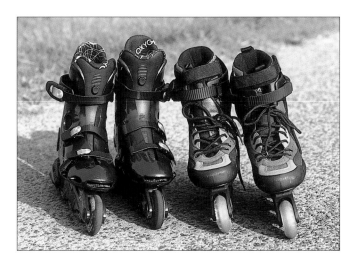

hard or soft boots depends on ability, your feet and their comfort, and proposed use. The best way to make a choice is to try the boots on, compare them and then choose.

Shell/outer boot

The shape and material of the outer boot determine their proposed use. In soft boots the external material is either leather or synthetic material. The durability of the boots depends on the use of high grade external materials. The first stages in skating are renowned for the wear and tear to the external boot since it often comes into contact with the ground. Unlike hard boots, soft boots are not as well ventilated and therefore do not offer a good foot environment.

If you have decided to buy a hard boot, a polyurethane shell is more than adequate for the leisure skater. Committed skaters often move onto high-tech materials such as "Duralite" or "injection molds" because their shells are lighter, more stable and more robust. You are well advised to give boots with PVC shells a wide berth. PVC shells are less elastic than polyurethane shells and are therefore more quickly worn out.

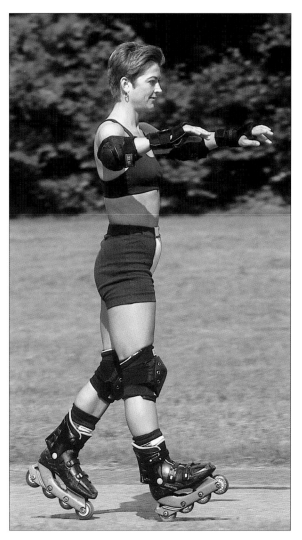

Inner boot

The inner boot is made of soft foam-based material. It cushions the foot against the hard shell and provides a hold. In terms of hygiene a removable inner boot has the advantage that it can be taken out and aired after use. Some manufacturers even

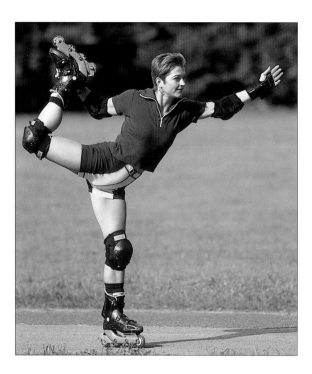

offer replacement inner boots. Various models come with anatomical insoles. Cheaper models come with hard card or thin plastic instead of the high comfort soles.

Wheel base/frame

The wheel base welds the boot to the wheels. The lighter and firmer the frame, the better the skate will be. Frames on cheaper skates are easily distorted and therefore offer less stability. Wheel bases are made of a range of materials such as synthetics, aluminum, nylon, fiberglass, carbon fiber, kevlar, titanium and other compounds. Pure nylon bases can be found frequently on cheaper skates and titanium and carbon fiber-kevlar frames on the top-of-the-line skates. On most leisure skates the frame is welded to the boot. If you want to leave yourself the option of tuning your boot at a later stage, you should rather think about buying detachable frames.

Bearings

As with any components there is a wide range in quality. The bearings are the key to quality. Good quality bearings allow the skater to hone his skills. You need two bearings for each wheel. Skaters have adopted the American industry norm of the ABEC (Annular Bearing Engineering Committee) as the quality standard. Non-ABEC bearings should be treated with caution and generally are of poor quality. If you buy a boot with low grade bearings you may tune the boot by changing the frame. In any event, you should always exercise great care when buying bearings. There are ABEC 1, 3, 5, 7, 9 models – the higher the number, the better the quality of the bearing. ABEC 1 or 3 bearings are entirely adequate for skating beginners. The two bearings in the center of the wheel are separated by what is known as a spacer. The spacer reduces friction. Plastic spacers are used in cheaper versions and sometimes none at all are used. Find out if your boots have aluminium or steel spacers. They may be more expensive, but they are more durable.

Rockering

The term rockering refers to the adjustment of the wheel height. Rockering enhances the turning capacity of the boots and therefore increases the range of their possible use. In almost all boots, the wheels are positioned at the same height (known as flat-rockering). This is the ideal setting for leisure skaters. The boot can perform more turns when the central wheels are set lower (known as positive rockering). This setting is appropriate for hockey. Stunt skaters heighten the setting of the central wheels (known as negative rockering). In this way, they can leap more easily over obstacles and objects such as steps, park benches and stairs and work on the frames (known as grinding). Specialists can even put on small performances during a tournament.

Wheels

Wheels usually differ according to size, profile, hardness and design. The wheel size (external diameter) is usually expressed in millimeters. Most in-line skates bought in shops are set with all-round wheels between 70 and 78 mm in diameter. Speed skating usually requires 76–82 mm wheels. However, foot comfort will suffer because the wheels become less stable as a result of the reduced contact area. On the other hand, stunt and trick skating actually require smaller wheels. The hardness is measured in durometers – in a range of 72 to 100 A. The higher the measurement, the harder the material. Leisure skaters prefer 76 to 82 A. With this level of hardness you can achieve a compromise between sensible wheel behavior and good road grip.

When you look at the various wheel widths, you will also notice that there are considerable differences. There are extremely fine wheels well-suited to speed skating because of their reduced contact surface. Wheels with larger contact areas offer correspondingly greater stability. Fitness wheels can be recognised by their medium width. With this special covering they are fast and clean running. When you buy new wheels, consider carefully how you propose to wear your boots. Since you are confronted by such a large range of wheels and specifications in material, you should not shy away from asking for some tips from a specialty dealer.

Brakes

Most in-line skates brake according to the "stopper principle." This means a small rubber or synthetic stop at the heel of the boot. It is used by stretching the leg and digging the heel into the ground. Provided you do not remove the stop for image reasons and use the stop in accordance with the right braking technique, the system will prove cost-effective and reliable. Various manufacturers have already developed new systems which reduce braking distance. Other systems are undergoing development.

Protective equipment

Even the best skaters fall at least once. In-line skating therefore requires complete protective equipment. Make it rule number one never to go skating without protective equipment. The standard equipment consists of a helmet and knee, elbow and wrist protectors. Many beginners tend not to want the helmet when buying their equipment. Although the skating helmet or replacement cycling helmet takes a bit of getting used to in the beginning, a fall without helmet protection can be very dangerous. The various types of skating disciplines each have their own protective equipment. So take advice when you buy.

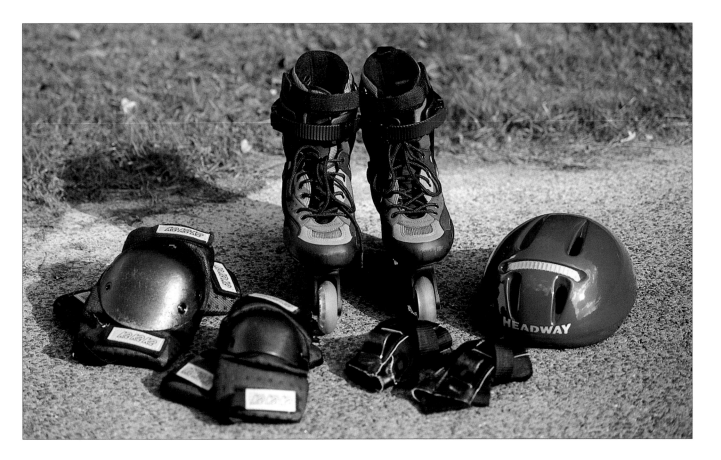

Techniques

Body posture/basic position

As with all sporting activities, successful skating depends on correct body posture. The wrong posture will result in a loss of balance. Try to stand up as straight as possible and distribute your weight evenly across the two skates. Look straight ahead. The skates should be placed a foot's breadth apart and parallel to each other, the knees slightly bent. By a slight movement in the hip, the weight can be brought further forward. Avoid at all costs pushing your weight backwards.

Basic step

From the basic starting position place your heels tightly together so that your feet form a V-shape pointing forwards. Your upper body should be inclined slightly forwards, and the knees should be slightly bent, and to kick away you should shift your weight onto your right leg. The left skate is then moved backwards and outwards along the inside. With this movement, you will roll onto your right foot which now bears your full body weight. The left skate is then brought forward and brought to the ground parallel to the right skate. Your body weight is therefore shifted onto your left foot and the right foot pushes backwards and outwards along the inside. This description should clearly show that the basic step involves pushing one leg back and out, while the other leg is moved forward.

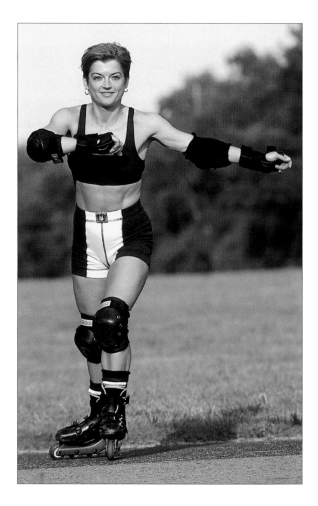

Arm posture

As in walking or running, the arm movement is usually quite automatic in in-line skating. The arms swing opposite to the thrusting leg and then they swing right. If the right leg kicks off, you will then swing your arm to the left, if you push away with your left leg, then your arms will swing right.

The arms perform the function of giving the body balance and providing thrust. For this purpose they move out and away from the body. Wild windmill movements are counterproductive and should be avoided at all costs.

Speed techniques for advanced skaters

Once your basic technique has become better and safer, you may try to introduce some dynamism and pace into your training by using the speed technique. There is an immediate optical difference between the speed and basic techniques by virtue of the different aerodynamic positions of the body.

Whereas in normal forward skating the upper body leans slightly forward, the speed skater adopts a much more pronounced upper body forward lean. The ideal position is achieved when an imaginary diagonal line can be drawn from head to foot through the body.

As in the basic technique, the body weight at the start is first placed on the thrusting leg. The right leg is, however, bent further and the push off from the whole right foot is firmer than in the basic technique. In order to maximize thrust, the thrusting leg must be straightened from the bent position to almost its full extension. You will easily feel the leverage movement over the larger range of movement. The sideways (not backwards) push-off position is particularly important. During push-off all the wheels should be equally used where possible. Professionals place their weight on the instep of the push-off leg and the outstep of the trailing leg. The arms swing opposite to the push-off leg to the left. In this way arms and legs work in harmony together and guide the skating rhythm. The body weight is shifted onto the left leg. The right foot leaves the ground and is brought to the ground again under the body, parallel to the left skate. The arms swing downwards from the left and are now in front of the body. Try to bring your skates with their outstep to the ground and lift your body weight onto the right. By alternating in this way, the left leg will become the push-off leg. The left leg, almost at full stretch, provides the powerful thrust to the side. For this reason, you must try to use all of the wheels on this side for as long as possible.

At high speed you can now slide on the outside of the right skate. While the arms swing from the right ahead of the body, you pull the left skate forward and bring it to the ground. The push-off

Braking technique

There are many interesting skating techniques which can be learned. Some are real crowd spectacles, others give the skater a tremendous amount of pleasure. However, the most important of all are the braking techniques. Skating can only be fun if you can control your own speed. The better you can brake, the more fun you will have skating.

The most appropriate braking technique for beginners is the heel-stop. This method may not be the most spectacular, but it involves a straightforward technique and is very effective. If you do not yet have any braking experience, try the technique described here without in-line skates to start with. Another preliminary exercise for practice is the grass stop. Here, you brake with the skates under your body. Under these simpler conditions you can acquire your first sense of this movement and a sense of braking security.

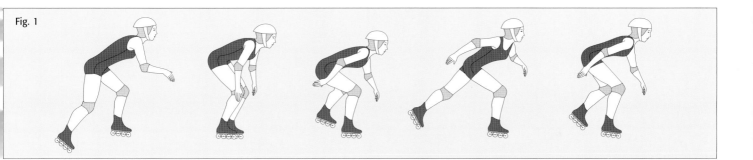

Fig. 1

starts again from the right foot. Your first speed thrill with this technique, if not sooner, will make you realize just how worthwhile it was to learn this technique (Fig. 1).

There are different arm movements in speed skating. The most appropriate arm swing for sprints and starts is the double swing described above. However, in speed skating the swing movement of the arms is more powerful and the movement range is greater than in the basic technique.

In the case of long-distance skating the single-arm swing is the most appropriate. This technique involves placing one hand with out-turned open palm on the lower back/pelvis. In order to reduce wind resistance to a minimum, the arm should be held close to the body. The free arm swings just like the two-arm technique, opposite to the appropriate push-off leg.

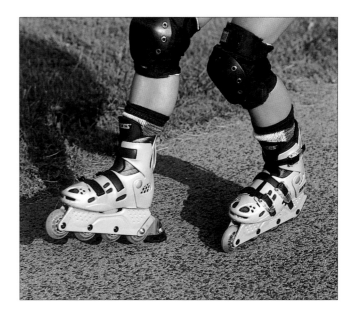

Techniques

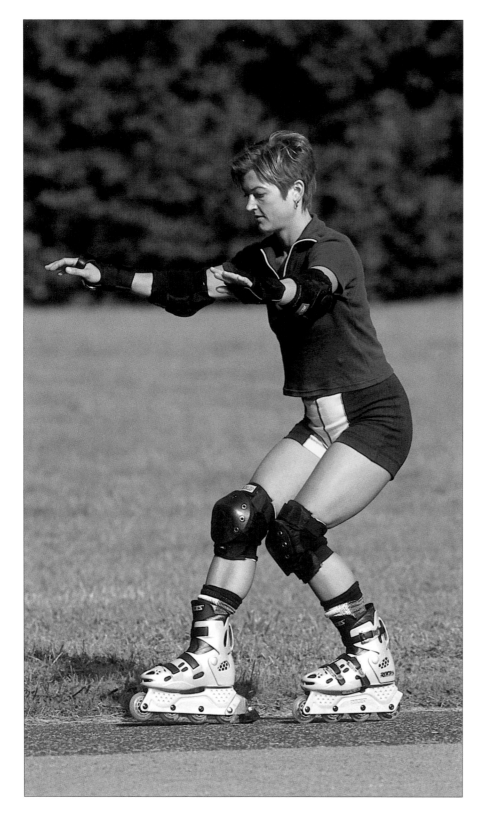

If you should practice on tarmac you will quickly notice that correct braking has to be learnt. Practice the stopping technique as often as you can. Adjust your speed to the terrain and your braking capacity. Without sound braking there can be no safe skating.

Heel stop

From forward travel the boot is pushed forward with the stopper, the knees remaining slightly bent. The tip of the boot of the foremost foot are raised until the stopper makes contact with the ground and brakes speed. Throughout the entire braking maneuver the body weight is placed on the trailing leg. As soon as the stopper has made ground contact, more pressure is placed on the heel stop and the knees straightened. The greater the pressure on the brake, the faster you will come to a halt.

Grass stop

If there is grass alongside the asphalt track then the grass stop can also be used as a braking option. Here, the skater leaves the asphalt and skates onto the grass, using it to slow him down. This may be a less elegant form of braking, but is appropriate for emergency situations and less as a standard maneuver. It can also clearly be advantageous for beginners to have heard of the "ride the grass" braking option when they take to their skates for the first time. A number of manufacturers have already introduced patented braking systems which greatly increase the safety of the skate while making braking easier. Seek advice from the sales assistant about the various brake systems and try them out to see if you can cope with the system.

Training Plan

In in-line jogging we use wheel movement specifically in order to enhance our endurance capacity. Aside from accidents arising from falls, in-line jogging is recommended for medical reasons. Unlike jogging, the skater is relieved of the flight and impact phases of jogging in which joints at times must endure high impact forces.

Before you take up training with in-line skates, you really must be totally familiar with running and braking techniques. For training purposes, find a good asphalt track without too many traffic lights, cyclists or pedestrians. Start with a moderate intensity 20 minutes relaxed in-line jogging. This can be calculated as a percentage on the basis of the Maximum Heart Rate (MHR). Every four weeks you should increase the training range by a few miles. Once you have achieved a training unit of about one hour you can increase intensity by planning out your training according to the interval principle. This involves high and moderate exertion phases.

	weeks 1–4	weeks 5–8	weeks 9–12
Training heart rate	60–75% of MHR	60–75% of MHR	60–75% of MHR
Training time per training unit	20–30 mins	30–40 mins	40–60 mins
Training units per week	2	2–3	3

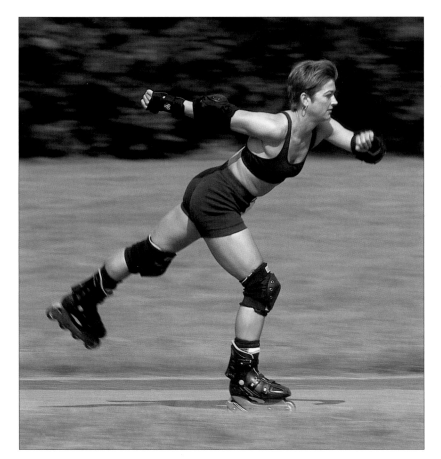

Guidelines for In-line Skating

The Federal Transport Ministry places skaters in the same category as pedestrians because skates are still considered sports or games equipment. For this reason, skaters are allowed to skate on pavements, but not on cycle paths or on public roads. Normally in-line skaters are tolerated on cycle paths, however. Always keep to the right and give sufficient safety margins when overtaking pedestrians on the left. Reduce speed on overtaking so that you can stop without causing injury to either the pedestrian or yourself. For safety reasons you should avoid hills in the beginning. The best training grounds are the carparks of large department stores after closing hours. Skating gives you particular pleasure on tarred pathways or streets near lakes, rivers or reservoirs. However, for safety reasons, do not skate in deserted areas without a partner.

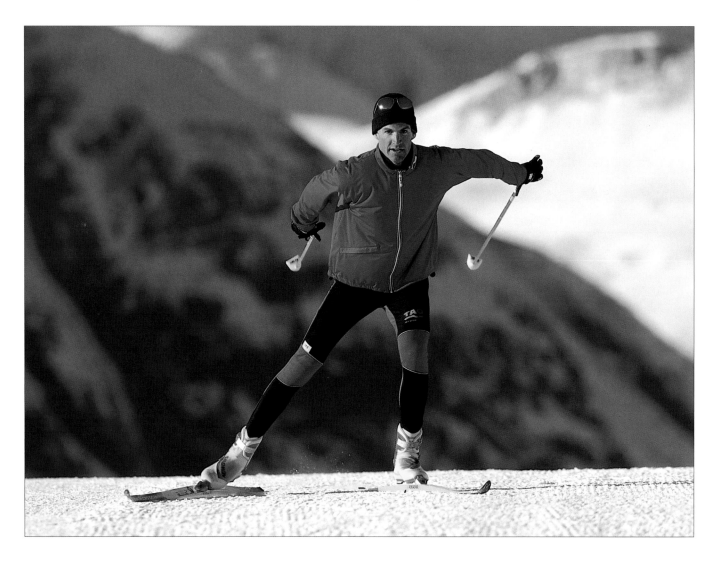

Cross-Country Skiing

From cliff face drawings and archaeological ski finds in northern Europe, Russia and Asia it is known that skiing is a form of travel stretching back over thousands of years. Our ancestors used skis as everyday equipment for traveling, warfare and hunting. In the mid-19th century, skiing, known as a "cultural technique," became a competitive and leisure sport. Today millions practice this winter sport, its pleasure made all the richer by stunning snow landscapes and the crisp clear air. Skiing is also a form of endurance sport which is particularly kind on joints since it involves a gliding forwards motion. As in jogging, training can be extremely effective in terms of endurance. The entire body is trained due to the complex movement involved. In addition to the dynamic use of the legs, the arm, chest and back muscles play a key role in maintaining body balance.

Choosing the Right Equipment

Cross-country clothing

Clothing for cross-country skiing purposes must protect the skier from cold, wind and precipitation and should also be breathable. In order to reduce wind resistance the clothing should fit snugly to the body. It should also be comfortable and allow the greatest possible freedom of movement. It is more expedient to use several thin layers of clothing as opposed to one thick layer. The "onion look" has distinct advantages when it comes to regulating heat.

Cross-country skiers wear a one- or two-piece running suit which affords great freedom of movement despite its snug fit. In order to prevent locking in too much heat, the clothing should be breathable. One-piece suits have the advantage that the top and bottom do not slip. In this way the body remains covered throughout and is not exposed to damp or cold. Some of the various suits offer additional support in the lumbar region and knees. Your underwear should be made of thermofabric. By virtue of these special fabrics sweat is quickly transported to the outside so that the body remains dry. Knee-high, thin socks protect the feet and lower legs from cold. If necessary, you can use two pairs of thin socks on top of each other. However, you would do better to forget grandma's old knitted socks with that chunky knit since they will only cramp the foot, creating the danger of blistering. There are anyway special shoe protectors available which offer protection from cold and wetness. In order to keep your ears and hands from freezing, you should wear a cap which protects the ears and warm gloves. On warmer days you can use a sweatband on the forehead to absorb the sweat. A typical skiing glove is the breathable, water-repellent fingered glove with added support between thumb and forefinger.

The right kind of cross-country skis

There is a wide range of equipment options on the market. Below you will find some basic information about equipment which should help you when you buy. It goes without saying that this brief advice can only offer guidelines and is not a substitute for the specialist guidance a specialty salesman can provide. If you are put off by the costs of new equipment, you could always hire it from ski schools and good sports shops on a weekly or daily basis.

The choice of skis is very much dependent on their proposed use. Beginners and inexperienced skiers require different skis from advanced cross-country skiers. In addition, the choice depends on the technique to be used – either classic or skating. In very general terms, the basic ski types are known as wax, no-wax, all-round or skating skis.

For advanced cross-country skiers who use classic techniques (such as the diagonal step or two-pole plant), the wax ski (WAX) is first choice. The ski comes with a smooth covering which

enhances the glide and thrust characteristics in the gliding areas (front and rear) with gliding wax and in the camber area (in the center of the ski) with adhesive wax. Other functional characteristics include the flex zone and ski hardness.

The name Nowax-ski is frequently misunderstood. The Nowax-ski must also be cleaned periodically, its wax removed and smoothed. The ski is designed for beginners, ski ramblers and leisure skiers who are well versed in the classic techniques but do not necessarily wish to be involved in waxing their skis. The use of special coverings and covering structures in the camber area of the ski (the push-off resistance) is designed to secure good push-off resistance without the use of adhesive wax. For this reason, no wax is required. However, to date it has not proved possible to develop a covering structure which can compete with a well-prepared wax ski in any snow conditions and temperatures. The skis do not always possess the best thrust and glide qualities. Still, they do offer the beginner a good compromise.

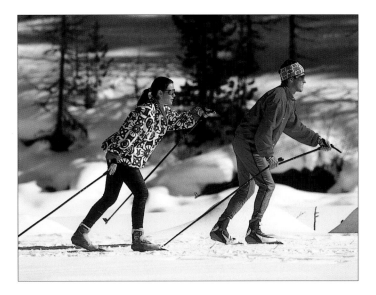

Beginners and leisure skiers who can use both skating and classic techniques are better advised to buy a set of all-round skis as a compromise. In terms of its structure, these are the classic adhesive wax skis, only about 2 to 4 inches shorter than the traditional classic ski because the latter makes skating difficult because of their length. There are nowadays a great many people adept at skating techniques (i.e. any form of skating movement). By virtue of their special technique, skating skis are sometimes

Equipment

shorter and firmer and have protected edges. Depending on the snow conditions, they may also be softer and have a different flex line. In addition, the skating ski is provided with a functional adhesive wax zone. The choice of the ski length depends on the height and weight of the skier, and on performance capacity and proposed use.

Ski poles

In years gone by people tended to use the longest possible ski poles. Today, shorter poles are being used since these are biomechanically better and allow higher movement frequency. The choice of ski poles depends on the arm and upper body strength of the skier and his personal skiing technique. For this reason, well-trained skiers who wish to perform at the highest level generally use longer poles than less trained skiers. Even in relatively level courses longer ski poles are used. The following rule of thumb can be applied to pole choice: poles for the classic techniques should be no longer than six inches less than the body height of the leisure skier. Skating poles are somewhat longer and should be four inches less than body height. When your body weight is low you are advised to go for stiff, break-resistant poles. Here, cross-country skiers are advised to opt for aluminum or carbon/kevlar-fiber-composite poles. Carbon-fiber poles are lighter than aluminum poles, but are also expensive.

Footwear and binding systems

Nowadays, most leisure skiers opt for half-length cross-country ski boots. These boots enable an optimum push-off

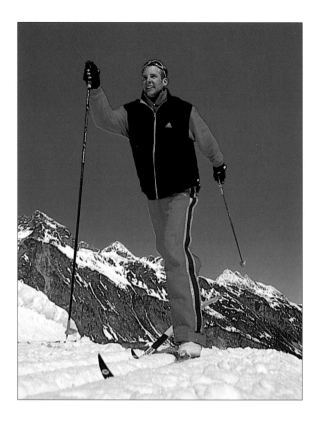

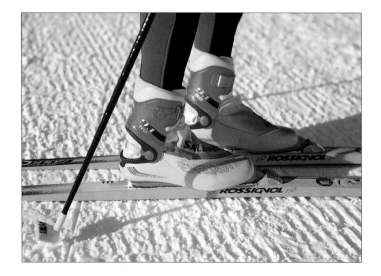

movement, protect the ankles and provide a firm foothold. A good boot should have soles which insulate your foot from the cold. A comfortable foot environment is guaranteed by a breathable and watertight boot. Advanced skaters tend now to opt for special skating shoes which are said to enable better power transmission.

Cross-country ski bindings secure the ski to the boot. The skier transfers his weight to the ski through the binding in order to move forwards and travel direct. The best bindings provide a high degree of directional stability without compromising the freedom of movement in lift. In Germany, the Salomon system and the Norwegian Rottefella-NNN bindings (also known as Rossignol-tie) are preferred. Both companies have adopted the principle of the "rubber-cushioned push-off movement" and developed it further. Due to the cushioned effect of the rubber buffer following impact, the ski quickly returns to the sole of the skier. In this way the ski can be more easily controlled. The attachment can be altered through various degrees of hardness to suit the individual techniques and preferences of each skier. In classic techniques the binding is loose, in skating, it is firm.

Techniques

Diagonal step

The most popular technique among leisure skiers remains the diagonal step. It is used at all levels. Due to its proximity to everyday movement (the cross coordination of arms and legs), this classic technique is relatively easy to learn. A further advantage of this technique is its wide-ranging applicability. Unlike skating techniques, the diagonal step technique is not necessarily linked to special cross-country ski courses. This original form of skiing is therefore the focus of the following pages.

In this way the push-off force of the leg can readily be converted into forward movement. In the basic position the legs are about one foot's width apart. In order to prepare for the push-off, the skier bends his ankles, knees and hip joints slightly. The upper body is hunched slightly and thus pushes body weight forward. The push-off phase is initiated by what is known as "adopting the pressure point." This involves a slight downwards movement by means of bending the right push-off leg. This, in turn, produces a redistribution of body weight to the right impact

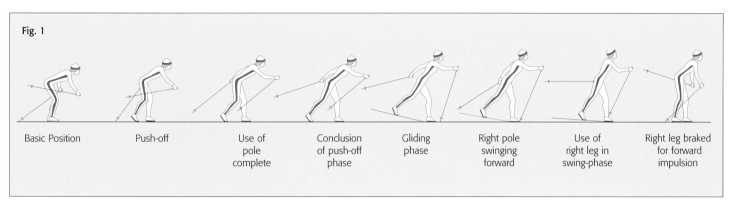

Fig. 1

| Basic Position | Push-off | Use of pole complete | Conclusion of push-off phase | Gliding phase | Right pole swinging forward | Use of right leg in swing-phase | Right leg braked for forward impulsion |

The diagonal step derives its name from the diagonal work of arms and legs (see Fig. 1). For those who ski as a hobby, this technique is suitable both for level courses and easy to intermediate climbs. An important principle is that the ski must be treated with wax before skiing (or equipped with climbing setting).

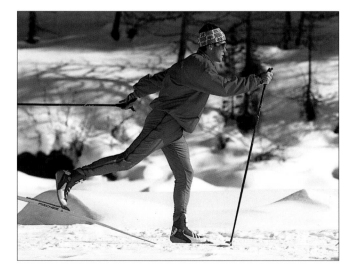

leg and a greater contraction of the front upper leg muscles. The push-off occurs through an explosive kicking motion to the rear from the hip, knee and ankle. This must be keenly felt since a push-off without the required effort would result in the ski sliding backwards. At the end of the movement, the upper body and the push-off leg form a continuous line. At the same time, the skier lifts himself on the left side with the aid of the ski pole. The use of the pole is already complete before the right leg is fully outstretched. During the push-off phase the body weight is shifted from the right lifting leg to the left trailing leg. As soon as the ski lifts from the snow, the push-off phase is concluded. The gliding phase can now begin. The skier glides without any support from the poles on a slightly bent left leg. The right lower arm has swung forward with a slight bend at the elbow, the arm to the rear now swings automatically outwards after the use of the ski pole. This phase demands a good sense of balance from the skier.

The passive gliding phase ends when the right pole swinging forward with the arm is used. Depending on speed, it will be planted in the snow either at the tips of the feet or just short of them to the side (at a slight angle). At this stage, the right arm enters the pulling phase and the right leg the pre-swing phase. During the swing phase the right leg is brought forward about as far as the gliding leg, pushed past it and suddenly braked in order to produce new forward impulsion. Only when this is carried out to perfection can this impulsion be harnessed. If you have either no or little experience of this technique then take a short break until you come to a standstill before starting push-off with the left leg and pull with the left arm. The movements always alternate and together form a fluid motion.

Small and intermediate climbs can easily be negotiated with the diagonal technique. Here, however, the gliding phase is shorter while the push-off phase is longer and should start earlier. Thanks to the shorter gliding phase the poles have to perform less work and the pole range is reduced. Note that at push-off the body weight is shifted slightly forwards in order to offer optimum support to the movement.

Arm and pole movement

Arm and pole work are especially important in the diagonal technique. The poles are used parallel to the body and planted in next to the track. When the poles are planted in the snow they form a slight rear-pointing angle. While the hand works to the front of the body while pushing the pole, we can refer to the pull phase. As soon as the hand reaches the body, the push phase begins. During the biomechanically more exacting pull phase the elbow is slightly bent. In the push phase the arm becomes increasingly outstretched. The pole handles run over the back of the hands. They must be so positioned along their length that when flipped back, the ski pole can be fed only between thumb and forefinger. Once the pole has passed the body, the hand can be closed and firmly grip the pole handle.

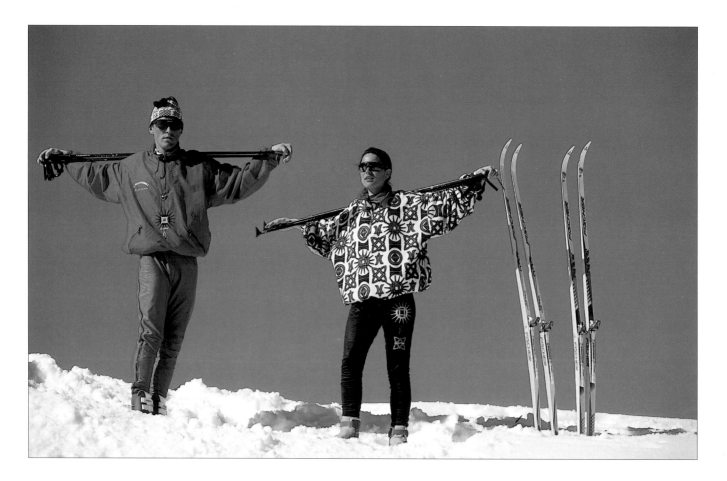

Training Plan

The skiing season for fitness skiers is normally restricted to a few weeks during winter vacations so longer-term skiing training does not make sense. Nonetheless, the following training recommendations can be made:

- Calculate your target heart rate range (= 70% of MHR) for the proposed training units (70% of 220 – age).
- First start with short skiing trips. In this way you can become better acquainted with the skis and achieve the required ski security.
- Even if you are on vacation and want to use every day for your training, you should also plan for recreational phases and rest days in your training.
- Gradually lengthen the training courses without leaving the training heart rate range.
- Keep fit outside the skiing season by practising other endurance sports such as running, cycling, skating, swimming, etc. In this way you will reduce the risk of personal injury and can prepare perfectly for the following skiing training. Almost all the sporting activities set out in the table are well suited to the main aim of summer training, which implies ensuring a good basic endurance. Endurance training for fitness and leisure purposes should be as varied as possible and involve as many sporting activities as possible.

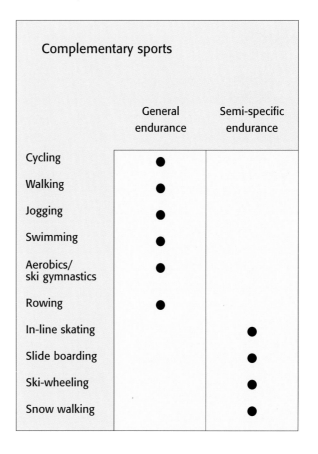

Complementary sports	General endurance	Semi-specific endurance
Cycling	●	
Walking	●	
Jogging	●	
Swimming	●	
Aerobics/ski gymnastics	●	
Rowing	●	
In-line skating		●
Slide boarding		●
Ski-wheeling		●
Snow walking		●

The endurance and technique transfer of semi-specific sporting activities and training instruments to cross-country skiing techniques is higher than in other sports because partial movements and the whole movement alike are very similar to the cross-country skiing technique. In months without snow, semi-specific instruments and endurance sports help to retain and improve acquired technical capacity.

Semi-specific training instruments

In-line skating: by virtue of the similarity of movements between in-line skating and ice skating, the summer variant can be an ideal preparation for the winter sport. Before starting in-line training, ensure that you master the running and braking techniques first. Locate a well-asphalted training course for your training.

Slide aerobics: slide aerobics trains the push-off and gliding movements and body weight shifting. The movement is very similar to the step in ice skating. (The movement technique is set out in detail in the section on aerobics.)

Snow walking: walking, preferably on hillsides, with the occasional use of poles. In this way the arm and body muscles and the cardiovascular system are specifically exerted according to long distance conditions.

Ski-wheeling: as the name suggests, ski-wheeling involves skis on wheels. Ski-wheels are designed so that ski-wheeling corresponds as closely as possible to the specific conditions of skiing. There are special models depending on the purpose (skating ski-wheelers, classic ski-wheelers, etc.). Depending on the proposed area of use, the skis are between 23 and 35 inches in length and weigh between 21 and 24 ounces. The ski-wheel makes sports specific training possible all year round. With ski-wheels various cross-country skiing techniques can also be trained. Both the technique and coordination training with ski-wheels are very close to real skiing conditions. In performance in particular, ski-wheels are a notable semi-specific training instrument by which to prepare yourself for the following skiing season. However, it cannot replace real ski training.

Aerobics

The term "aerobics" means an aerobic form of fitness gymnastics. It originated in the USA around 1982 and has differentiated into step-, slide- and box-aerobics, becoming an extremely popular sporting activity for both sexes.

Aerobics aims primarily to improve the general performance of the organism (cardiovascular system), but motor elements such as power, movement and coordination capacities are also significantly developed. Aerobics is therefore an ideal complement as well as an alternative to such endurance sports as cycling, swimming and also jogging.

With exciting music, group motivation and qualified instruction, you can learn the most important basic rules about the step combinations or even choreographies.

If you already have your own suitable equipment, you can, of course, do your aerobic training at home. By training at home you do not need to observe any course timetables. However, you do miss out on corrections in your technique and the motivation which comes from the group experience.

The Right Equipment

To secure pleasure and foot protection, aerobic training requires cushioned footwear. You should never perform aerobics barefoot, in stockings or thin gymnastic shoes without cushioning and foot protection. A good aerobics shoe provides ample support without cramping or pinching the feet. So seek advice from

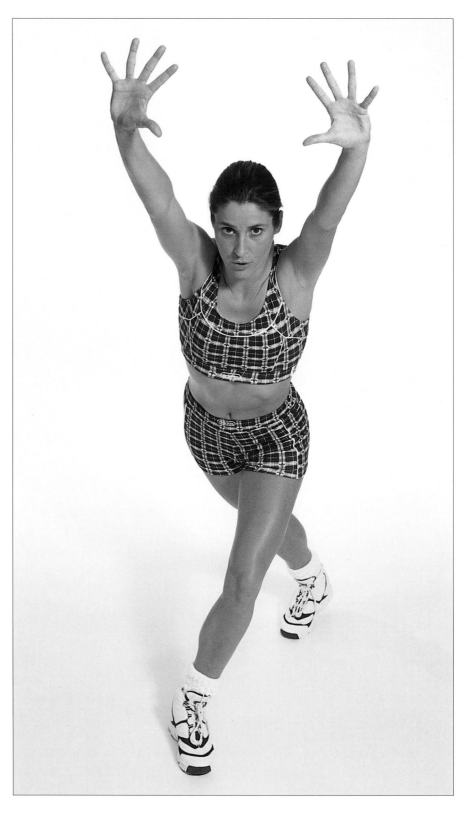

specialists in the sports shop before buying your footwear. The following checklist details the key features of a pair of appropriate aerobics shoes:

- foot stability, ankle-height
- good impact cushioning, arch support
- good foot environment, good ventilation
- light weight and comfortable
- bending zone to the front
- support in the area of the Achilles tendon.

The choice of clothing depends very much on what is comfortable and what you feel good in. You should decide if you want to follow fashion trends or opt for a classic aerobics outfit. Anything is possible: leggings or shorts with T-shirts or body-hugging leotards which permit maximum body movement and do not slip.

The Choice of Music

Anyone who has been to a nightclub or has had dancing classes will know how closely related music is to movement. In aerobics, movement is heavily influenced by the rhythm of the music. The musical rhythm can perfectly regulate the intensity of endurance training. In addition, it can offer an incentive to the athlete and en-hance his performance motivation. Effective endurance training means essentially carrying out the exercises without interruption. So choose music that offers a regular beat and does not put too much strain on you.

In order to check the appropriateness of your choice of music for training, count the bass beats made in one minute. If the song contains between 118 and 122 beats per minute, then it is ideally suited to step and slide training. Commercial aerobics music players register beats as BPM (beats per minute). This figure registers the beat of the music and therefore also indicates the beat and intensity of the exercise. In practice, this means that a bass beat corresponds to a step. Avoid songs with high BPM since these easily lead to a neglect of the movement techniques of the exercises and to an increase of injury. Moreover, your individual exertion limit will easily be exceeded.

There are no step movements in the conventional sense in slide aerobics. In the period of two beats you have to move from side to the other. Wait for a further two beats and then push out to the opposite side again. Alternate in this rhythm. Should you wish to exercise at higher intensity, cut down the number of breaks and glide from left to right without interruption with every second beat. Use this beat variation with care since the higher speed involved increases the risk of injury. Moreover, it is difficult to perform this technique "cleanly." If you observe these basic rules, then you can start training on your own.

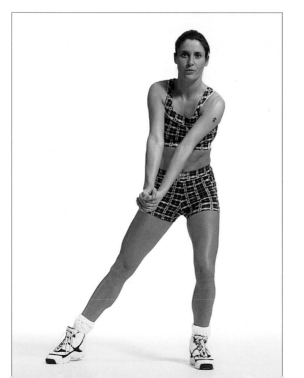
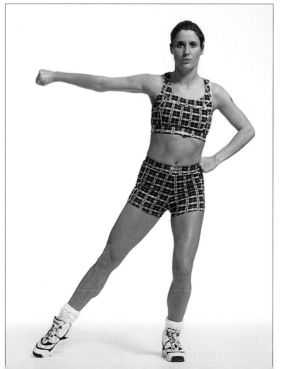

Step Aerobics

Step aerobics is suited to both men and women, old and young, beginners and advanced. It is particularly popular with men by virtue of its powerful and athletic movements. Step aerobics is a recent form of training which developed from traditional aerobics in the USA at the onset of the 1990s. Step training involves varied stepping movements up and down on height-adjustable and skid-resistant platforms much like a step. Arm movements can also be carried out. Step training involves combining various step sequences, arm movements and limited choreography. In order to reduce to a minimum the strain on tendons, ligaments and joints, you should perform only walking movements when stepping up and down. This is known as a low impact form of training. You should always avoid high impact jumping or hopping. Since the platform height is adjustable, this form of training is suited to any condition. Step aerobics is multi-faceted and is perfectly suited to the training of endurance, coordination, power and movement.

The Right Technique

Before starting step training, check first that the step adjustments are correctly inserted. Remember that a good step technique reduces the risk of injury and increases step safety. As soon as you feel the quality of your down- and up-stepping diminishing, take a short break or conclude your training in order to avoid accidents. For effective and varied endurance training, you are advised to combine the steps described below.

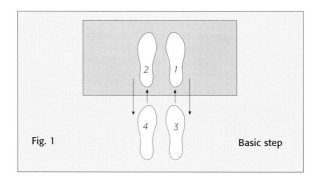

Fig. 1   Basic step

Basic position and basic step

In the position known as basic step single lead, the feet are placed about a foot's breadth apart, the toes pointing forward. In order to ensure the correct position for the spine, the knees and hips are bent slightly and the stomach and backside muscles are tensed. The upper body is held straight and the head forms a continuation of the spine. It is from this position that you start your first steps. You should stand at a distance of about 9–13 inches from the step placed crosswise in front of you. Slightly incline your upper body and tense all the body muscles. Place first the right foot in the center of the step. Be sure to place the full sole on the step. In order to protect your joints, the knee should be directly above the ankle.

Now with the left foot step onto the platform at a distance of about one foot's breadth the right foot. To resume the starting position, step backwards with first the right foot and then the left

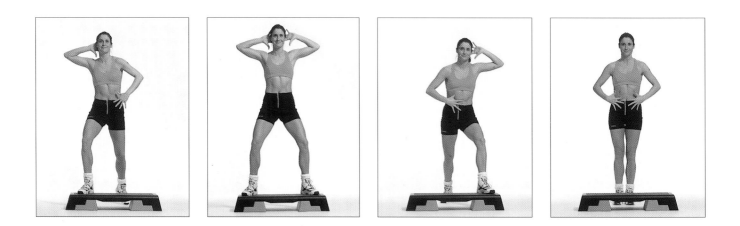

(Fig. 1). Step down with the ball of the foot first and then roll through to the heel. Throughout this movement the slightly bent arms can swing with the legs in order to support leg movement. As a variation, the arms with slightly bent elbows can be pushed forward to about shoulder height. Here, the arms swing forward together with the appropriate leg. As the right foot steps up, the right arm swings forward; as the right foot steps back, the right arm follows suit. To increase exercise intensity the arms can be thrust more powerfully. The coordination element of the exercise is increased by using various arm movements.

So that the movement does not become too repetitive, the leading leg should be changed after a planned interval. Start by lifting the right leg and then, after four to eight repeats, start with the left. There is a further pleasant variation on the basic step. This is the basic step with alternate lead. For this variation, step up onto the middle of the step, as in the basic step, with the right foot, and then with the left. The feet step down one after the other to the starting position – first the right and then the left. However, unlike the basic step, the left foot is brought alongside the right foot but only just touching the floor without pressure. After this light contact, it is the left foot which assumes the lead. Then the right foot follows. In the step down the left foot is grounded first, followed by the right which just touches the floor. The legs now work alternately and with equal strain.

An additional variation is the V-step. Here, the feet perform a V-shape during the step (Fig. 2). From the basic position, place your right foot as far as possible on the right of the platform and the left to the left in the same way. In the same sequence step down into a closed foot position. However, it could be too much to perform all the variations. This should be left to the choreographers (see photo sequence).

Basic Rules at a Glance

- The height of the step should always be adjusted according to individual performance capacity.
- Check that the parts of the step are properly inserted.
- The upper body leans slightly forward, the spine remains in its physiological form.
- The knees are always slightly bent.
- The whole foot is placed gently in the middle of the step.
- Do not perform any turning movements on the carrying leg.
- When stepping down, use the ball of the foot first and then roll through the rest of the foot to the heel.

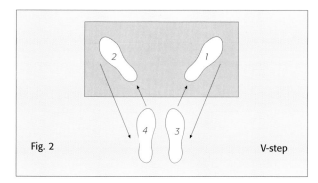

Fig. 2   V-step

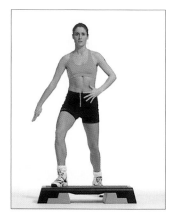
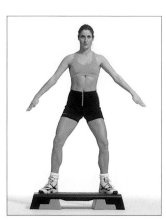
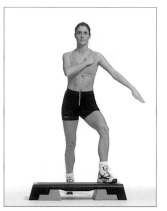
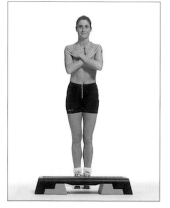

Slide Aerobics

A full hundred years ago Scandinavian winter sportsmen used slide-like movements as training movements by nailing planks to the sides of a waxed barn door set in the ground and then carried out the typical speed-skating movements. Since the 1950s too, this form of training has been used by physiotherapists in the treatment of ankle, knee and hip joint injuries. In fitness clubs, however, slide aerobics is a much more recent variant which, unlike other training movements, focuses on the training of sideways movements. In the traditional sports, such as football and tennis, most injuries occur through sideways movement or by lateral collisions. Slide training therefore helps to prevent injuries. The sideways movements on the slide effectively train body, backside and the entire leg muscles. In addition, endurance and stable stance are improved.

This kind of movement program requires a slide mat and special sliding socks or booties made of nylon. These slide socks are simply pulled over normal sports shoes. For safety reasons, the slide mat is covered with a skid-free coating on its underside. In order to make sliding possible, the top surface is covered with a special resin-based polymer. The sides of the slide mat are finished with two small buffers which make it possible to initiate and brake the slide movement. On closer inspection, the buffers have a ten-degree taper towards the top and a offset position of four degrees (a slight V-form). With this taper, the stopping movement is gentle and cushioned so that the joints are protected. The offset position of the buffers is important for the positioning of the foot, knee and hip joints.

Should you wish to use the slide for training at home, then you will need to place it on a skid-free surface with sufficient distance from furniture and walls. For a mat measuring 63–71 inches in length and about 20 inches in width, you will require about 22 to 33 square feet space. Performance sportsmen buy mats of up to 94 inches in length. The equipment can be rolled together with ease and easily carried in the car or stored in a cupboard. When buying, you should decide if you wish the edge buffers to be adjustable in terms of length or welded onto the mat. With adjustable buffers the equipment can be adjusted to suit individual leg length and the training condition of the participant. However, wrong setting can lead to injuries. For the purpose of private use, where one and the same person will be using the mat, a mat with non-adjustable buffers is recommended.

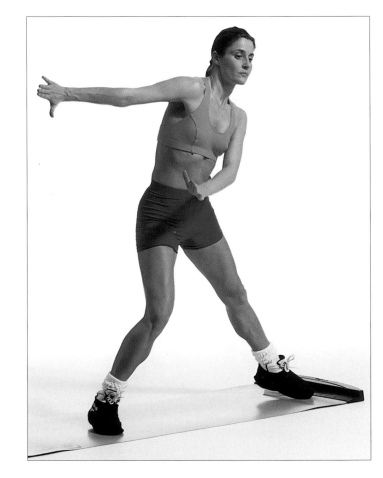

The Right Technique

Preparing for the basic step

In order to increase familiarity with the mat, movements are trained slowly and are performed in a controlled way at first. Make sure that the buffers are set open to the front (in the slight V-position). Stand on the left of the mat. Your left foot should be placed against the inside of the buffer and should push off with low to medium force. By pushing off from the buffer, both feet will slide towards the opposite buffer without hitting it.

During the slide, body weight remains centered on both feet. The body assumes a slightly forward-leaning posture. During push-off, knee and hip joints are slightly bent. Repeat the movement two to three times from the left before doing the same from the right buffer with the right leg. Once you have mastered this leg movement you can use your arms as support. In each push-off and sliding phase raise your arms to approximately shoulder height and lower them when the legs close.

Basic step

Gradually you will strengthen the push-off until you can slide without effort from one side to the other. It is important for your training that you push off from one buffer so that the trailing leg can easily reach the opposite buffer. This means that the whole body must be tense. By suppressing the interval, the basic step becomes faster and more dynamic than the pre-exercise. So your arms will need to be adjusted to the new pace: if you push off from the left buffer, raise both arms to the left to about shoulder height. By sliding to the opposite end both arms will harmoniously swing through past the body to the height of the right shoulder.

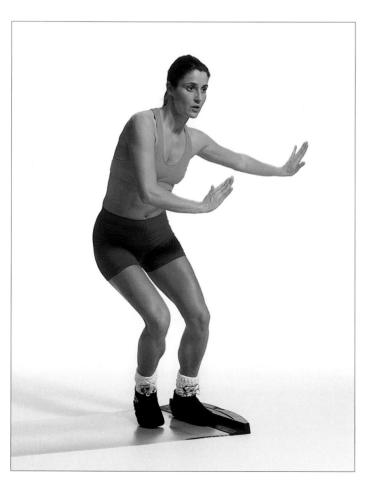

Basic Rules at a Glance

- In the beginning, your eyes look at the equipment; once the movement becomes automatic the head is positioned in a line with the spine.
- Build up and keep full body tension, especially in the stomach, body and rear.
- Knees and feet should point forwards during the movement in a slightly outwards pointing position.
- In order to increase stable body stance, the legs remain open as long as possible during the slide.
- During the slide the knee joints are bent, when the legs close the knees are straightened without fully extending them (high-low movement).
- During the slide body weight is centred on both legs.
- Speed is controlled by the trailing leg.

Box Aerobics

In the recently introduced box aerobics, simple elements of classic aerobics are combined with basic punches and steps from boxing. Training involves an emphasis on balanced upper body stance and legs. For fitness sportsmen box aerobics training has a significant impact on basic motor abilities. It is straightforward and trains endurance, power, speed and coordination while offering complete joint protection. Unlike boxing, box aerobics does not involve direct contact and so reduces the risk of injury. Using the technique of harmless shadow boxing, box aerobics trains all the specific hit movements (punch, jab, uppercut, etc.) and step movements (V-slip, shadow, etc.) of conventional boxing without actually injuring anyone.

By combining the various hit and step movements you can achieve your first box aerobic choreography. House music, with a beat of between 120 and 130 bpm, offers the ideal musical accompaniment. This music allows about two steps per second and means that movements can be evenly carried out. This guarantees that movements can be performed safely so the risk of injury is reduced. In the beginning it is not at all easy to adjust arm and leg movements to the music. However, with practice, the movements easily become automatic.

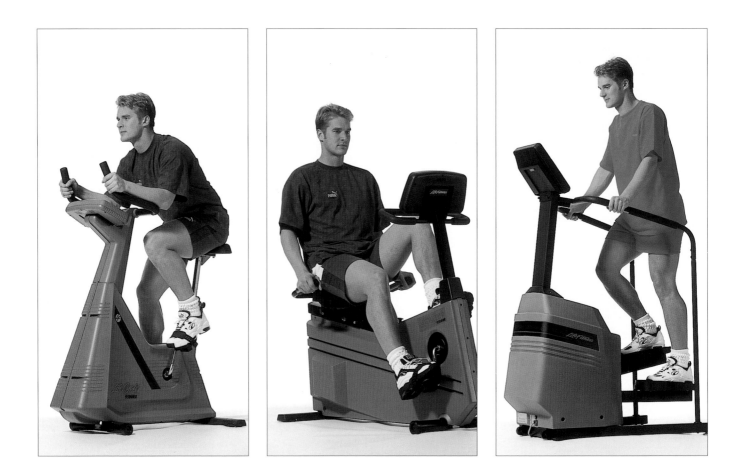

Cross-Training

In the area of fitness training, cross-training is not identical to its original meaning in medical therapy. In medicine, the effects of cross-training (also known as crossing effect or cross-lateral transfer) is used to improve the functional condition of injured muscles. For example, if the left arm is placed in a cast as a result of injury, special training on the healthy side can reduce the functional loss (such as atrophy, power, coordination) in the plastered arm. In high performance sport this technique is used to improve the technique of sportsmen and women.

In the context of fitness, cross-training involves interval training with various exercises. Exercise variations are made possible so that the various basic motor abilities can be trained. This form of training is particularly applied to endurance and power training.

In group training, the participants are oriented by a trainer throughout the course. His task is to motivate the group and correct errors where necessary. In individual training the trainer does not normally accompany athletes over the entire training unit. As a result, athletes in individual training often assume a greater individual responsibility by checking their own training criteria (training heart rate, weights, repetitions, duration, etc.).

Indoor cross-cardiotraining

Traditional endurance training based in a fitness studio is usually carried out as stationary training on cardio-fitness equipment. In cross-cardiotraining the focus is placed on the interval method known for its planned variation of exertion and relaxation phases. The exertion phases take place on various cardio machines. Here, the athlete is given the necessary relaxation breaks which occur when the instruments are changed. For example, an athlete can cycle for ten minutes on the ergometric cycle, take a two- to three-minute (active) rest while he changes to the ergometric rowing machine, where he rows for a further ten minutes in accordance with the established training heart rate, calculated in turn by the maximum heart rate (MHR). By changing instruments in this way, shorter rests can produce higher general muscle relaxation. On account of its exercise diversity, this kind of training is short and highly motivating. In addition, the risk of injury on account of one-sided exertion is considerably reduced.

Training recommendations assist the goal groups in the choice of appropriate cardio-instruments.

Training with Cardio-Fitness Equipment

● only slightly appropriate ●● appropriate ●●● highly appropriate

Type of equipment	overweight people	sedentary people	people with back problems	beginners/ inexperienced
Cycling machine	●●●	●	●	●●●
Stepper	●●	●●●	●●●	●●
Treadmill	●	●●●	●●	●
Rowing machine	●●●	●●●	●	●
Climber	●●●	●●●	●●●	●●
Horizontal cycle	●●●	●	●●	●●●
Crossrobics	●●●	●●●	●●	●●
Gymnastics/Aerobics	●●●	●●●	●●	●●
Skitrainer	●●●	●●●	●●●	●●
Arm crank ergometer	●●	●	●●	●●

Group training is conducted in exactly the same way. Course participants divide themselves among several different cardio-instruments and change to a new machine on completion of the pre-established interval duration. The choice of training machines and the setting of exertion range such as training range, intensity and interval use, depend on the training condition and objectives of the participants. The two tables presented here facilitate training planning for various groups.

Aspects of Training Planning

	beginners/inexperienced	experienced	advanced
Training method	extensive interval work	extensive interval work	extensive and intensive interval work
Choice of possible ergometric combinations	cycle/stepper cycle/crossrobics treadmill/stepper ...	cycle/stepper cycle/skitrainer treadmill/stepper ...	rowing machine/ skitrainer climber/crossrobics stepper/ rowing machine skitrainer ...
Duration of exertion	10–20 mins	20–30 mins	30–60 mins
Exertion intensity	60–70% of MHR	60–75% of MHR	60–85% der MHR
Exertion intervals	2–4 intervals of 4–5 mins each, 1 min break between intervals	2–6 intervals of 5–10 mins each, 1–2 min break between intervals	2–8 intervals of 5–15 min. each, 1–3 min break between intervals

This rough table should assist the individual goal groups in setting out individual training plans. The recommendations on training method and exertion standards should be adjusted according to individual performance levels.

Indoor Cross-Cardiotraining

Training example

	instrument combination (ergometer)	exertion intensity	1st exertion interval	break	2nd exertion interval	
Beginners/Inexperienced	cycle/stepper	60–70% of MHR	4 mins cycle	1 min	4 mins stepper	
	cycle/crossrobics	60–70% of MHR	5 mins cycle	1 min	5 mins crossrobics	
	treadmill/stepper	60–70% of MHR	5 mins treadmill	1 min	5 min stepper	
Experienced	cycle/stepper cycle/skitraining	60–75% of MHR	7 mins cycle	1–2 mins	7 mins stepper or skitraining	
	treadmill/stepper	60–75% of MHR	9 mins treadmill	1–3 mins	9 mins stepper	
	cycle/stepper/rowing	60–75% of MHR	10 mins cycle	1–3 mins	10 mins stepper	
Advanced	cycle/stepper	60–85% of MHR	10 mins cycle	1–3 mins	10 mins stepper	
	stepper/climber/ horizontal cycling	60–85% of MHR	5 mins stepper	1–3 mins	15 mins climber	
	skitraining/crossrobics/ rowing machine/ climber	60–85% of MHR	10 mins skitraining	1–3 mins	10 mins stepper	

The training plans above are only recommendations. Depending on your training condition and aims, more than three model intervals are possible. Provided you ensure during a training unit that you are neither being over- nor under-exerted by the exertion standards given, you should change them in accordance with your individual condition and proposed aims.

break	3rd exertion interval	break	4th–8th exertion interval	break	training duration
1 min	4 mins cycle	1 min	...	...	15 mins
1 min	5 mins cycle	1 min	...	...	18 mins
1 min	5 min on treadmill	1 min	...	...	18 mins
1–2 mins	7 mins stepper or skitraining	1–2 mins	...	...	approx. 27 mins
1–3 mins	9 mins stepper	1–3 mins	...	...	approx. 36 mins
1–3 mins	10 mins rowing	1–3 mins	...	...	approx. 39 mins
1–3 mins	10 mins cycle	1–3 mins	...	...	approx. 39 mins
1–3 mins	15 mins horizontal cycle	1–3 mins	...	...	approx. 54 mins
1–3 mins	10 mins rowing	1–3 mins	10 mins climber	1–3 mins	approx. 52 mins

Outdoor Cross-Cardiotraining

In outdoor cross-training the relaxing effect of contact with nature is greater than in indoor training. Moreover, movement in fresh air also strengthens the immune system. In accordance with the basic principle of cross-training, here, too, typical endurance sports such as walking, running, cycling, swimming, rowing and skating, etc. are combined. The training recommendation set out here demonstrates which endurance sports are appropriate for the various goal groups.

Cycling is particularly well-suited to overweight people since the wheels bear the weight of the body. Since it reduces impact, cycling also offers appropriate exercise for people with problems in their joints by the relaxed position adopted. By virtue of the simple control of exertion cycling is also perfectly suited to inactive people who want to take up a sport. Groups of people who for professional reasons are confined to sedentary positions, should however opt for sports other than cycling, such as walking, jogging or swimming. These sporting activities provide a counterbalance to the long sedentary periods at work.

Inline skating is another complex sporting activity since it trains endurance in addition to power and coordination. As a fun sport with low impact strain, it is therefore also ideally suited to counterbalance those long days spent in the office. Do bear in

mind, however, that inline skating is a potentially dangerous form of sport because of the danger of falling.

Because of its extremely high training effect, cross-country skiing is a seasonal sport restricted to the winter months. To learn the various techniques you are best advised to book into a skiing course at a recognized ski-school. Outside the skiing season you should keep fit by means of other forms of sport in order to avoid injuries and excessive strain.

Training recommendation

● only slightly appropriate ●● appropriate ●●● highly appropriate

Discipline/	overweight people	sedentery people	people with back problems	beginners/ inexperienced
Cycling	●●●	●	●	●●●
Jogging	●	●●●	●●	●
Walking	●●	●●●	●●●	●●●
Rowing	●●●	●●●	●	●
Swimming	●●●	●●●	●●●	●●
Cross-country skiing	●●●	●●●	●●●	●
In-line skating	●●	●	●●	●●

The training recommendation helps the goal groups in the choice of appropriate endurance disciplines.

Training examples

	combination of endurance sports	exertion intensity	1st exertion interval	break	2nd exertion interval
Beginners/ Inexperienced	walking/jogging	60–70% of MHR	5 mins walking	1 min	5 mins jogging
Experienced	cycle/in-line skating	60–75% of MHR	10 mins cycle	1–3 mins	10 mins in-line skating
Advanced	swimming/cycle/ jogging	60–85% of MHR	15 mins swimming	1–3 mins	15 mins cycle

Rowing is an endurance sport which provides great fun in summer. However, the rowing technique is extremely complex and makes great demands on the coordination and condition capacities of the rower. Whereas the complex total exertion of the entire body musculature is to be seen as something positive, inexperienced people or people with back problems are better advised to opt instead for sporting activities such as walking or swimming, since they protect the spine. If you do wish to learn this fine sporting activity make sure that you learn the technique from a fully competent trainer.

The rough table should help individual goal groups to set up individual training plans. The recommendations on training method and exertion standards should be set according to individual performance levels.

Elements of training planning

	Beginners/Inexperienced	Experienced	Advanced
Training method	extensive interval work	extensive interval work	extensive and intensive interval work
Choice of possible endurance sport combinations	cycle/walking swimming/ walking walking/jogging	walking/jogging cycle/jogging in-line skating/ cycle	in-line skating/ cycle swimming/ cycle/jogging
Exertion duration	15–20 mins	20–30 mins	30–60 mins
Exertion intensity	60–70% of MHR	60–75% of MHR	60–85% of MHR
Exertion intervals	2–4 intervals of 4–5 mins each, 1 min break between intervals	2–6 intervals of 5–10 mins each, 1 min break between intervals	2–8 intervals of 5–20 mins each, 2–4 mins break between intervals

The proposed training programs for outdoor training, unfortunately, have to be tailor-made for the individual. Consequently, more than the given three examples are possible depending on the individual's condition and objectives.

break	3rd exertion interval	break	4th–8th exertion interval	break	training duration
1 min	5 mins walking	1 min	N. A.	...	18 mins
1–3 mins	10 mins cycling	1–3 mins	...	...	approx. 39 mins
1–3 mins	15 mins jogging	1–3 mins	...	...	approx. 54 mins

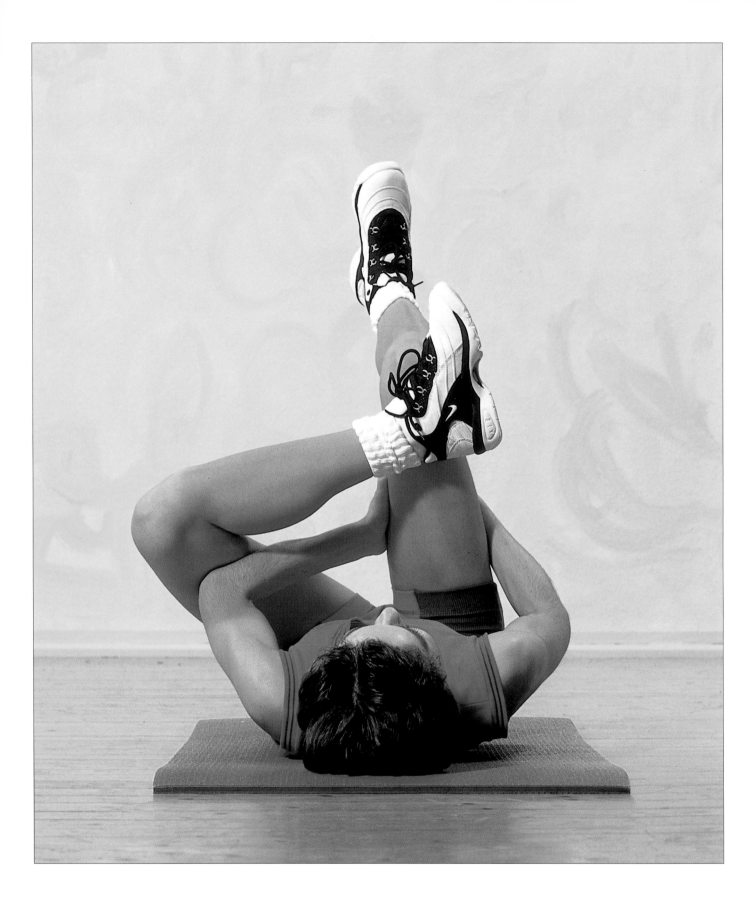

Mobility training – How does it work?

Developing mobility is an essential part of a comprehensive fitness program. Stretching is particulary important after strengthening exercises, in order to prevent the freshly exercised muscles from contracting.

Mobility is defined as the capacity to carry out movements in one or more joints with great rotational breadth, either voluntarily or under the influence of external forces. The mobility involved is made up, in equal measure, of the ability of musculature, sinews, ligaments and the joint capsule system to stretch and the suppleness that comes from the structure of the joint itself.

Several kinds of mobility can be distinguished. Active mobility is where a muscle is stretched only by the agonist contracting. In passive mobility, on the other hand, the muscular system is stretched by external forces, for example the weight or force of a partner. Depending on whether the stretch is held or alternatively is effected in seesaw or bouncing fashion, a further distinction is made between static and dynamic stretches. Stretching produced by the force of an antagonist is a smaller-scale movement than passively supported stretching. In fitness training, passive, static stretching, sometimes loosely called just 'stretching', has been favored in recent years.

Although the healthy, preventive use of regular stretch training is not seriously questioned by anyone, it still lurks in the wings for many sportsmen and women. This is probably due to the fact that they often do not have positive, practical knowledge thereof. The reason for this is that non-functional exercises are still being taught everywhere. Nonetheless, the situation is slowly improving. Correctly applied, stretching can offer the following benefits:

- Tenseness is eased enormously, thus enhancing greatly the sense of general well-being.
- Limitations on mobility because of age can be prevented in the long term.
- Improved mobility and suppleness improve our body awareness.
- Stretch stimuli promote blood circulation and the metabolism of the musculature and connective tissue.

- The danger of injury is lessened due to the fact that musculature, sinews and other structures of the mobility system acquire increased elasticity.
- Due to greater scope of movement in the joints, muscles can be trained for strength over a greater period of time.
- Stretch exercises after training promote regeneration by normalizing *muscle tone* and improving circulation.

How stretch reflexes work

As described in the case of training for strength, the following correlation is all-important: the individual muscle's job is to bring two bones, linked by a joint, closer together by moving the insertion of the muscle towards the origin. The corresponding muscle is stretched simply when its function is reversed; that is, the insertion is removed as far as possible from the origin.

If stretching is carried out with force or great speed, the human body has a mechanism to protect the musculature from pulling or even tearing. This is a reflex mechanism between the spinal cord and musculature. It is made possible by small organs of measurement called *muscle spindles.* These are distributed in the musculature and register both the speed and extent of muscle stretch. If either the speed or strength of muscle stretch exceeds the spindle's set value, the latter triggers off a reflex-type contraction in the stretched muscle fibres, hindering further stretching. In the case of more rapid and intensive stretching, this protective reaction or *reflex contraction* of the muscle is precipitated that much more forcefully. Consequently, it becomes more and more difficult to stretch the muscle further.

This reflex contraction has incidentally saved the lives of many of us. If, for example, you nod off while driving, the protective reflexes of the muscle spindles return you to wakefulness, thus considerably improving your chances of survival. The moment you fall asleep at the wheel, the support musculature of your head relaxes. The weight of the head causes it to drop sharply to one side, and the musculature opposite is stretched with a jerk. This triggers off the reflex contraction, which pulls the head violently backwards and jolts you awake.

The stretch sensitivity of the muscle spindles is incidentally not constant. It can be 'adjusted' to different levels of sensitivity across the nervous system. Factors influencing sensitivity include the surrounding temperature (cold = sensitive, warm = less sensitive) or your level of psychological tension (stressed = sensitive, relaxed = less sensitive). In stretching, the sensitivity of the muscle spindles is reduced by your even, relaxed breathing as well as the duration of the stretch (20–30 secs), so that stretching becomes easier.

Moreover, the muscle spindle is neurologically linked with the antagonistic musculature. Thus a contraction of the thigh extensors sets off a reflex relaxation of the thigh flexors (hamstrings).

It is not only the musculature that has monitors of stretching and length, in the shape of muscle spindles. Tendons also have a tension gauge called the *Golgi synovial organ,* though, it has precisely the opposite effect of a muscle spindle. If tension values in the Golgi organ exceed the threshold, they trigger relaxation in the stretched muscle. This is to prevent particularly high tension values in the stretched muscle which could create an even greater

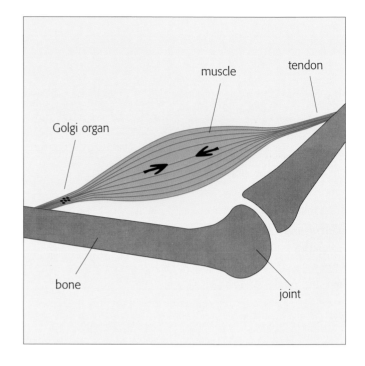

With fixed bones, the tension in the tendon and Golgi organ is increased by voluntary tensing of the muscle.

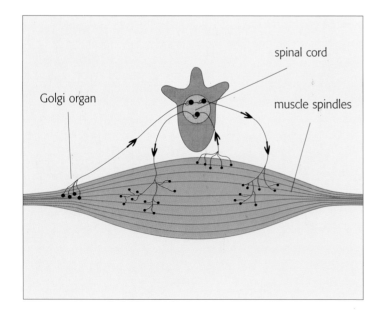

The interaction of nerves and muscles in the simple reflex curve – information is processed without intervention from the brain.

risk – of pulling or tearing – in its protection reflex, that is, contraction. Such high tension values in the tendon can arise either from a particularly strong tug at the stretched end position of the muscle and tendon, or if the muscle tenses very strongly prior to stretching. The tendon is pulled in both cases, but from different directions.

Methods of stretching

For fitness-minded sports enthusiasts, three common methods of stretching can be derived from the aforementioned stretch reflexes. Bouncing dynamic stretch is here deliberately ignored. Although it occasionally makes its comeback in competitive sports, it is not to be recommended as a leisure and fitness activity as it is hard to control and therefore carries the danger of potential injury.

1. Active, static stretch – for example, reaching backwards with the arms at shoulder height, employing the force of the back muscles to stretch the chest muscles – takes advantage of the relaxation of the antagonists. The final position is held for 10 to 15 seconds, while breathing steadily.

2. Passive, static stretch reduces the stretch sensitivity of the muscle spindles by adopting the stretch position slowly and measuredly. The deliberate relaxation effect is reinforced for the 20 to 30 seconds of stretch by calm, steady breathing. Pain-free intensification of the stretch or extending the end position can be attempted during the breathing-out phase or the pause between breathing in and out.

3. Post-isometric stretch, also known as tensing-relaxing-stretching, takes advantage of the tension-dampening effect of the Golgi organ. To do this, the muscle to be stretched is brought to the end position by a sustained passive stretch until a slight give is experienced. The stretched muscle is then tensed strongly against the passive resistance for six to eight seconds. After that, the muscle is relaxed for two to four seconds, before being further stretched beyond the previous end-position by passive stretching.

All of the stretch exercises shown in the exercise catalog can be carried out as both passive stretch exercises and post-isometric stretching. Post-isometric stretching is counter-recommended only for exercises involving stretching of the muscles of the neck and nape. In the course of an optimal fitness training unit, stretches can be carried out as preparation directly after your warm-up, between strengthening exercises, or in a block after your strengthening exercises. Always make sure that the particular muscles strengthened in training are subsequently stretched to prevent them from contracting.

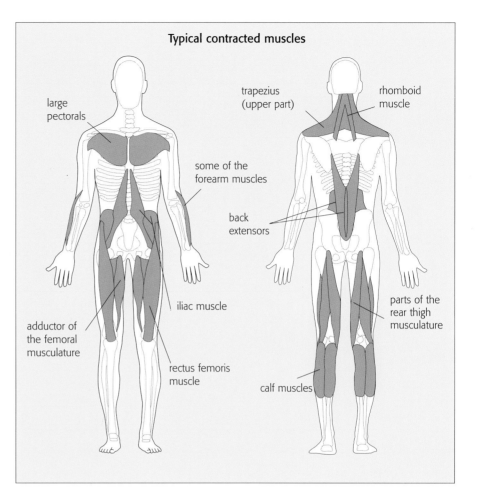

Typical contracted muscles

large pectorals

trapezius (upper part)

rhomboid muscle

some of the forearm muscles

back extensors

iliac muscle

adductor of the femoral musculature

rectus femoris muscle

calf muscles

parts of the rear thigh musculature

Muscular imbalance

As you already experienced in the chapter on *Strength training,* along with the phasic muscles under the skeletal musculature, which effectively form a dynamic musculature and are susceptible to loss of tension, are the tonic muscles, whose function is principally to hold. These muscles are prone to contract. The uneven weighting that can arise between phasic and tonic muscles in the case of unbalanced loading or incorrect or excessive strain is called muscular dysbalance, and can be evened out either by specific strength exercises for the phasic muscles or specific stretch exercises for the tonic muscles. An account of which individual muscles are prone to contract is given here. You can find out in the following exercise catalog how these muscles can best be stretched.

Just as with groups of muscles prone to weakening, contraction of the muscles concerned can be counteracted by stretch exercises, even if the likely cause of the contraction has not yet been identified. However, irrespective of the reasons such as lack of exercise, an unbalanced work posture, protracted, frequent sitting, psychological strain or other factors, the long-term eradication of muscular imbalance is only possible if the circumstances are recognized and eliminated or improved.

Arrangement of exercise catalogue

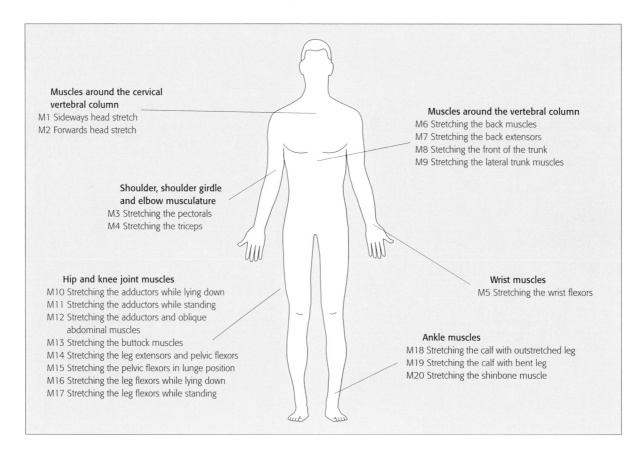

Muscles around the cervical vertebral column
M1 Sideways head stretch
M2 Forwards head stretch

Muscles around the vertebral column
M6 Stretching the back muscles
M7 Stretching the back extensors
M8 Steching the front of the trunk
M9 Stretching the lateral trunk muscles

Shoulder, shoulder girdle and elbow musculature
M3 Stretching the pectorals
M4 Stretching the triceps

Wrist muscles
M5 Stretching the wrist flexors

Hip and knee joint muscles
M10 Stretching the adductors while lying down
M11 Stretching the adductors while standing
M12 Stretching the adductors and oblique abdominal muscles
M13 Stretching the buttock muscles
M14 Stretching the leg extensors and pelvic flexors
M15 Stretching the pelvic flexors in lunge position
M16 Stretching the leg flexors while lying down
M17 Stretching the leg flexors while standing

Ankle muscles
M18 Stretching the calf with outstretched leg
M19 Stretching the calf with bent leg
M20 Stretching the shinbone muscle

For many individuals, it is especially their predominantly seated work posture that contributes to the contraction of muscles not used in this position. These include the hip flexors, which consequently pull the pelvis into a hollow-back posture even during standing, and the pectorals, the contraction of which causes stooping and drooping shoulders. To deal with the cause of this kind of muscle contraction, a frequent change of seated posture is advisable and, if possible, alternation of sitting and standing. Contraction of the muscles can also result from unbalanced athletic effort in sport. Sportsmen and women of sundry disciplines will therefore find tips in the chapter on *Programs* as to how a balance can be effected with complementary stretch exercises.

Golden rules

In order to improve your mobility while enjoying yourself and sparing your joints, bear the following hints in mind:

1. A thorough warm-up is necessary even before starting the stretch exercises.

2. Never stretch into a painful area.

3. Do not stretch in a seesaw or bouncing way.

4. If you carry out stretch exercises before muscle strengthening or between strengthening exercises, hold the stretch position for a maximum of 10 to 15 seconds. If you do your stretching after the strengthening exercises, always maintain the stretch position for 20 to 30 seconds.

5. In every case, breathe in and out deeply and evenly while stretching. This reinforces the relaxing effect.

6. The muscle being stretched should be relieved of weight.

7. In a stretch exercise, stretch into the end position until you feel a slight give in the muscle being stretched, and intensify the stretching during the breathing-out phase as long as the stretch position remains pain-free.

General structure of exercise catalogue

The diagram on the opposite page will make it easier to put together your own exercise program sensibly. If possible, pick out at least one exercise from each muscle area, paying particular attention to muscles prone to contraction and any muscles you have strengthened in your preceding weight training.

As in the strength section, the stretch exercises in the following catalog have been arranged according to muscle groups and joint affiliation. Again, classification goes from the top of the body to bottom; that is, from the shoulder/nape of the neck down to the ankle muscles. While the starting position and the actual exercise in the catalog of strength exercises are treated separately, the catalog of mobility exercises describes the correct stretch position in the basic position. If your mobility is somewhat limited, use a towel in some exercises as an extension of the arm, to get into the correct basic position. To spare your joints in standing exercises, you have to adopt the following uniform basic position:

Stand four-square (feet slightly apart, at hip-width), with your feet parallel to each other and knees slightly bent. Tighten abdomen and buttock muscles slightly, to lock the upper body. Hold your head upright between the shoulders in a straight line with the spine. The shoulders should be parallel. Breathe quietly and evenly. In stretching double-jointed muscles, note that one joint is in the end position while the muscle is stretched over the free joint. Every exercise is described in the following basic layout.

M-number and description of the exercise:
Use the numbering as a quick and handy reference to the various exercises in your training program.

Variants:
These help to add some variety to the basic exercises in your training program.

Basic position:
This describes how to get into the stretch position correctly. Particular emphasis is placed on doing the exercise in a way that is kind to the joints. Time and again, special reference is made to a natural posture for the vertebral column and knee joint.

Tip:
The tips can help you, even in the short term, to pay attention to details which can help to increase the effects of the exercise.

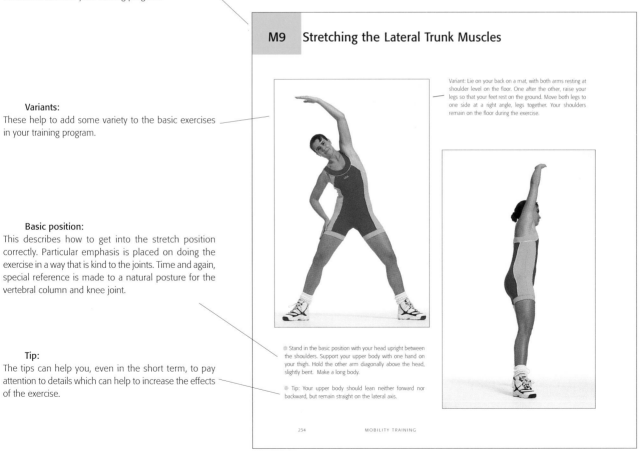

M9 Stretching the Lateral Trunk Muscles

Variant: Lie on your back on a mat, with both arms resting at shoulder level on the floor. One after the other, raise your legs so that your feet rest on the ground. Move both legs to one side at a right angle, legs together. Your shoulders remain on the floor during the exercise.

● Stand in the basic position with your head upright between the shoulders. Support your upper body with one hand on your thigh. Hold the other arm diagonally above the head, slightly bent. Make a long body.

● Tip: Your upper body should lean neither forward nor backward, but remain straight on the lateral axis.

234   MOBILITY TRAINING

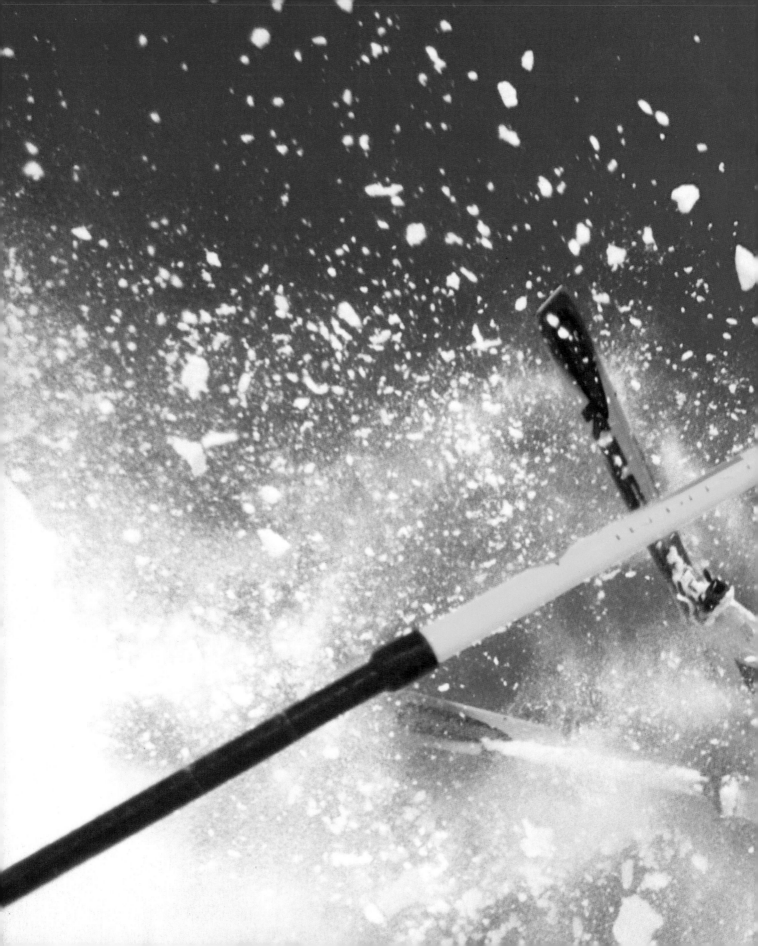

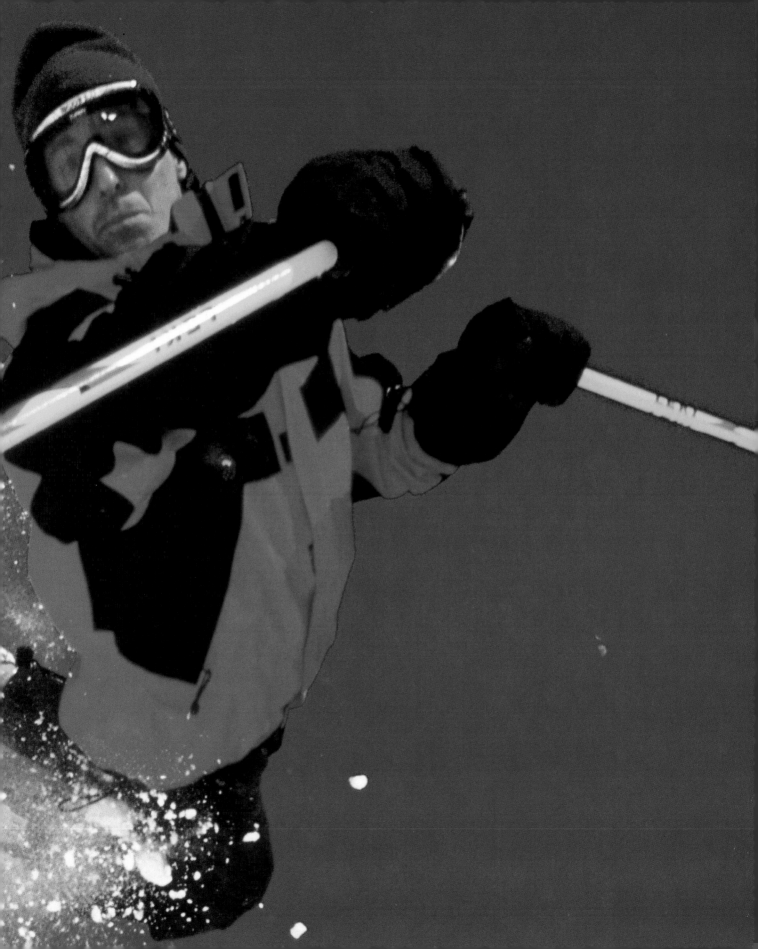

VARIANT

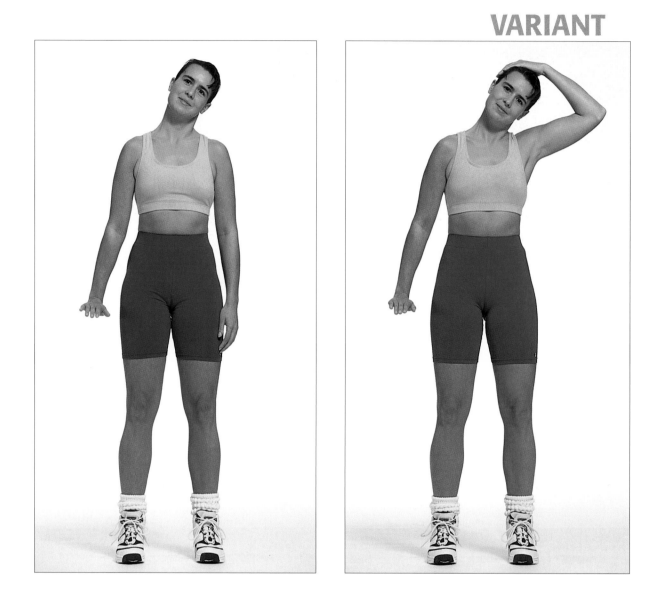

▷ Stand in the basic position. Make a long head (head extends towards ceiling) and tilt it sideways. Take care that you do not raise your chin. Push the right hand on the stretch side into a right angle so that, in the end position, the palm of your hand faces downwards. The fingertips will point forward, so that your arm and hand do not twist outwards. Throughout the exercise, let the other arm hang loose. Pull both shoulders downwards evenly.

Variant: Stretching the lateral neck muscles can be stepped up by grasping your head with your free hand. Rest the palm of your hand lightly on your head without touching your ear, then press the head carefully sideways. Take care to pull your elbow sideways, not letting it slide forwards.

⓵ Tip: Consciously push your shoulders back a little so that your upper body remains upright and you do not lean forward.

▷ Return to the four-square basic position. Remember to tense your stomach and buttock muscles. To stretch the rear neck muscles, take your head in your heads, spreading your fingers just above the rear hairline and resting the thumbs just below the jawbone. Press lightly with your fingers, while pulling your head slowly forward and upwards at the same time.

Variant: To intensify the exercise, bring your chin as close to your body as possible. Once you are practiced, touch your body with your chin.

⓵ Tip: During stretching, hold your shoulders and elbows slightly forward.

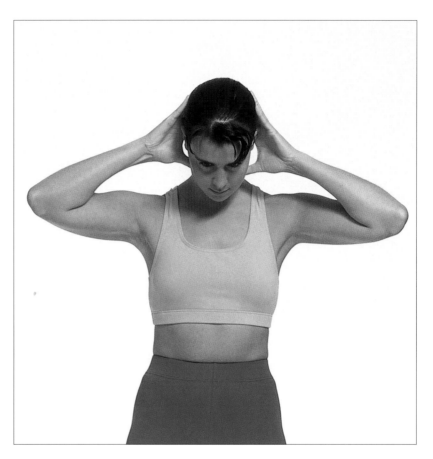

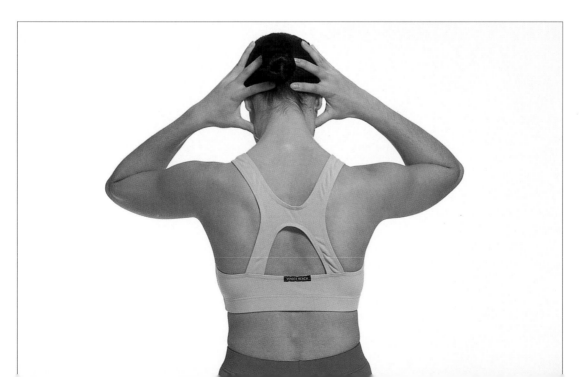

M3   Stretching the Pectorals

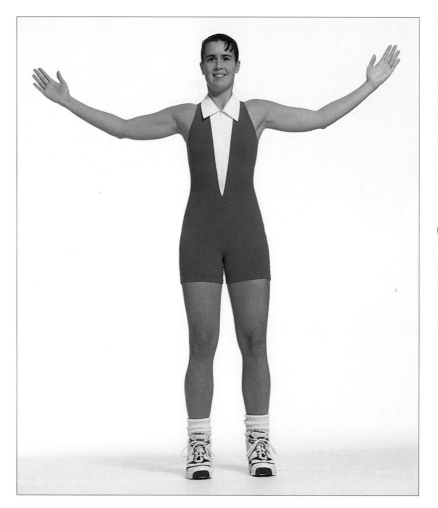

Variant: Get down on all fours, leaning towards the floor as if to do push-ups. Now stretch out one arm flat on the ground, to make an extension of the shoulder-girdle, supporting yourself meanwhile on the other arm, which almost forms a right angle. Look towards the supporting arm, but keep your head off the floor. Now ease the shoulder of the supporting arm upwards.

❗ Tip: Make sure to keep a long neck and that your head is held to form the natural extension of your spine, aligned to the axis of the shoulder. Under no circumstances should you pull the head between the shoulders.

▷ Stand in the basic four-square position. Raise your arms to shoulder height, slightly bent, until you feel your pectorals stretching. In the end position, the palms of your hands should face forward, and the fingers should be loosely spread. Remember to maintain your basic tautness throughout the exercise so that your upper body remains locked upright. Pull your shoulders slightly downwards.

VARIANT

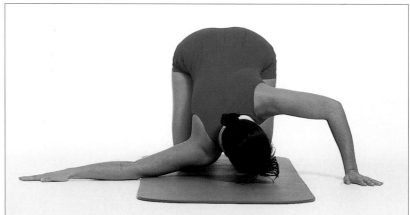

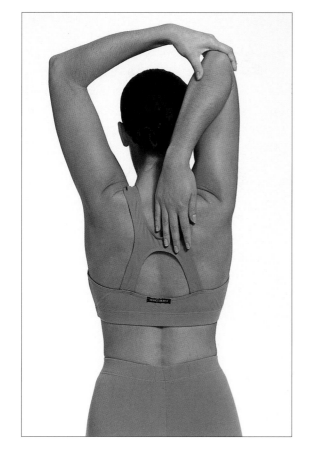

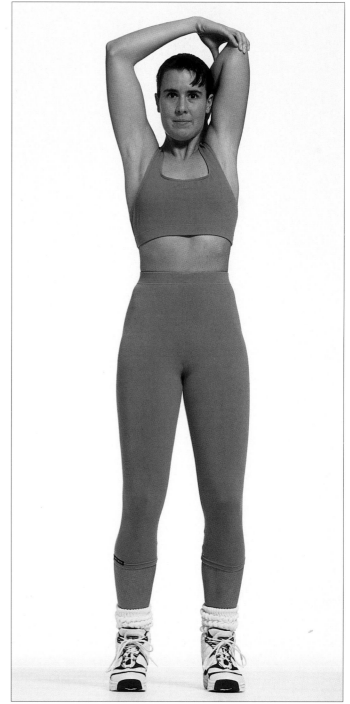

▷ Stand in the basic four-square position. Stretch one arm upwards, bending it downwards, if possible, to touch your shoulder blade. Your upper arm remains vertical, with the elbow pointing at the ceiling. Grasp the elbow with your other hand and pull in a direction parallel to the shoulder opposite. The upper arm is often pulled too far off the vertical towards the shoulder opposite. This position overtaxes the shoulder capsule of the arm being stretched.

❶ Tip: If the forearm of the arm being stretched does not move down by itself during the exercise, press it down with your thumb while your hand is grasping your elbow.

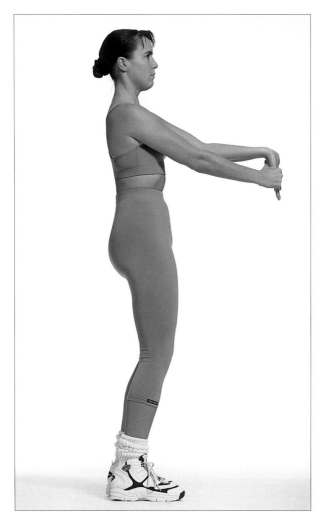

▷ Stand in the basic four-square position. Stretch out in front of you the arm to be exercised, turning the inner arm upwards. With your free hand, clasp the other hand and wrist. The thumb rests in the crease formed by your hand and wrist, the other fingers on the palm of your hand. With your fingers, gently press the hand of the arm to be exercised downward until the fingers and thumb of the stretched arm are in the end position parallel to the body.

❶ Tip: Remember to press the thumb of the stretched arm downward as well.

Variant: Get on all fours on a gym mat. Twist the arms outwards so that your fingertips face your legs. Ease your upper body back until you feel the stretch. Particularly remember during the exercise to tighten your stomach and buttocks muscles so that the upper part of your body remains firm and does not droop into a hollow back. Your head should form a natural extension of your spine.

VARIANT

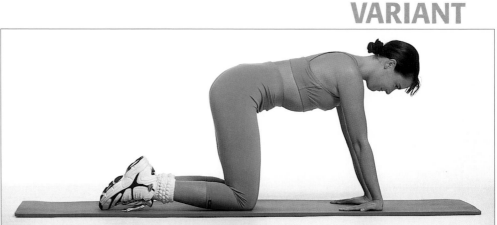

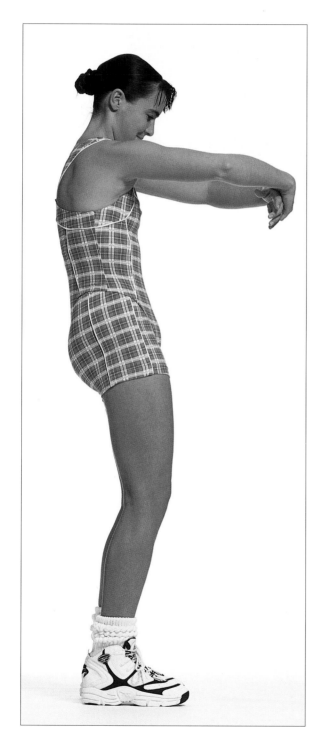

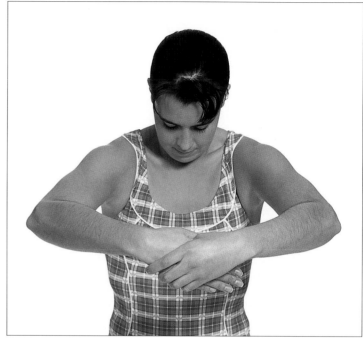

▷ Stand in the basic position with your pelvis tilted forward slightly. One hand grasps the back of the other. Now move both arms forward as if in an embrace, so that your arms are level with your shoulders. Pull your shoulder blades outwards and your chest slightly inwards. Your head will be pushed outwards somewhat, forming a natural extension of the spine. Look forwards and downwards at the floor.

Variant: Get down on all fours, with your buttocks directly above your knees and your shoulders above your hands. Make your shoulders as round as possible, pulling the shoulder blades outward.

❗ Tip: Make sure that, seen from the side, your shoulder, hip and knee joints form a straight line. Adopt the forward tilt of the pelvis only after you have attained this position.

M7   Stretching the Back Extensors

▷ Sit on the floor with legs loosely bent and apart. Your feet remain loosely angled forwards throughout the exercise. Tilt your pelvis forward and then bend over, rounding your back. Now place your hands between your legs, reaching outwards under your lower legs until you can clasp your feet. Make sure your back is as round as possible. Tighten the stomach muscles and thrust out the dorsal vertebrae. Your shoulder blades are also pushed outwards.

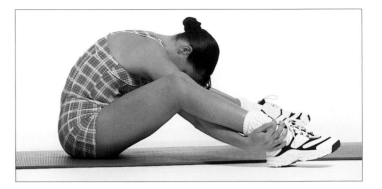

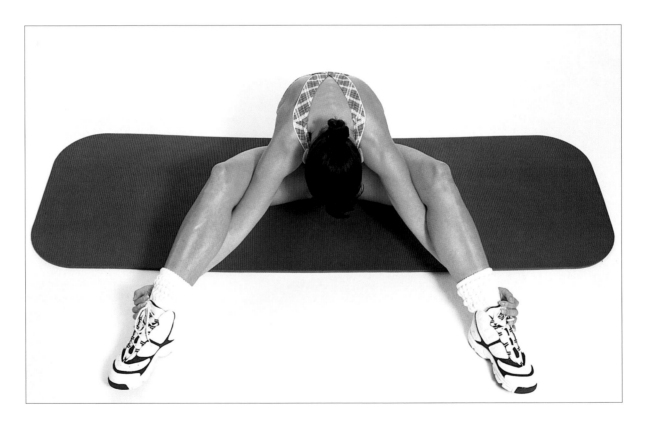

Variant: If you have a chair, box or training bench available, you can also do the exercise sitting on the edge.

🛈 Tip: To relax the tension, put your hands on your thighs and uncoil your back vertebra by vertebra until you are upright.

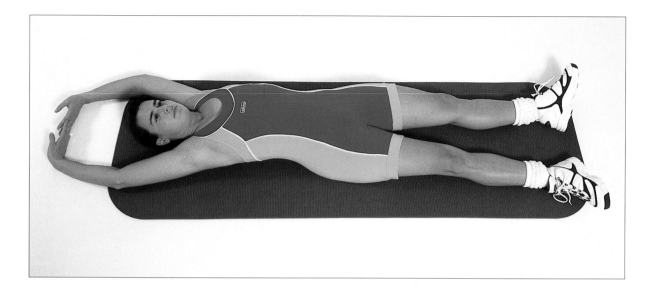

▷ Lie on your back on a gym mat. Stretch out your arms full length behind your head. Leave your legs slightly apart and your feet tipping slackly outwards. Stretch into a long body. Your fingertips should be touching.

Variant: For a more demanding front-trunk stretch, place a rolled-up towel under the lumbar vertebrae. Proceed to do the exercise as described.

❗ Tip: Hold your hands so that the backs face your head. This hand position ensures that the arms rotate outwards and thereby lift the thorax.

VARIANT

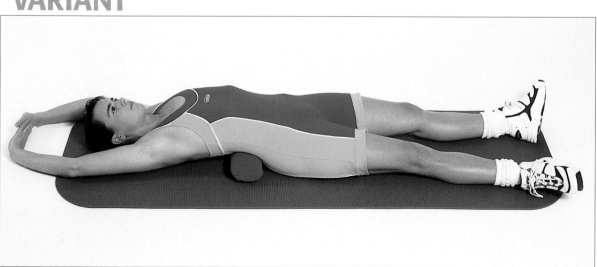

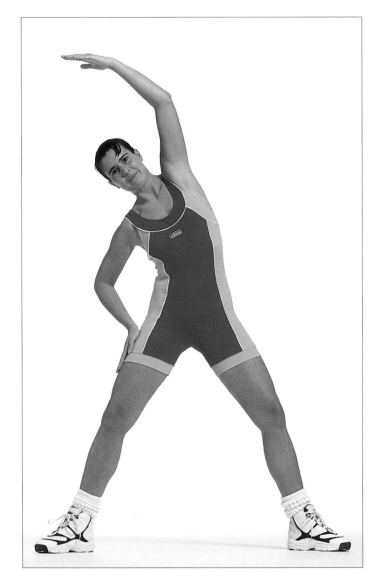

Variant: Lie on your back on a mat, with both arms resting at shoulder level on the floor. One after the other, raise your legs so that your feet rest on the ground. Move both legs to one side at a right angle, legs together. Your shoulders remain on the floor during the exercise.

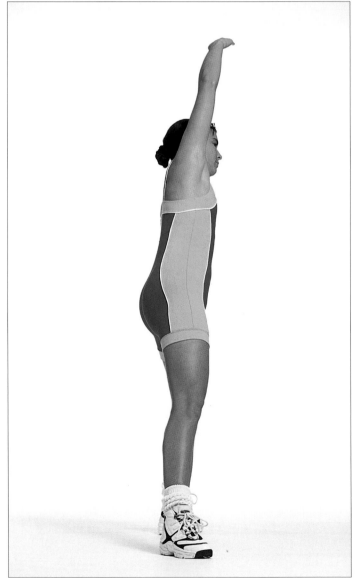

▷ Stand in the basic position with your head upright between the shoulders. Support your upper body with one hand on your thigh. Hold the other arm diagonally above the head, slightly bent. Make a long body.

⚠ Tip: Your upper body should lean neither forward nor backward, but remain straight on the lateral axis.

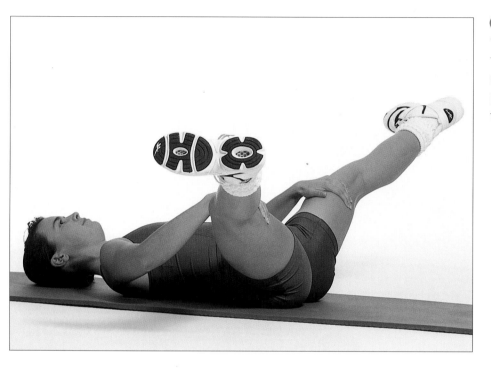

Tip: Make sure that your lumbar vertebrae remain on the floor throughout the exercise. As the adductors are very sensitive, ease slowly out of the stretch position by carefully pushing your legs together with your hands.

VARIANT

Lie on your back on the floor. Stretch your legs vertically upward and then spread them as far as possible. Rotate the thighs outwards, drawing up your feet slightly as you do. Keep your legs somewhat bent so that your feet are parallel to the floor. Rest your hands loosely on the side of your thighs beneath the knee joints.

Variant: You can also bend your legs slightly while stretching so that your feet are in front of your buttocks while doing the exercise.

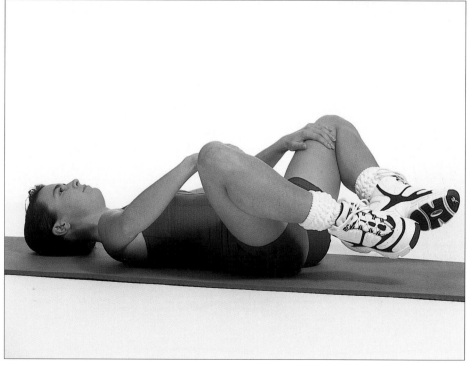

M11 Stretching the Adductors while Standing

▷ Stand in the basic position with feet wide apart. Bend one leg, leaving the other leg more or less outstretched. Your hips and center of gravity will shift towards the bent leg. The toes and knees of the bent leg should point in the same direction. Make sure that the angle of the bent knee is not less than 90°, so the knee is not overly strained. The head forms an extension of the spine, erect between the shoulders. The upper part of the body remains upright.

Variant: Sit on the floor with feet sole to sole. Now press your soles against each other, pulling the knees towards the floor. Your hands should lightly clasp your ankles. Make sure you hold your back straight throughout the exercise. Hold the shoulders slightly back to support an upright position.

❗ Tip: In the basic exercise, place your hands on your bent thigh to support yourself, fingertips pointing forwards. In this position, the thorax will straighten up and the shoulders will be pulled back. You can reinforce the stretch by leaning forward somewhat with the upper part of the body. Remember to remain erect while doing so.

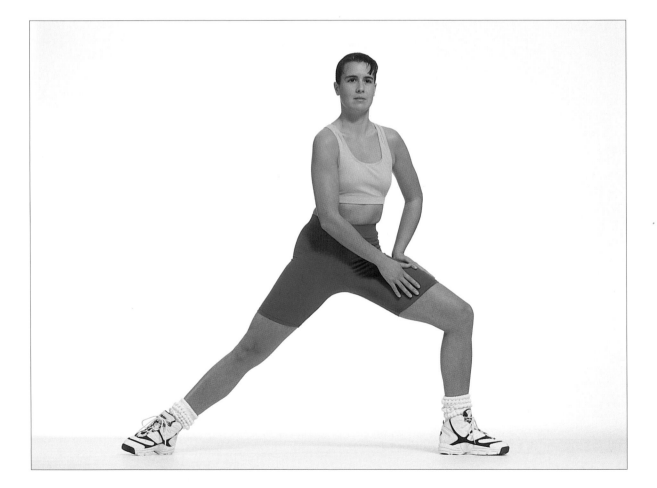

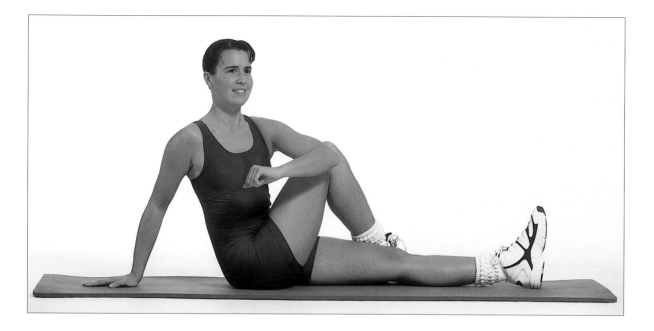

Sit on the floor, legs outstretched. Leaving one leg outstretched, raise the knee of the other and place the foot on the outside of the outstretched leg at knee height. The upper part of your body will turn in the direction of the raised knee. Press the raised leg with the back of the opposite upper arm, which is bent. Meanwhile, hold your head erect, as a natural extension of the spine. Take care that your back remains straight throughout the exercise.

Variant: Lie on your back with both knees raised. Place one leg on the opposite thigh, with the ankle bone just above the knee. The knee of the crossed leg should face outwards. Clasp the erect leg with both hands and pull it towards your head, leaving the lower part of it hanging loose. Your elbows will be pulled slightly outwards.

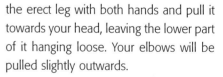 Tip: In the basic exercise, the forearm of the pressing arm should be held horizontal to the floor. This will prevent your shoulder falling forward, and keep the upper part of your body erect.

VARIANT

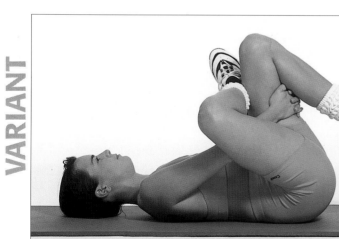

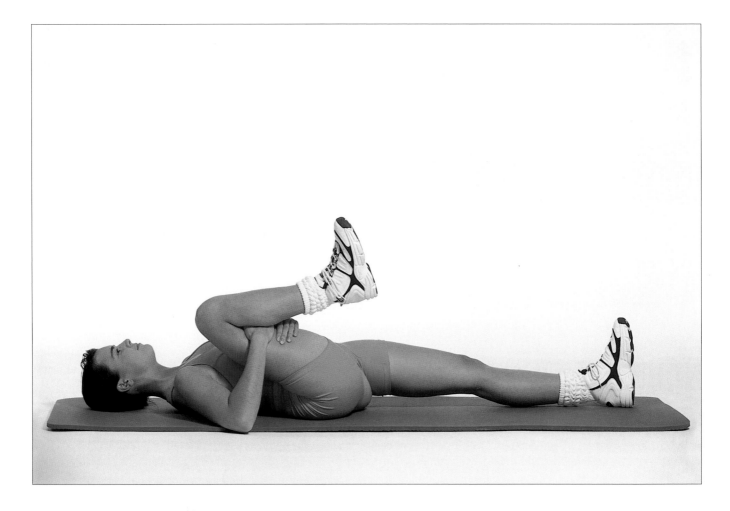

▷ Lie flat on your back. Keeping one leg outstretched, bend the other up towards your upper body. Clasp the raised leg around the back of the thigh below the back of the knee, and pull it towards you, lifting your elbows outwards while doing so. The lumbar vertebrae should remain on the ground throughout the exercise. Your head should lie straight between the shoulders. Pull with the back of the head gently on the axis of the spine, in order not to strain the cervical vertebrae.

Variant: Lie on your back, legs outstretched. Leaving one leg loosely outstretched, raise the other knee and place your foot on the floor. Using the opposite arm, clasp the bent leg just above the knee on the outside thigh and pull it downward over the outstretched leg. During the exercise, both shoulders should stay in contact with the floor.

❶ Tip: Tighten stomach and buttock muscles to prevent a hollow back from developing. Always grasp your leg by the back of the thigh. If you hold it by the shin, the knee will be too compressed.

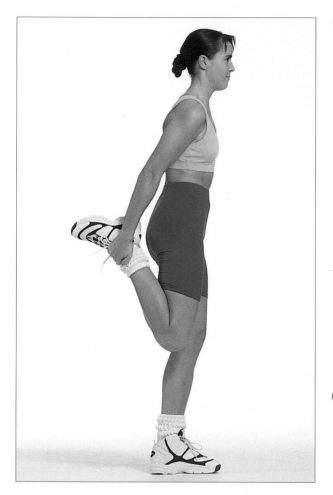

▷ Stand in the basic four-square position. Bend one leg backwards and grasp it at ankle height, using the hand on the same side. Pull the foot towards the buttocks and the leg backwards. To avoid losing your balance and making compensatory movements, prop yourself against a wall or machine. Your hips should remain parallel to your shoulders. A common mistake is to allow the raised leg to 'spread' sideways. Remember to hold it straight. Here too it is important to keep stomach and buttock muscles tight, in order to lock the upper body.

Variant: Lie on your side on the floor. Your head should lie relaxed in a straight line with the spine on the outstretched arm. The under leg is bent at the hips and knee into a right angle. The top arm clasps the top leg by the ankle and pulls it towards the buttocks. Pull the leg backwards as far as is possible, tighten the abdomen and buttocks. Take care with this exercise and remember not to raise the bent leg out-wards but keep it in line with your body.

❗ Tip: Do not over-extend the pulling arm. Keep it slightly bent throughout the exercise.

VARIANT

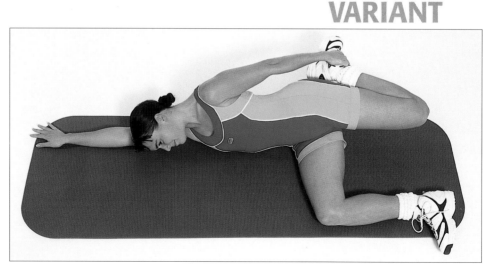

M15 Stretching the Pelvic Flexors in a Lunge

▷ Stand in the basic four-square position. Take a big lunging step, then rest your back leg from knee to foot on the ground. The forward knee should not be directly above the front foot. Your upper body should form a straight line with the back thigh, and your head with your spine. Balance yourself with one arm on the bent leg and place the other arm on the ground. Pelvis and shoulder girdle should remain parallel, while the pelvis is pushed forwards and downwards. A common mistake is to let the upper body sag into a hollow back. You should therefore make sure that your stomach and buttock muscles are tightened.

Variant: One leg is bent at an angle, while you kneel with the other. Your upper body is erect, but tilted forward slightly. Lift the foot of the kneeling leg and grasp its ankle with both hands, pulling the foot towards the buttocks. Remember to keep your hips parallel, and do not let a hollow back develop. To counteract it, remember to keep your stomach and buttock muscles tight. Always hold the ankle, that is do not pull the foot by the heel or twist your foot.

⓵ Tip: Your weight should not bear frontally on the kneecap of the back leg but on the upper part of the knee. Further reduce the strain on the knee by placing a towel under it. If the angle of the front leg is less than 90°, take a bigger step forward.

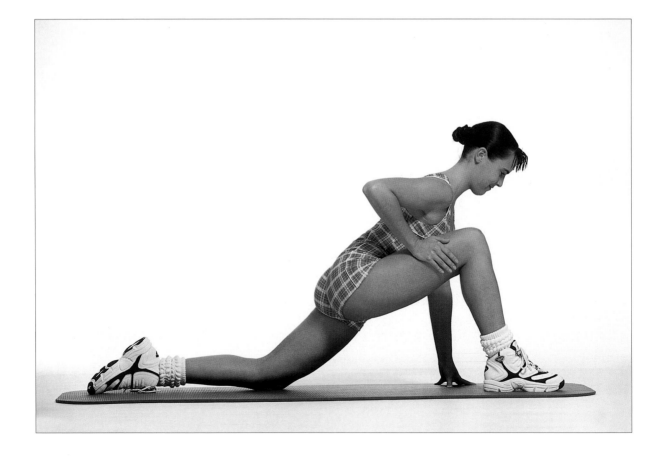

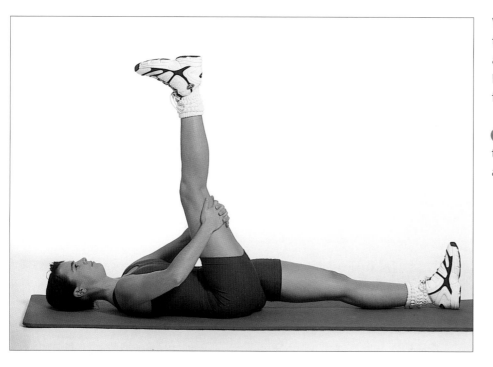

Variant: If you are not yet stretched enough to clasp your leg relaxedly, wrap a towel around the calf of the leg to be stretched. Pull the leg towards you with it until you feel the stretch.

⚠ Tip: To reinforce the stretching, keep the leg being stretched almost straight, if at all possible.

VARIANT

▷ Lie on your back on a gym mat. Leave one leg outstretched on the ground, while raising the other leg towards your upper body. Grasp the (slightly bent) raised leg with both hands immediately below the back of the knee, at the back of the thigh. The toes of both feet should be pointing forward, with the sole of the raised foot facing the ceiling. Pull the leg towards the stomach. Make sure your pelvis remains parallel to the shoulder girdle throughout the exercise. The buttock of the outstretched leg should also not leave the ground. Keep the outstretched leg straight until you complete the relaxation process. Remind yourself throughout to hold your head and shoulders down.

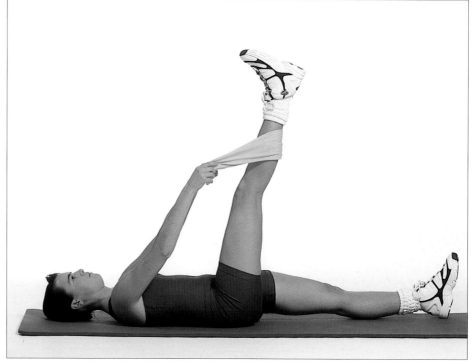

VARIANT

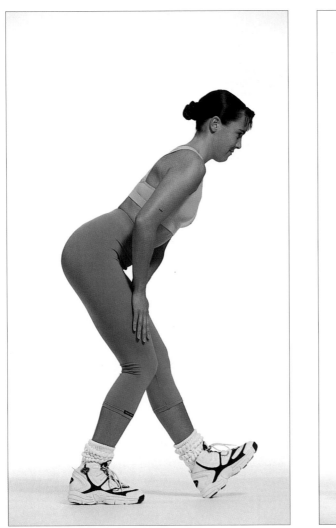

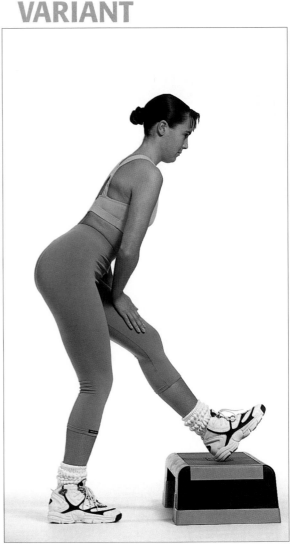

▷ Stand in the basic stepping position. Bend the upper body forward from the hips, keeping the back straight. Place the hands on the back leg for support, keeping the pelvis and shoulder girdle parallel. The front leg remains more or less outstretched, with the toes drawn up. The foot points forward throughout the exercise. Remember to hold your head straight, an extension of the spine, to avoid straining the cervical vertebrae. Look forward and downward.

Variant: If you have one available, you can do the exercise on a step or box. The exercise remains the same, but the leg to be stretched is placed on the step. Include your hips in the stretch, keeping them parallel.

! Tip: Place your hands so that the tips of the fingers point downwards on the outside and inside of the outstreched thigh. This position stops the back getting round. Pull the shoulders back in support.

▷ Stand in the basic long-stepping position. The upper body leans forward in a straight line with the back leg. Make a long neck, holding the head in a straight line with the spine. Support your upper body by placing your hands on the front thigh. Do not let the knee of the front leg hover directly above the front of the foot, or you will strain the knee. The back leg is stretched out, and both feet point forwards. Take care that the hind foot (on the stretched leg) does not leave the ground.

Variant: Basic stepping position on a step. The front leg is slightly bent, the hands rest lightly on the thigh. Place the ball of the back foot on the step, leaving the back leg outstretched. Now flex the leg with the heel in the direction of the ground. Remember to point the knee and toes in the same direction.

❗ Tip: The fingertips resting on your inside and outside thigh should point outwards. To ensure that the upper body is erect, consciously push your shoulders back.

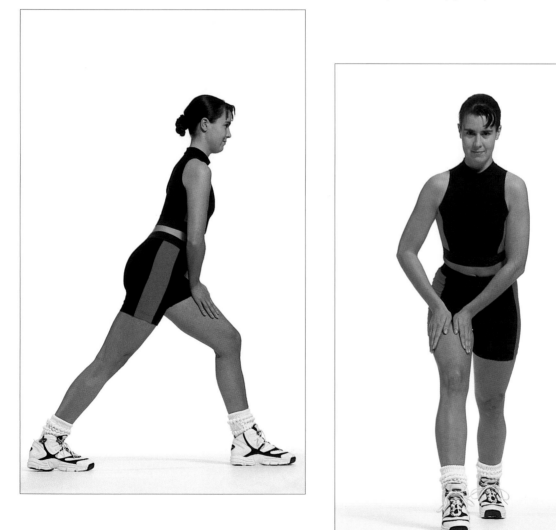

M19 Stretching the Calf with Bent Leg

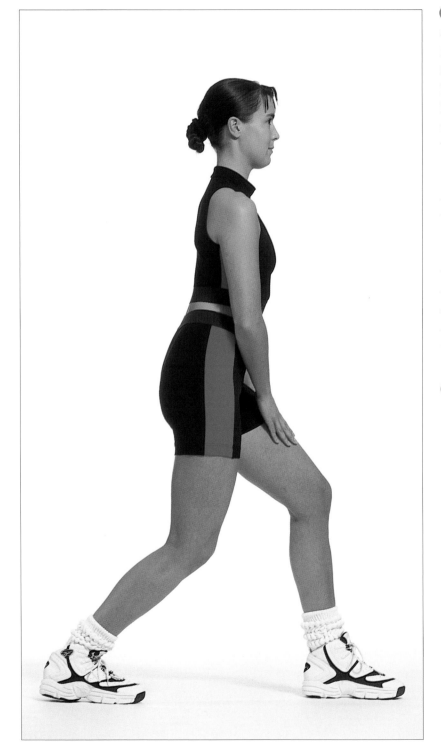

▷ Stand in the stepping position as in M20, but make a smaller step. Both feet should be parallel, pointing forwards. Bend the knee of the leg to be stretched, allowing the body to sink until you feel an unmistakable stretching sensation in the back calf. The upper body remains erect. Remember not to raise your head or chin. They must form an extension of the spine. Throughout the exercise, the heel remains firmly on the floor.

Variant: Basic stepping position on the step. Do the exercise as above, though this time only the ball of the back foot rests on the step. The heel points towards the floor.

❗ Tip: If the heel rises, reduce the size of the step.

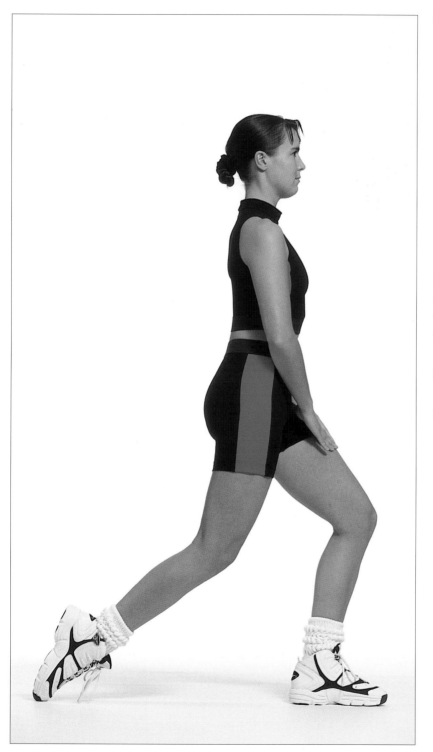

▷ Stand in the stepping position. Place your hands on your front thigh for support, holding your shoulders back. The tip of your back foot rests on the floor, keeping the foot stretched. Leg and foot form a straight line, but do not let the ankle tilt outwards. Now pull the back of the foot slowly towards the ground until you get a stretching sensation.

Variant: Sit on a chair or bench. Both legs should be bent, with the feet parallel and four-square on the ground. Raise one leg on its toes. Bend your toes and back of the foot towards the floor.

❶ Tip: If you do not get maximum stretch in training shoes, do the exercise barefoot.

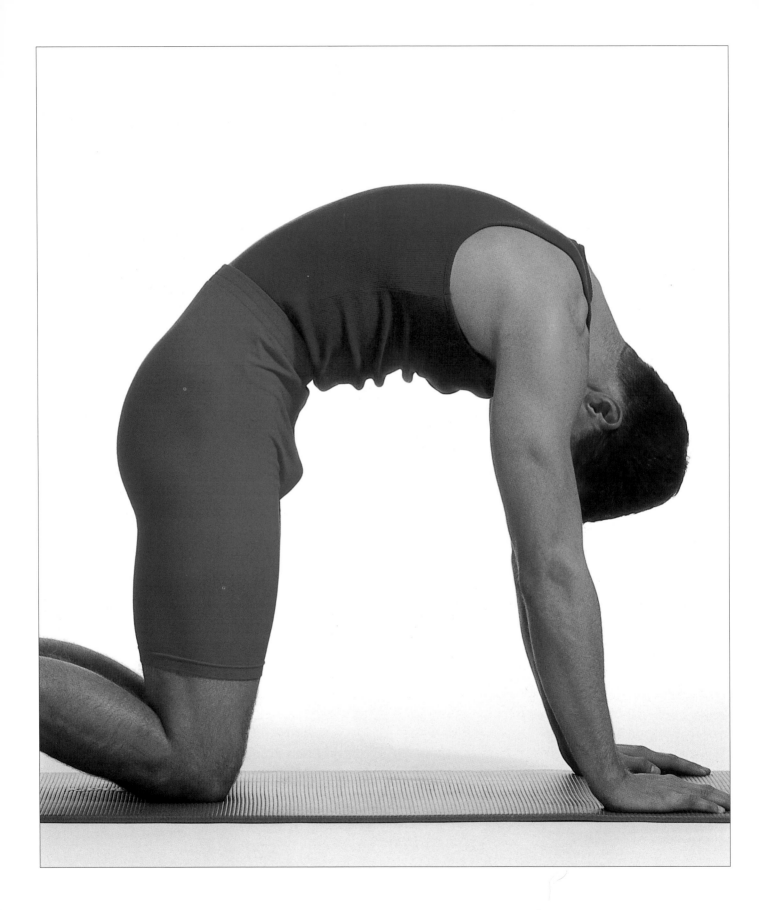

Flexibility

Exercises that serve to keep the joints flexible, especially the vertebral column and its various sections, are unspectacular compared with all the other exercises presented in this book. Usually they are noticeable for their absence in most training programs used by sports and fitness enthusiasts. Their beneficial effects can be directly felt even during the exercises themselves. Yet as exercises for flexibility serve to improve neither strength nor endurance or speed, and do not even do much for mobility, they are easily dismissed as superfluous. If anything, the best that can be directly adduced for them is improved coordination, but this can be achieved in other ways just as effectively. What then is the benefit of the flexibility exercises presented here?

In order to appreciate the most important demonstrable benefits, it is essential to understand how the various body tissues are nourished. Whereas nutriment for the muscles is supplied directly via the vascular system in a rapid exchange rhythm, there is no such active supply system for the cartilage tissue covering the ends of bones in joints. Cartilage instead is fed by the migration of particles from the joint fluid surrounding it, known as synovial fluid or *synovia.* To be able to absorb this synovial fluid optimally, the cartilage has recourse to an alternation of pressure and suction forces. It is precisely this regular rhythmical exchange optimizing the supply to the cartilage that is achieved with flexibility exercises. Imagine a cartilage that is short of fresh nutrients as a dirty sponge. The dirt in the sponge represents the nutrients already used up. If you then hold the sponge in a bucket with fresh water representing the synovial fluid containing nutrients and squeeze it, you will see how the dirt from the sponge is distributed in the clean water. Relax the pressure, and the sponge expands back to its original size, absorbing clean water.

Along with improved cartilage nutrition, flexibility exercises loosen up your whole connective tissue. They have a relaxing effect and improve bodiy awareness. It is this enhanced sensitivity that constitutes one of the most underrated effects of flexibility. Whereas beginners doing strength exercises in particular are inclined to concentrate on mastering the weight more than

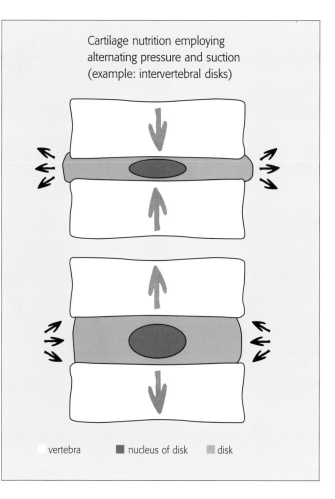

Cartilage nutrition employing alternating pressure and suction (example: intervertebral disks)

☐ vertebra   ■ nucleus of disk   ▨ disk

their own bodies, in flexibility exercises inward concentration is both possible and necessary. As flexibility exercises are carried out without great effort and a continuous change of situation is effected in the parts of the body moved, your use of particular muscles, especially those that affect the position of the vertebral column, becomes bit by bit more conscious. In addition, if you do the flexibility exercises while monitoring yourself in the mirror, you will soon be in a position to adopt any given vertebral column position consciously and actively.

Sideways Head Flex

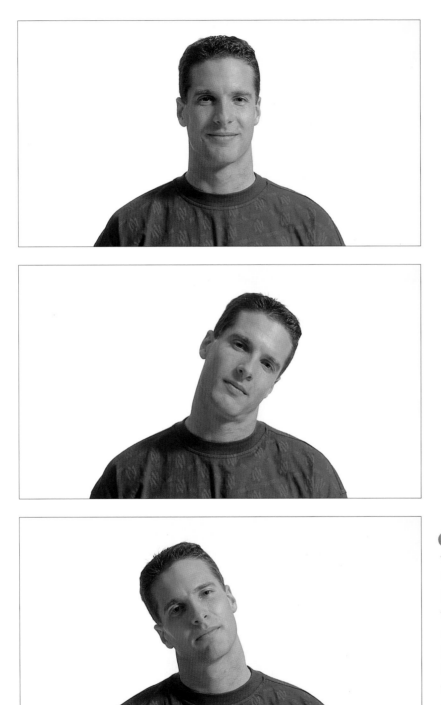

▶ Stand in the basic four-square position, with your feet parallel. Extend your spine. In the initial position, the head is erect between the shoulders in a straight line with the spine. Now incline your head slowly towards one shoulder, then return it just as carefully to the initial position. Carry out the exercise in the same way in the direction of the other shoulder. Take care that your shoulders remain relaxed and at the same height throughout the performance of this exercise.

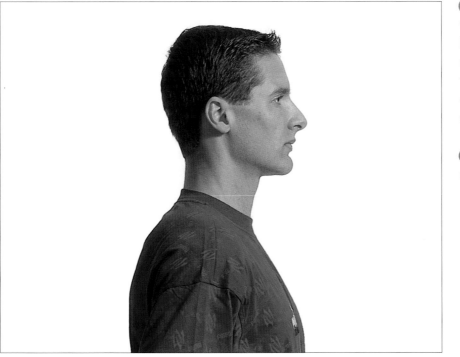

▷ Stand in the basic four-square position. Make sure that your head is erect between your shoulders. In this variant, move your head slowly backwards from the initial position. Remember to keep it erect, imagine you are balancing a book on your head.

❗ Tip: Tighten your stomach and buttock muscles in order to lock your upper body.

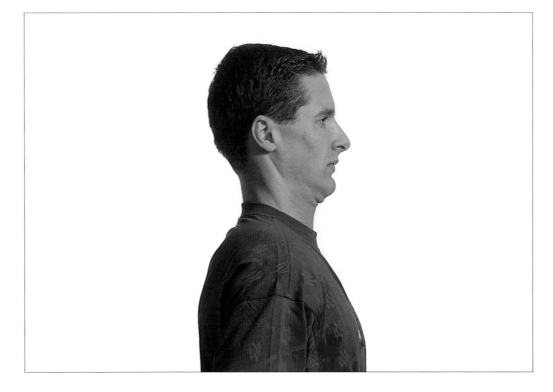

Turning Your Head

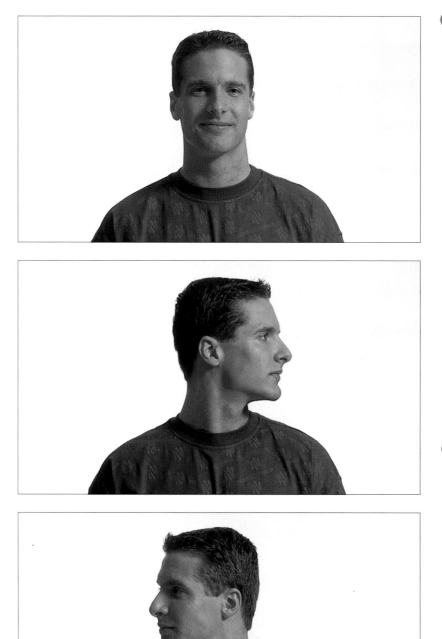

▶ Stand in the basic four-square position. Holding your head between your shoulders as an extension of your spine, make a long neck. Now turn your head slowly from one side to the other. As before, remember in this exercise to hold your head straight throughout the exercise and keep your chin at the same level. Imagine you have to draw a line with your chin on a horizontal board.

Variant: Quarter turn of the head. Stand in the basic four-square position. In the initial position, look straight ahead. To do the exercise, bend your head forwards. Your chin will now point at your chest. Now rotate the head, chin first in a quarter turn towards the shoulder (see clockwise picture sequence opposite). Return to the initial position and carry out the rotation movement in the same way on the other side.

❗ Tip: Do all the rotations slowly and carefully, to avoid straining the spine.

VARIANT

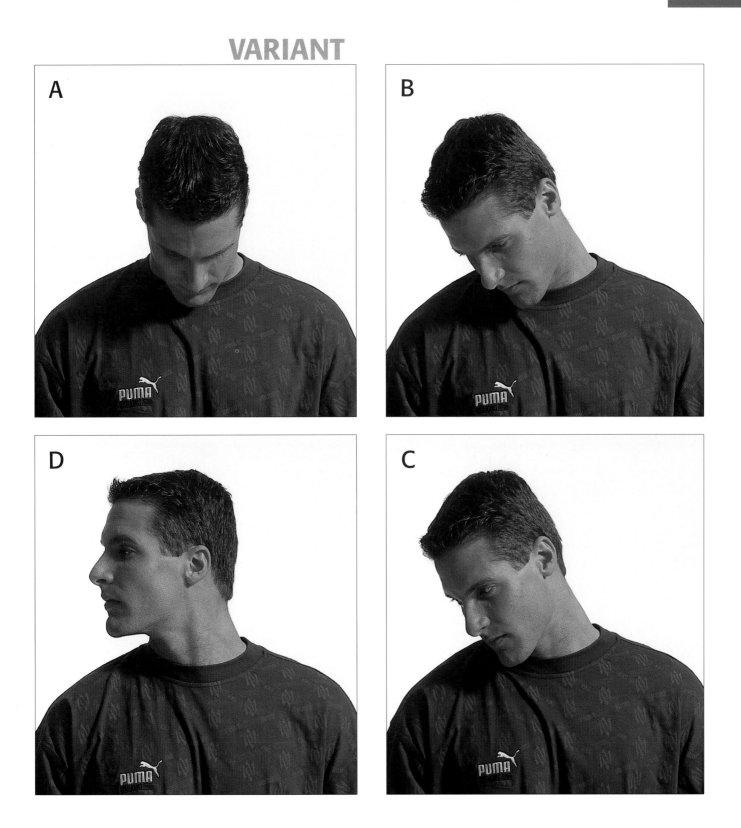

A

B

D

C

Arched Back on All Fours

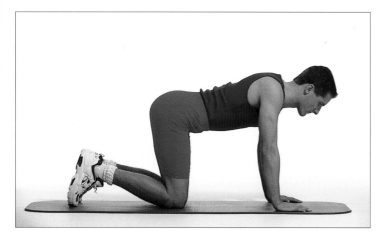

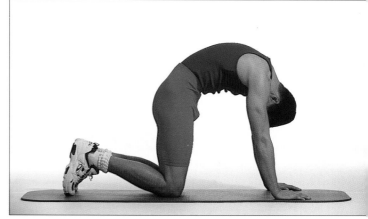

▷ Take up the basic position but on all fours. Locate your hips directly above your knees, your shoulders above your wrists. The fingers should point away from the body, straight ahead. Hold your back straight in the initial position. Your head should form a straight line with your spine, between the shoulders. Now lower your chin towards your chest and slowly arch your back, as if your thoracic vertebrae were being pulled upwards.

❶ Tip: For all exercises involving kneeling, make sure you have a suitable base (e.g. a practise mat or on carpeting), to reduce the strain on your knee joints.

Variant: Arched back in forearm position. The exercise position resembles the all-fours position, except this time place your forearms on the floor. Your head still forms a straight line with your spine, between your shoulders. Now pull it towards your chest, at the same time pressing your lumbar vertebrae towards the ceiling.

❶ Tip: Hold your head in the initial position in a straight line with the spine, so as not to put your cervical vertebral column at risk.

VARIANT

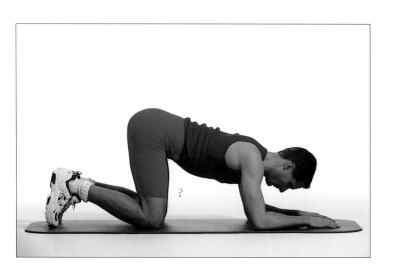

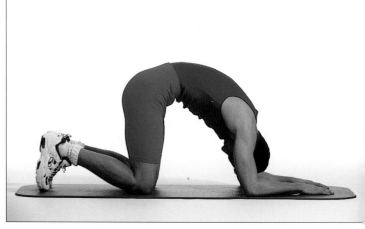

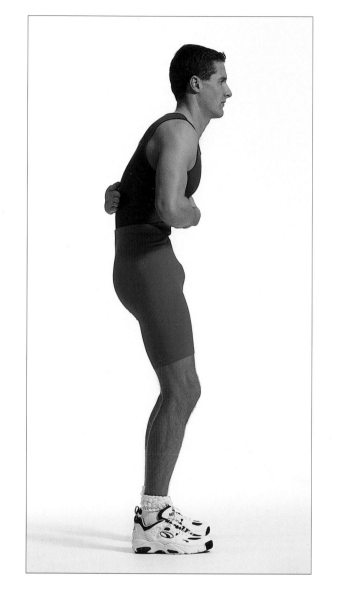

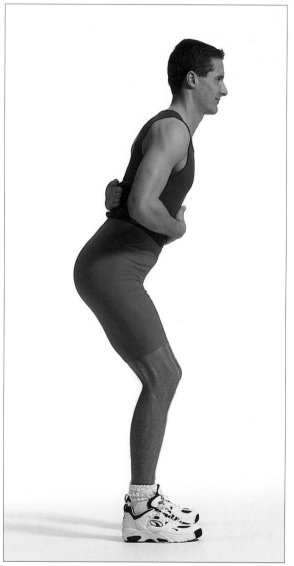

▷ Take the basic position standing four-square, with the feet parallel and the knees slightly bent. Stomach and buttocks should be tight. Hold your head straight between your shoulders, and take care to keep your head upright throughout the exercise. Now slowly tilt your pelvis forwards and back as far as you can. Take care that buttocks and stomach also remain tightened during repetition.

❗ Tip: To reinforce self-awareness and carry out the correct movements, you can either put your hands behind your back or stand with your hands on hips.

Pelvic Shift Lying down

▷ Lie down on your back. Make sure you have something smooth to lie on, so that the pelvic movement during the exercise is not hampered by non-slip material. Hold both legs outstretched, lying apart so that the feet are parallel with your hips. Place your arms loosely on the floor beside your body. Now push your pelvis towards your upper body, alternating left and right sides, without raising your lower body from the floor.

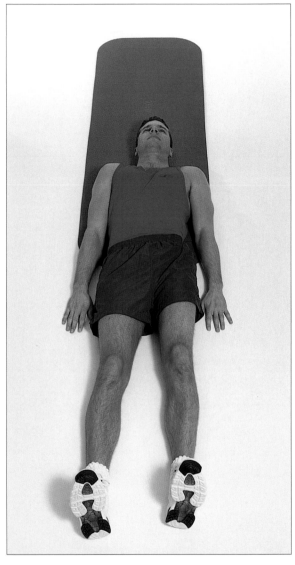

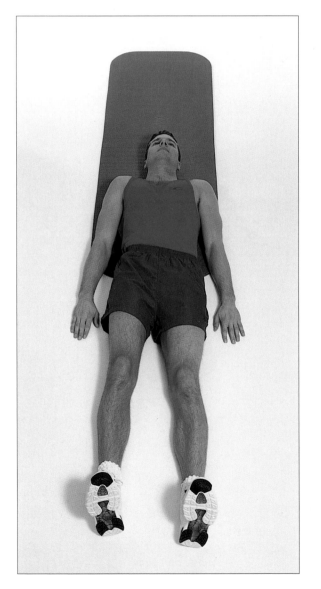

❗ Tip: You can reinforce the exercise by drawing one side downwards away from the trunk while pushing the other upwards.

▷ Lie on your back with your shoulders resting on the floor. To stabilize the shoulder girdle, stretch out your arms beside your body on the axis of the shoulders. Bend your legs, with the feet resting on the floor parallel to your shoulders. Now twist your hips and both legs to the right until the right leg almost touches the floor. Now do the same on the other side.

Variant: Sit on the edge of your gym mat and support your upper body with your hands on the floor. The legs are bent, the feet somewhat wider apart than shoulder-width, resting flat on the floor. Now twist your hips slowly from right to left.

❗ Tip: If, in the end position, the knee of one leg touches the other leg, you have not placed your feet far enough apart. Increase the distance between the feet and begin again.

Note: This exercise must not be carried out in the case of previous orthopedic injury to the back.

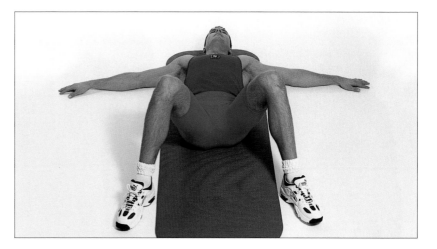

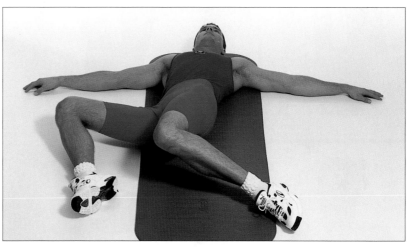

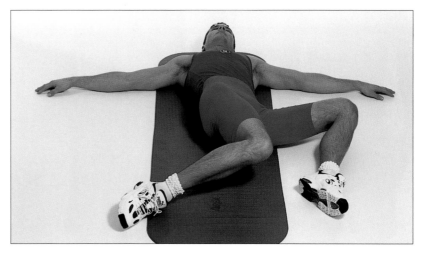

Shoulder Revolutions and Turns

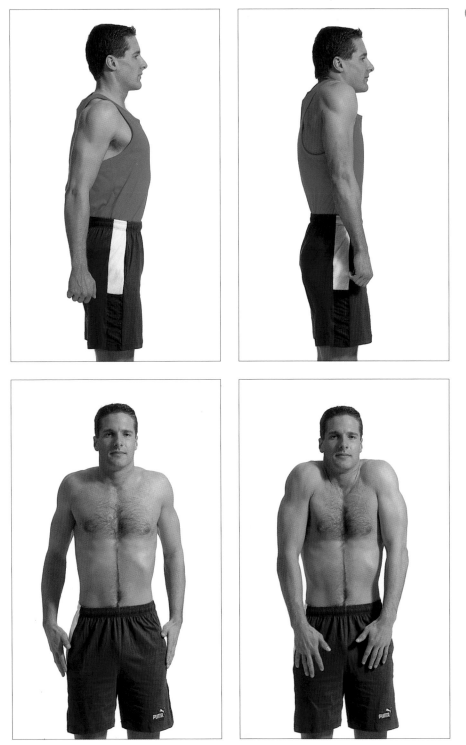

▷ Stand in the basic four-square position, with the feet parallel. Keep your head erect between the shoulders in a straight line with the spine. Hold your arms slightly bent, with hands and fingers dangling loosely. Now let your shoulders revolve slowly from the front to the back.

Variant: You can do this exercise in both directions or rotate your shoulders one at a time. Alternatively, you can include your upper arms and elbows in the circular motion.

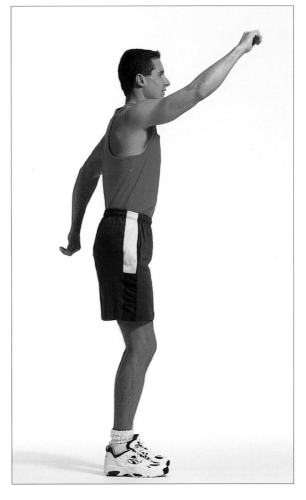

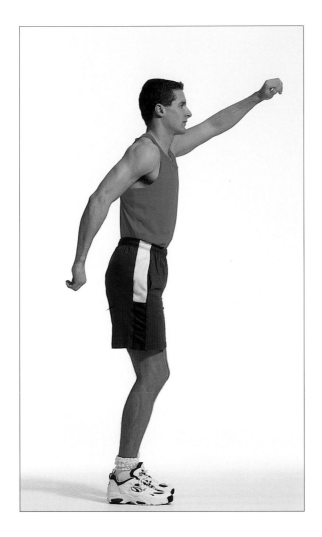

your legs in the end position (rocking). Take care to keep your shoulder girdle straight while performing the swinging movements.

Variant: You can also swing both arms together forwards and backwards with the same rocking motion. Here too the shoulder girdle must remain directly above the hips.

⚠ Tip: Remember to keep your stomach and buttock muscles tightened, in order to lock your upper body during the swinging movements.

▶ Basic position standing four-square. Adopt a slight forward-lean position from the hips. Your feet should be parallel to each other and the arms slightly bent. Now let your arms swing alternately backwards and forwards. Your hands should dangle loosely throughout the exercise, the arms slightly bent. The swinging movement is started in the middle position by making as if to squat, then stretching

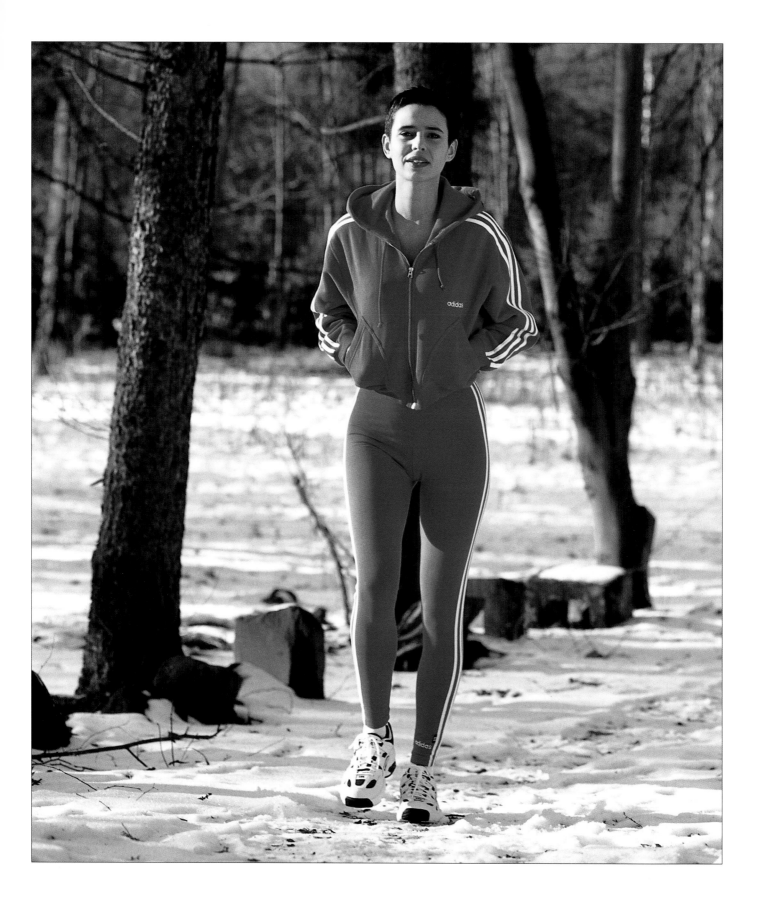

COOL-DOWN

Cool-Down –
The Perfect Ending

You should finish a training session by cooling down, by slowing down the pace of the exercise and preparing the body for rest and relaxation after the hard work. By slowing down the pace, we mean that the aerobic activity increases again but you are no longer demanding a competitive pace. Cooling down has more to do with forestalling the period of exhaustion and results in super-compensation, where increased energy storage provides a basis for improved training performances.

The cyclometer, treadmill and other aerobic equipment are suitable for cooling down, as they provide increased circulation in the muscles, which quickly delivers more oxygen via the bloodstream. This then continues processing the lactic acid (lactase) present in the muscle cells and builds up new stocks of energy. In fact, if enough oxygen is available, all the energy can be extracted from the lactic acid, in which case, the resulting water and carbon dioxide are expelled via the urine and lungs.

Together with running and cycling, stretching exercises (mobility) also have an important part to play in the regenerative process. Increased muscle tone and less extendibility mean that the muscles are less robust and therefore more liable to injury. Stretching, on the other hand, reduces muscle tension – which increases measurably during training and may reduce suppleness in the muscles by 5 to 13 per cent – therefore allowing the muscles to recover quickly. Gentle stretching also helps the circulation and therefore contributes to the process of breaking down the by-products of the metabolic process. In addition, stretching makes a great contribution to the relaxation process and encourages relaxation and recovery after the exertion of the training.

Energy Supply

Energy is required to contract the muscle's cells. The only energy which can be directly utilized by the body is called ATP (adenosine triphosphate). This chemical energy is produced in the cells by breaking down foodstuffs into their component parts and is for the most part carried by the blood in the form of heat. Only a small proportion is temporarily stored and used for movement by the cells of the muscles. This energy reserve is, however, limited and therefore soon used up. "Filling up" for more work by the muscles can be done in two ways. For short-term competitive bursts such as a 100-meter race, the muscles use creatine phosphate to reconstitute ATP. Breaking down carbohydrates (glucose), on the other hand, creates the energy required for longer-term work from the muscles. If the blood carries enough oxygen, aerobic energy is produced and the oxygen reacts with the metabolic by-products produced by the breaking-down process. This process releases energy, which fills the ATP stocks. Long-term work, such as long-distance races, uses aerobic energy almost exclusively. With exercise such as longer distance sprints, where high levels of energy are consumed very quickly, glucose is broken down in several intermediate phases, without the involvement of oxygen, that is, anaerobically, into lactic acid salts, which collect in the cells and over-acidify the muscles. The result is that the chemical processes responsible for preparing more energy in the muscle cells, now cease to operate, which you perceive as fatigue. In fact, nature set up this method of producing energy because it is faster than complete combustion and also works when there is a shortage of oxygen. This way, unused energy is not wasted but is stored as ATP in the lactic acid and may be released again when oxygen is available. Lactic acid is therefore a by-product very rich in energy and in no way a waste product of the metabolic process. So we have an explanation for shortness of breath after short-term, intensive exercise such as the 400-meter sprint. This is how the body obtains the oxygen it requires to process the lactic acid, and therefore to break down the acidity. ATP is responsible not only for flexing the muscles, but also for relaxing them so that they soften again. Because less ATP is present in the muscles after an intensive training session, there is limited suppleness. This is why you must not try to increase the suppleness of your muscles during the cooling down session, but just stretch each group of muscles for no longer than two minutes.

Regenerative Measures: Rest and Recovery

The cooling-down process is when the regeneration of physical resources starts again. This is the phase when the heartbeat and breathing return to normal, the lactic acid is broken down completely, and the empty energy stores are replenished. It is precisely this regeneration of energy-producing processes which makes cooling down an important part of the training cycle that

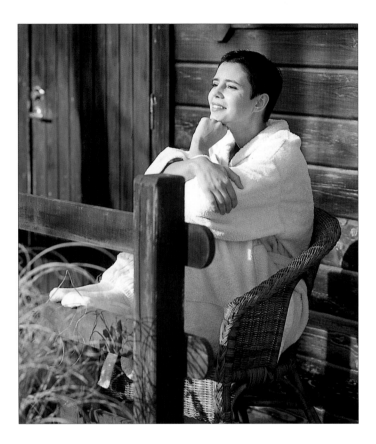

should not be neglected. If fresh training activity is initiated at too early a stage, before sufficient energy reserves are available, performance may not meet expectations.

The recovery process is working if you are able to improve your performance in the long term. It is in this regard that we speak of "over-regeneration" (super compensation). This is when we not only compensate for the consumption of the building blocks and vital components needed for the muscles, but the increased storage capacity will enable you to build up greater energy reserves, and performance will therefore increase beyond the initial level.

There are various ways of helping your own recovery. A diet rich in carbohydrates, for example, will speed up the reconstitution of energy supplies. You should drink plentifully to maintain water and mineral levels at a constant level. Minerals such as sodium, potassium and magnesium will, among other things, ensure that muscles are able to contract and remain ready for work – a lack of minerals can lead to weak muscles and cramp, forcing you to cut short your training.

Therapeutic treatments like massage, showers and saunas improve the blood supply so that the body's waste products are carried away and eliminated more quickly. Activation of the metabolic process means that the energy stores are re-filled as quickly as possible and cell regeneration is stimulated. In addition, hot and cold showers and saunas reinforce the body's defenses and make you less liable to training injuries.

Techniques such as relaxation through breathing techniques and progressive relaxation of the muscles also increase the recovery rate. Learning to relax quickly is an effective way of reducing muscle tone increased by training. This means the muscles recover earlier

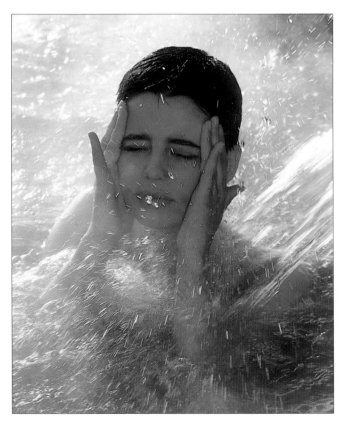

and are therefore less liable to injury. And not least, you can use these methods as an aid to falling asleep. Healthy sleeping patterns regenerate physical and mental resources: while we sleep we produce the growth hormone required for cell growth and rapid regeneration of the muscles' energy reserves.

Nevertheless, you must not think that everything can be learnt correctly and efficiently in "do-it-yourself" mode. A qualified teacher is absolutely necessary for certain relaxation techniques: *Autogenic Training, Feldenkrais, Eutonics* or an introduction to imaginary trips and mental training systems should only be undertaken with specialist trainers.

Relaxation through Breathing Techniques

The diaphragm is the most important human muscle for breathing. Its up-and-down movement when we breathe in and out has the effect of an internal massage of the heart, lung and stomach/intestinal area. This stimulates the circulation, and thus the vital functions of all the organs are stimulated by the improved circulation and increased resources.

Correct Breathing Techniques

Breathe in through the nose. This encourages deep breathing, since the resistance created by the air coming through the nasal passage causes deeper breathing and this, as a side effect, provides training for the breathing muscles. Breathe deeply into your stomach. To check whether or not you are breathing properly, place your hand on your stomach, over your navel and you will feel how your stomach rises and falls. Let your breath out and leave a small pause after breathing out, until the need to breathe in through the nose takes over naturally. Breathe in again through the nose.

Breathing Exercises

Do these exercises for ten minutes at least once a day – twice or three times is best. Lie or sit down in a comfortable position. If sitting, rest your open hands on your upper thighs. Place your feet flat on the floor and, where possible, do not support the upper back (unless you have back problems). Close your eyes and breathe in and out six times through the nose. Do not force your breathing; allow yourself to breathe normally. Follow the feeling of the air coming in through the nose and traveling down to the chest, then

the stomach, and flowing out again. Concentrate on the chest and stomach areas and be aware of how the stomach rises and falls. Do not worry if your mind wanders. Be aware of your thoughts and let them go: imagine they are butterflies you can see flying off. You can concentrate better on your breathing if you count (1 for breathing in, 2 for breathing out, etc.). Enjoy the rest and relaxation. Finally, stretch yourself to prepare for further activities.

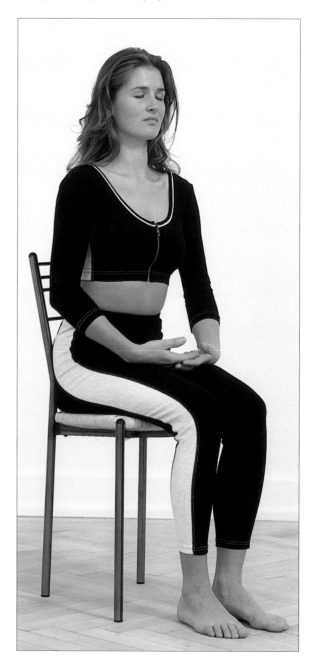

Progressive Muscle Relaxation

During the nineteen thirties, Edmund Jacobson developed an effective program of muscle relaxation, known as *Progressive Muscle Relaxation.* This method of relaxation provides training to enable the subject to consciously create an inner sense of repose at will, whatever the physical situation, by consciously controlling the muscle groups, with the result that tension and feelings of anxiety and stress are quickly dissipated. This relaxation technique is easy to learn and is suitable for all those for whom other relaxation techniques such as Autogenic Training or meditation are difficult. In this case the term "progressive" refers to gradual relaxation throughout the body, until it is completely relaxed. It involves tensing the muscles as much as possible then consciously releasing them. The method is so effective because the subject becomes aware of the physical difference between tension and relaxation and in the end is able to take action against stress and tension by moving into a state of deep relaxation within a very short space of time.

Initial Comments

Progressive muscle relaxation is an active method for training the muscles by subjecting them to intensive stress, that is, all the precautions discussed in the chapter *Training Guide* will apply here too. Exercise only when you are fit and healthy. If you have a health problem, consult your doctor about whether this type of muscle relaxation is suitable for you.

Basic Rules

Exercise on a regular basis. If you leave more than four days between training sessions, it will take longer for your muscles to achieve complete relaxation.

- Set aside about half to three-quarters of an hour when you will not be disturbed.
- Dress warmly and comfortably (jogging gear, thick socks, etc.).
- Black out the exercise area and make sure it is warm enough.
- If you are relaxing in a sitting position, sit down comfortably so that your clothing and position do not in any way obstruct the circulation in your legs.
- Relax your breathing (see "Breathing Techniques").

Exercise Guide

Lie down comfortably. Place the arms alongside the body, with the legs hip-width apart and your feet falling loosely outwards. Close your eyes and breathe calmly and regularly through the nose. Tense each muscle group for between two and six seconds. If you have not yet started your training, keep the muscle-tensing phase down to two seconds at first. Then relax for 15 to 20 seconds. At the beginning it is best to tense each muscle group twice in succession and then relax. After the second time, pause for 30 to 40 seconds. Then compare the difference between tensed and relaxed muscles and concentrate on the increasing feeling of relaxation. It is often helpful to think of a key word or phrase you can concentrate on at the moment you release the tension (for example, let go, relax or something similar). If you do these exercises regularly, just the thought of the key word or phrase will be enough to induce a deep and refreshing state of relaxation.

To train your physical responses, we recommend you start with the extremities, for example the right side only, then change over to the left. Later you can tense and relax both arms or both legs at the same time.

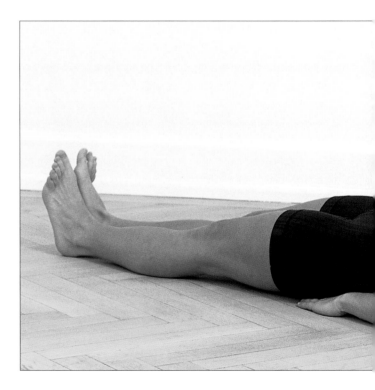

The sequence below is simply a suggestion of how to do your training. You can vary the sequence of exercises according to your own requirements.

Legs: Pull back your toes towards your body. Make them as tense as you can. Relax. Bend the toes and pull the soles of your feet down towards the floormat. Hold and then release. Stretch the leg across the knee joint and bend the foot up and in towards the body. Tense as much as possible then relax. Before going on to the left leg, compare the difference in tension between the right and left legs.

Pelvis and Buttocks: Squeeze the buttocks together, tense the pelvic muscles, hold and release.

Stomach: Tense the stomach muscles by drawing in the stomach, hold and release.

Arms: Clench the fist as tightly as possible. Bend the elbow and try to touch the right shoulder with the wrist. Lay the arm down again. Stretch the arm and hand as far as possible, and release. Repeat the exercise with your other arm.

Back and Neck: Press the back of the head and shoulders down firmly against the floormat, hold and release.

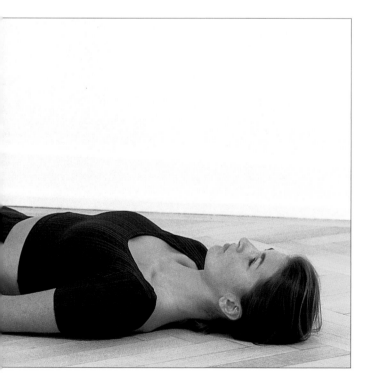

Chest: Press the upper arms against the rib cage while pulling the shoulders downwards and forwards at the same time, hold and release.

Shoulders: The best way of tensing the shoulders is to pull them down and back.

Neck: Tense the neck muscles by pulling the shoulders up and at the same time pulling the head down between them.

Face: Wrinkle the brow. Close the eyes and mouth and scrunch. Then clench your teeth and pull the corners of the mouth outwards, hold and release.

Lie there for a little longer enjoying the feeling of repose and relaxation. The exercise should end with you taking a deep breath and stretching your body out while still lying there, in preparation for activity. If you want to use Progressive Muscle Relaxation as an aid to sleep, leave out the stretching at the end. You can now also stretch your muscles, depending on how you feel (see *Mobility*).

If you suffer from arthritis, muscle contractions in the affected joints may be too painful. However, you can do the Progressive Muscle Relaxation if you leave out the groups of muscles concerned. On the other hand, if one or more of the exercises causes pain, you should apply less tension. If the problem does not subside, it would be advisable to see a doctor about it before training again.

Problems?

Sometimes tensing the muscles to the maximum can cause cramping. Stretch the muscle group concerned and shake it out. After that, change your technique by tightening the muscles for shorter periods and less intensely, to avoid tension and cramps.

Slight stiffness may occur in the muscles after these exercises, especially if you have not been training. You can prevent this by warming up and stretching the muscles slightly before you start the relaxation exercises. To speed up the regeneration of the muscles, you can also include the Progressive Muscle Relaxation exercise in your training program.

While training, some people occasionally feel uneasy. Change your training schedule to find a rhythm that helps you to relax better. When you exercise, have longer or shorter pauses between the phases of tension, to suit yourself, or vary the length of your training session. If necessary, try doing the exercises in a sitting position.

Sauna

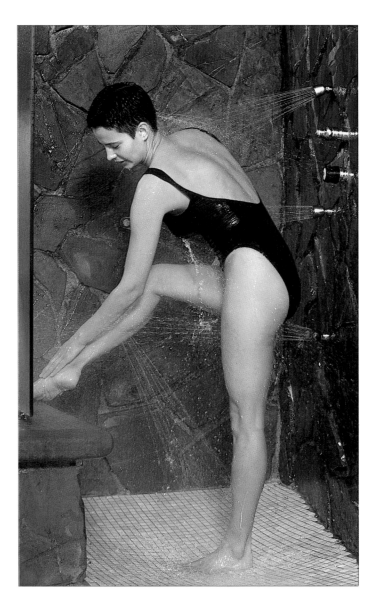

Ground Rules

• If you are ill enough to stay in bed, you should not use the sauna. If you have an acute condition, consult your doctor to make sure that your current state of health is not adversely affected.

• Take your time: a sauna consists of both a warming-up and a cooling-down period. The warming-up period should not take longer than twelve or at most fifteen minutes, as a longer sweating process at high temperatures puts too much stress on the heart and lungs. Even "withdrawing" to the cooler lower benches to be able to stay

longer serves no purpose from a health perspective. It is advisable to take as long to cool down as you spent in the dry heat room. This means that, if you go through two or three sauna cycles, you need two to two and a-half-hours for a full sauna.

• Do not take a sauna on an empty stomach or after a full meal. Because the heat in the dry heat room draws blood to the body's external surfaces, the additional need for blood in the stomach and intestines (caused both by appetite and a full stomach) could easily cause a lack of blood in the brain.

Please Note

Exercise first, then go to the sauna! If reversed, the restorative effect of the sauna is destroyed and the body will get tired. In addition, there should be enough time between the training session and the sauna for the pulse and circulation to return to normal.

Preparation

A shower before going into the sauna will remove cosmetics and body oils from the skin, so that the sweating process is not unnecessarily obstructed. Dry yourself thoroughly so that you start sweating quickly in the dry heat room. Any dampness on the skin produces condensation cooling and works against the effects you are looking for from the heat and the sweating process.

Dry Heat Room

Sit on the top or middle bench. The high temperatures in this area guarantee that you overheat as required in the short time you will be staying in the dry heat. If there is enough room, stretch out on the bench so that the muscles along your backbone receive the full benefit of the hot air and relax more quickly. If you are sitting, put your feet up on the bench so that the whole body is in one temperature zone and there is no risk of the blood sinking into the legs. Do not forget that the sauna is a place of relaxation: avoid any strenuous activity such as changing places often or talking (you are in danger of fainting). The last two minutes before you leave the sauna should in any case be spent sitting upright so that the body is prepared for the vertical position.

Cooling Off

First of all walk around the room for a couple of minutes to lower your body temperature a little and to prepare to cool down. Shower thoroughly with cold water. Multiple showerheads are absolutely ideal for this as the body is exposed to several jets of water on both sides. It is best not to have alternating hot and cold showers, as this would overload the circulation system (danger of collapse). Sit or lie down comfortably in the relaxation room and enjoy the increasing feeling of relaxation. After a sufficient recovery time, you can take one or more further sauna cycles.

Finish your sauna unhurriedly, by sitting or lying down again. This will help to restore the normal surface temperature of the body, before you get dressed. Getting dressed too soon increases the risk of heavy "after sweats" and catching cold as a result, especially in low temperatures.

It is only by regular visits that a lasting improvement to your physical and mental well-being will become evident. You should build one or two weekly visits into your schedule to maintain the effect of the sauna. Once you realize how effectively the sweating process can aid recovery and start to build on this to increase performance, you will find a permanent place in your training schedule to indulge yourself in the sauna.

If, in spite of everything, you do not feel well in the sauna, it could be attributed to the type of sauna involved: dry heat sauna is not suitable for everyone. Many saunas propose several alternatives, for example the steam sauna. The best way of finding out what suits you is to try them out or discuss it with the sauna management. Hydrotherapy clubs are also a way of finding like-minded people and doing something for your health in a relaxing and pleasant atmosphere.

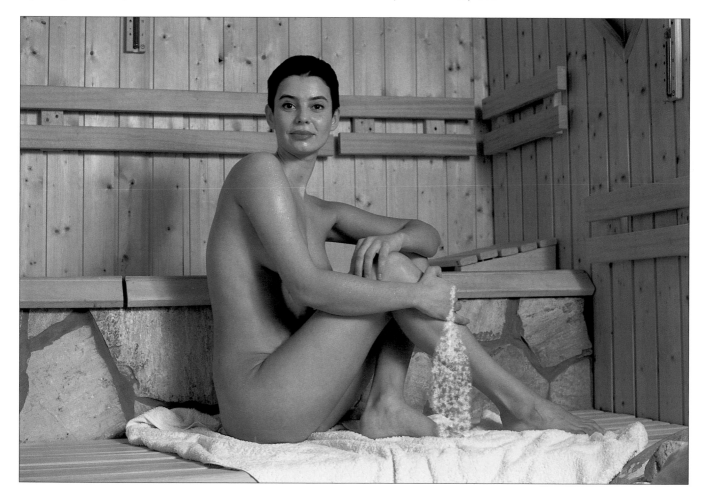

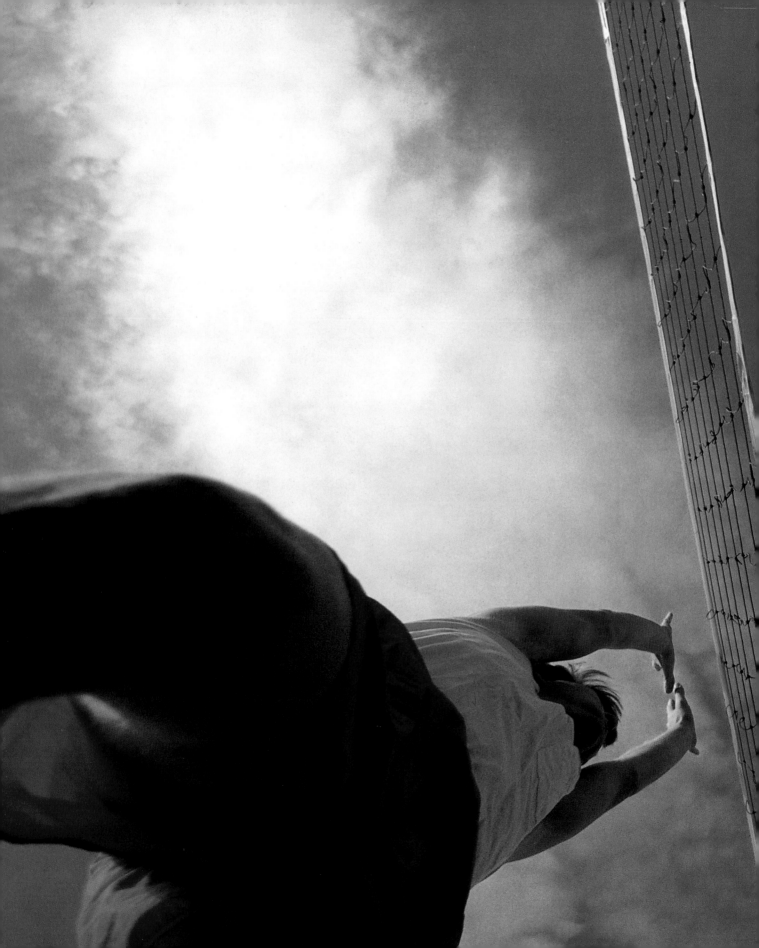

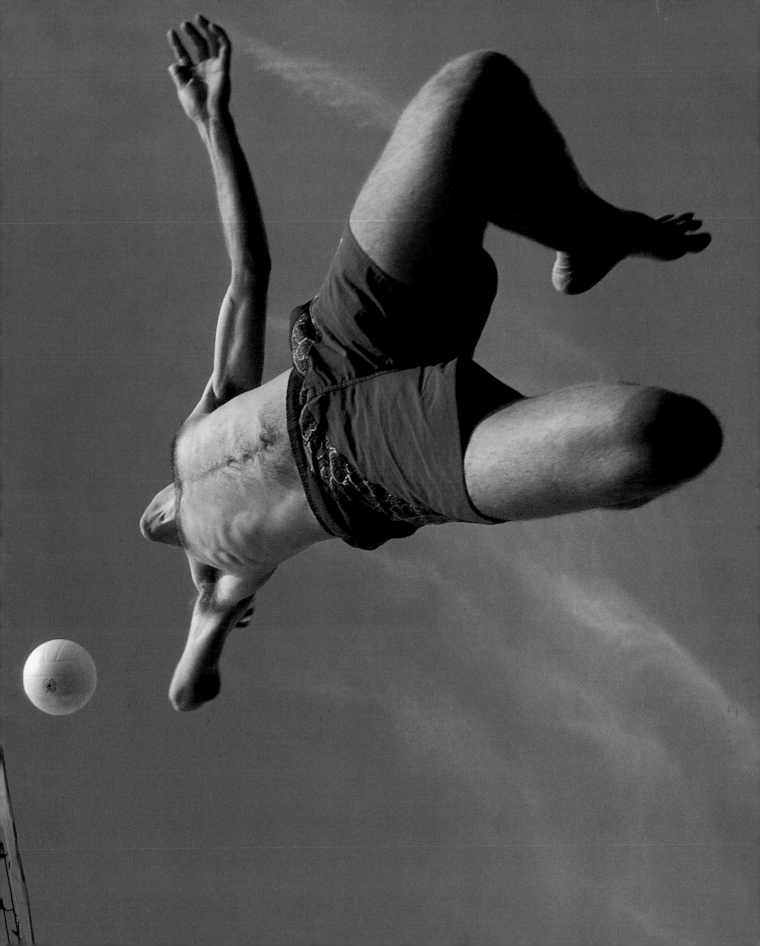

Weight Reduction

Are you happy with your figure? If your answer is "Yes," good. However, if this is not your answer, you could find this chapter extremely interesting.

Many people are unhappy with their figures. There is however no shortage of good ideas about how to shed a few pounds of excess weight. From the "Flat stomach in 3 weeks" program to the "Bikini Blitz Diet," various more or less useless methods are on offer. All of these "quick methods" have one thing in common – they exploit the impatience of those who want to lose weight. Some of them promise weight loss of a pound a day in order to

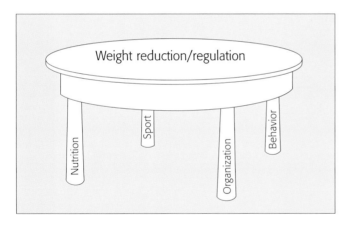

Any potentially successful, meaningful and long-term weight reduction program is based on four factors which complement each other.

achieve the dream figure as quickly as possible. Weight loss of this order is certainly possible in the short term, but involves not just fat, but muscle and water too.

There is certainly a large number of qualified specialist advisors on the subject of weight reduction, all with varying points of departure. Some concentrate on dietary considerations, others on a precisely controlled exercise program, yet others give tips on organizing your life, while still more see being overweight as a psychological problem and offer help in this area. For successful

long-term weight reduction a combination of these approaches is recommended. Imagine that each of the areas listed here: diet, sport, organization and behavior, is one leg of a heavy table. Each of these supports contributes to the stability of the table: if even only one of them is not strong enough, your table – like your idea of weight reduction – is standing on shaky legs. This chapter is not concerned with adding yet another to the extensive range of dietary regimes. It introduces the necessary elements of a successful weight reduction program and points out how these should, ideally, be combined if they are to lead you to lasting success. The initiative to put these elements into practice then lies with you.

The Metabolic Process

In order to understand why the body protects itself so strongly against any attack on its reserves requires a basic understanding of the metabolic process. The concept of the metabolism basically covers nothing more nor less than the whole range of biochemical reactions which occur in our bodies. In everyday language, the metabolism is repeatedly mentioned in connection with speed: "He has a high metabolic rate, she has a low metabolic rate, your metabolic rate will slow down with this medication," etc. It is clear that the speed of the chemical processes in our bodies can vary. The fact that the metabolism is indeed subject to variation like this means that it is somewhat more difficult to plan a specific weight reduction program.

In reality, the logic is clear: I absorb more energy than I need and my weight increases; I absorb less energy than I need, and it goes down. But our metabolism does not work like that. For an understanding of the parameters involved in weight gain or loss, we use the image of a bowl of water: to illustrate the variability of the metabolic rate, we look at the rate at which water enters the basin together with the rate it drains out. If the inflow of water drops (energy uptake), the outflow (energy consumption) automatically drops after a short delay. By how much it drops and when the choke occurs depends on the individual. The reverse process is, naturally, that when the energy up-take increases, energy consumption also increases after a short time.

Activation of the Metabolic Process

If we want to apply our newly acquired knowledge about the variability of our metabolism to the task of controlling our body weight, we should avoid behavior which slows down the metabolism. There are three practical ways of naturally stimulating the metabolism:

1. Muscle Building (hypertrophy)
2. Physical Activity
3. Eating More and/or More Frequently

A health-oriented, fitness aware individual would not even consider unreasonable and even illegal measures such as less sleep, exposure to cold, consumption of coffee or nicotine, drugs or doping to increase the metabolic rate. So we will look at methods of controlling the metabolism which are compatible with good health.

1. Muscle Building

Since muscle tissue has a prolific blood supply, its metabolic rate is higher in absolute terms than that of fatty tissue. In other words, the metabolic engine runs higher in muscles and increases fuel consumption. In modern gymnasiums and fitness training centers, muscle building is now almost outdated. But the question is: "What else is happening in weight training, if not muscle building?" The fact that many people have false expectations of their fitness training is often the result of stubborn prejudices where weight training is concerned, for example:

- Through training, the *problem areas* of fat can be targeted, and will melt away, tighten up and turn into muscle.
- Women will form big muscles through weight training.
- Weight training with light weights and high recovery rates tones the muscles and has a slimming effect.

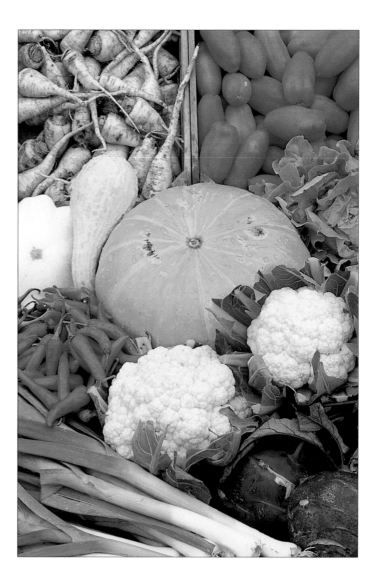

What is true is that, if it were, for example, possible to burn off fat from a targeted area of the body, it must also be possible to target fat to a specific body area by leaving that area inactive. The fat storage process is however laid down by genetic information stored in our body cells. Men are genetically predisposed to develop the so-called apple shape, that is to say that excess fat is stored mainly in the general area of the stomach. On the other hand, women develop the so-called pear shape, that is, excess fat is found on the belly, hips, buttocks and upper thighs. When we shed fat, we do so in reverse order to the order it was stored in.

The areas which gained weight most recently will be the first to slim down. The areas your first little rolls of fat developed will be the last to lose them. It makes no difference if we lose fat through a special training program, a diet or a change in eating habits. Nor is it possible to convert or achieve a lifting effect, because of the difference in structure between fat and muscles. Nevertheless, if the aim of getting rid of fat is translated into a change to the right type of foods and an active lifestyle, one does in fact see a percentage increase in the body's overall muscle mass.

But what can we say about the fear of building too much muscle? It is women who often have a certain fear of using the heavier weights in power training, because they do not want to look like a female Arnold Schwarzenegger. A less effective method is the widely accepted practice of training using lighter weights in highly repetitive sequences. In this case muscle strength and expansion is achieved – the prerequisite for stimulation of the metabolism – only if greater demands than usual are made. In addition to this, nature has set things up so that the figure of any woman involved in leisure time training could never even come close to that of Arnold Schwarzenegger. The simplest way of not gaining more muscle, if you have reached your "personal limit," is not to increase your training targets any further. You have already read about the basic

requirements needed to establish a training schedule for muscle building and increased power in the first chapter.

2. Physical Activity

With all physical activity, the metabolic stimulation is achieved not only during the training phase: it goes on for while after the end of the training. The more exhausting the training feels, the longer the metabolic rate is increased – for up to six hours after an intensive training session.

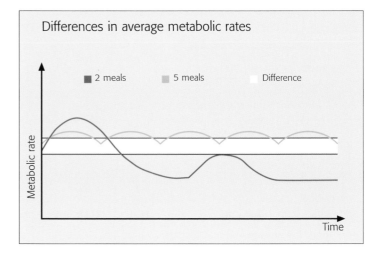

Differences in average metabolic rates

■ 2 meals   ■ 5 meals   □ Difference

Metabolic rate

Time

3. Eat More and/or More Frequently

The very people who tend to put on weight easily are often those who do not eat much. On the contrary: for days at a time they often eat less than they need for their actual energy requirements. They often try to reduce their calorie intake by eating less often. Small or greater sins during the weekend or at parties are compensated for with a meager diet over the next week. But the sins involved cannot be compensated for by eating less over the next few days. The fact that this is not the case is explained by the economy measures applied by the metabolism. These come into effect after not just a few days of poor diet, but after a few hours. If, for example, you miss a meal because of work pressure, all energy-consuming processes are at first slowed down. With two meals a day the average metabolic rate may therefore be much lower than with five meals a day at two- or three-hour intervals. It should also not be forgotten that the metabolism works slower at night than during the day.

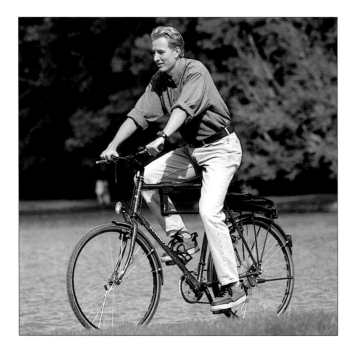

Energy Gain

Sport is one important element leading to successful weight reduction. However, the choice of a suitable sport poses the question of whether endurance training automatically involves burning off fat? Yes and no! Because burning off fat depends on adequate supplies of oxygen. Let us look at what happens with a burning candle when an (empty) glass is placed over it. Correct, it goes out. Exactly the same thing happens if you try to burn off fat by doing more intensive exercise. In principle, our bodies have the choice of absorbing energy from three, or strictly speaking, four different sources: sugar or carbohydrates, fat, protein and alcohol.

For all intents and purposes, alcohol should be set aside as a source of energy, particularly where weight reduction is concerned. The body only consumes protein to any notable extent during periods of fasting or intensive endurance work (such as a marathon). The muscles then serve as the protein source, that is, the body uses the protein content of the muscle tissue which has of course a far more important purpose than energy supply. Therefore, protein is also of little interest as a major energy supply in sport. Only sugars, also known as carbohydrates, and fats remain. In practice the two are always used together in a specific variable combination. When the body is at rest, the proportion of fats predominates, at almost 90 per cent, as adequate oxygen supplies are available over a long period. With very strenuous endurance work, the ratio is almost the opposite, because of the increased supplies of oxygen. One often hears that a not-too-intensive endurance training session can burn off fat efficiently after half an hour. This is only partly true. In fact, the carbohydrate-to-fat ratio changes from one minute to the next, right from the start.

In the graph below it is clear that the proportion of fat burned off in the first half-hour is very low compared with the second. In fact, with moderate endurance work, fat reduction increases progressively and almost reaches its peak after half an hour. It still

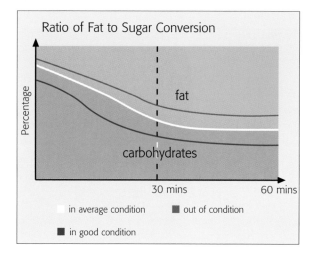

Ratio of Fat to Sugar Conversion

fat

carbohydrates

Percentage

30 mins   60 mins

■ in average condition   ■ out of condition
■ in good condition

Age	max. Pulse per min.	60% of Pulse per min.	65% of Pulse per min.	70% of Pulse per min.
20	200	120	130	140
25	195	117	127	137
30	190	114	124	133
35	185	111	120	130
40	180	108	117	126
45	175	105	114	123
50	170	102	111	119
55	165	99	107	116
60	160	96	104	112
65	155	93	101	109
70	150	90	98	105

remains to be explained what "moderate" and "not too strenuous" mean. You have already discovered the pulse range best suited to your heart and lungs for endurance training. The performance-related rule of thumb (pulse 180 minus age, plus or minus an allowance for fitness) is then reduced by 20 to achieve the best fat reduction ratio. So we have a pulse rate of 160 minus age. Then we have the same addition or reduction as indicated in the chapter *Endurance*. The table on this page gives an overview of the best range of pulse rates for burning off fat: endurance training, which aims to burn off fat as an energy store, must observe the following ground rules:

- It must last long enough (it only becomes worthwhile from half an hour onwards).
- It must not be too intensive (a pulse rate of about 20 less than for aerobic training).
- It must be uniform.

It is specifically the condition requiring uniformity in endurance training which is not fulfilled by almost any ball game such as volleyball, football and basketball, nor by squash, tennis or badminton. A major feature of this type of sport is a constantly changing pulse rate. One moment a player is standing quietly (for example during the serve), and the next moment he is running for the ball. These constant variations in the heartbeat mean that the body is mainly converting sugars, as the sugar structures contain relatively large amounts of oxygen, and fat has relatively little. Therefore, in situations where oxygen is in short supply, our bodies prefer to use a quickly available short-to-medium-term energy supply, namely sugar.

It is only with long-term, uniform exertion with a constant rate of oxygen supply that the metabolism turns to fats as a long-

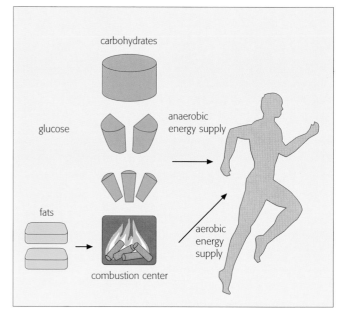

The sugar combustion (wood) requires less oxygen and thus burns quicker than the oxygen-intensive fat combustion (briquettes), which only functions optimally in the heated wood fire.

term energy source. The fast-track sugar supply is saved for emergencies, because of its oxygen requirement.

The difference in energy supplies is demonstrated by comparing sugar with thin slivers of wood and fat with briquettes. If you hold a lighter under the slivers of wood, they burst into flames, while the briquette shows no sign of catching fire. It is only once you have started a fire properly with the slivers of wood that you can throw your briquette onto it and it will also burn, after a certain length of time, for much longer than the wood (see illustration).

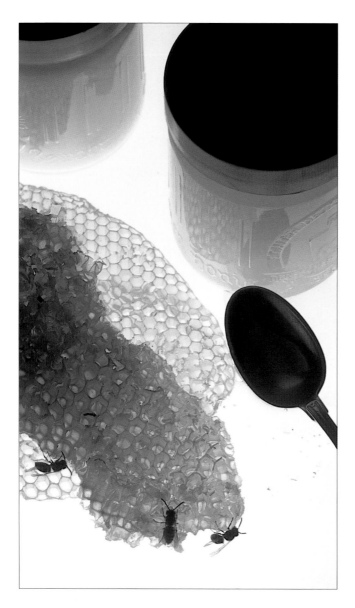

Perhaps you know one or two very sporty, active individuals who, nevertheless have weight problems. The explanation for this is almost obvious: even daily training sessions often only burn large amounts of sugar, depending on the type of sport, and this is often replaced at the next meal, because the appetite has been stimulated. Sports that encourage sugar consumption, pose yet another problem: each separate chemical reaction in the metabolic system is made possible by a specific *enzyme.* The enzymes required to burn fat are not identical to those used to burn sugar. With regular training of the sugar metabolic systems, for example in the above-mentioned ball games, larger numbers of the enzymes for sugar combustion are formed in preparation for similar workloads in the future. In other words, the original narrow track used for sugar conversion now gradually grows into a multi-lane motorway. The fat metabolism, on the other hand, continues to use the narrow track, as there has been no special training.

The logical conclusion we draw from these details about the metabolic processes favors the uniform, long-term and not over-intensive endurance or burn-off training. It is recommended in principle for weight and, especially, fat reduction. For beginners in particularly poor physical shape – you will certainly have found out long ago whether or not you are in this group from the tests in the first chapter – initial aerobic training using the relevant pulse rates is recommended for the first few weeks or months before you can start burning off fat. The plans provided in this section show the best method of burning off fat during training sessions.

Test your condition beforehand, for example with the Cooper Test. If your test result is lower than average, you can begin your training to lose fat with the training schedule for people with less than average fitness. If your test result is at least average, you can start immediately on the lower training schedule. From the list in the chapter *Endurance,* pick out any type of sport (for example, swimming, cycling, walking or jogging) which suits you best and which meets your current requirements. At the end of the twelfth week of training, measure your condition again. If by then you have reached at least average condition, you can proceed with the lower training schedule. Otherwise, you should continue with the type of training you have been doing over the previous three weeks and should be raising your pulse rate to 70 or 80 per cent of the maximum pulse rate during the training. Repeat the condition test every four weeks and transfer to the next plan when you achieve average results.

Training Schedule Below Average Condition

	Weeks 1 to 4	Weeks 5 to 8	Weeks 9 to 12
Pulse during training	60–70% of pulse	60–70% of pulse	60–70% of pulse
Training time per session	20 mins	30 mins	40 mins
Sessions per week	2	2–3	3

Training Schedule Average Condition

	Weeks 1 to 4	Weeks 5 to 8	Weeks 9 to 12
Pulse during training	160 minus Age	160 minus Age	160 minus Age
Training time per session	40 mins	50 mins	60 mins
Sessions per week	2–3	2–3	2–3

Nutrition

Everyone of us has a basic knowledge of nutrition. But it is not easy to process all the information you need for a healthy diet. At the same time, we all have a certain amount of basic knowledge about healthy eating. More information is given below.

You will learn that the classical diet for weight reduction, irrespective of how it is presented, always has a snag. You will get to know the relationship between the various appetite stimuli and food intake, as well as individual food components and their major features. With this knowledge you will be introduced to a framework for a nourishing and balanced diet.

This chapter has been deliberately included with the weight reduction topics, as knowledge of correct diet is one of the pillars upon which successful weight reduction can be built: in the end, diet and exercise are inseparable. But what is the use of the most expert knowledge in the areas of sport and diet if the practical application fails to establish a long-term, day-by-day link between the dietary and the sporting components of weight reduction.

Promises versus Reality

Every spring it's the same thing: winter fat becomes apparent in all its glory. The weather for the first light skirts and shorts is not far away. It is now that all the different methods for fast weight reduction become very tempting.

Let us assume that you, too, have decided on a fast method of shedding a few superfluous pounds. For fast results most of the so-called crash diets are based on an energy intake of less than 1000 *kilocalories.* But you already know that your metabolism is very economical with reserves. So, if you take in so little energy for a few days, your energy output will drop considerably. In spite of this, the reduced energy intake will indisputably result in a certain amount of weight loss, especially during the first few days. As we have already explained, weight loss in these cases only partially affects body fat. What is more, over half of the lost weight comes from protein-rich muscle tissue and the related water content.

To understand that a reduction in body weight of about one pound a day, as achieved by a crash diet, does not mean a loss of fat only, we need to make the following calculation: one gram of fatty food liberates 9 kcals on combustion, whereas by

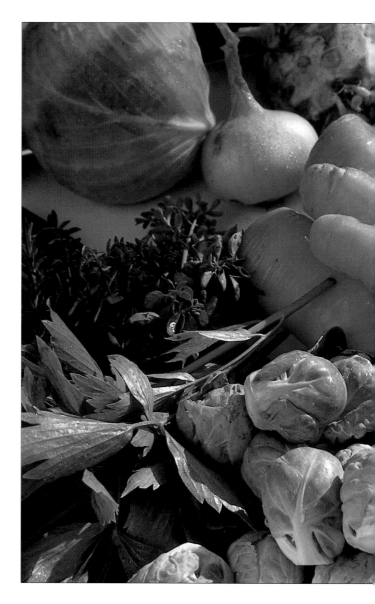

comparison, one gram of body fat produces 7 kcals. The energy content of body fat is lower since the body tissues contain, for example, connecting tissue which contributes nothing to its fuel energy. At best, one pound of body fat therefore releases 500×7 kcal = 3500 kcal on combustion.

The daily intake recommended by many nutrition institutes for a 25 to 51 year-old man is 2400 kcals and for a woman of the same age, 2000 kcals, assuming moderate physical activity. No special knowledge of math is needed to realize that it would be difficult to make savings of 3500 kcals from a basic requirement

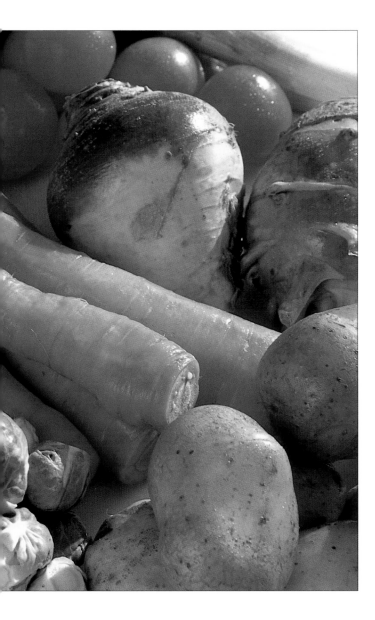

realistic result from any planned diet. It would be much more reasonable to follow this target without major reductions in energy expenditure.

From a health point of view, too great a reduction in energy intake, as for example with crash diets, also involves a restricted supply of various vital nutritional elements. This is why the low energy mixed diets proposed at the end of the chapter, as recommended by many nutrition institutes, are not only more effective but also provide a healthier alternative route to a slimmer form.

Dietary Principles

At this moment in time, several hundred different diets promise ready solutions to weight reduction. While at first the situation seems extremely complex, closer inspection reveals one common basic principle: together with fat loss, poor nutrition causes the body to consume muscle tissue. Considerable weight loss is then achieved because of the water content of the lost muscle tissue. However, this is soon regained after the diet has been discarded. In addition, most diets are so unbalanced that they manage to cause appetite loss after a certain length of time. This also quickly leads to weight loss.

The concept of a diet is generally understood to be a specially designed way of eating which is followed for a certain length of time. This demonstrates the most serious disadvantage of a diet: the energy and nutritional content are often not suited to cover the long-term needs of the human organism, so that whenever a diet comes to an end, the eating habits that were in place before the diet generally take over. Even if a loss of body weight is achieved by a strict diet, most diets do not give any information about how to continue with sensible eating in the future.

There are certain eating patterns which have neither the balance of the usual nutritional recommendations nor the short-term nature of a diet. These are described as alternative ways of eating. Among them we include *vegetarianism, macrobiotics* and the *Hays Diet.*

for 2400 or 2000 kcals. Then we also have to think about the diets providing about 1000 kcals. From the figures in our example, a reduction of one pound of body fat would mean a need to burn off 2100 to 2500 kcals through sport. This is the equivalent of a 5-hour cycle ride.

Looking at the calculations set out above, you have a practical demonstration that the usual promises about diets are impossible to achieve. If we include in our calculations the slowing down of the metabolism which occurs in any case after a few days of dieting, a loss of one pound of body fat per week is the maximum

Theories on Appetite

What drives the human body to ingest food? There are various theories about this, all of them with a greater or lesser scientific base. The most thoroughly researched of them is the relationship between the feeling of hunger and the blood sugar level. The further the blood sugar level falls, the stronger the feeling of hunger. But the degree of expansion of the stomach is also considered to be a stimulus for food intake. The set-point theory provides another point of view: it holds that stored in each individual's genes is a specific *ideal weight* and therefore a specific level for fatty tissue. If the stored weight is under- or over-achieved to any marked degree, the brain manages food intake so as to achieve it. However, research on twins has brought the results of this theory into question, as it can be proved that one twin can be overweight and the other slim, although they both carry the same genes. It is also assumed that there is a relationship between food intake and the levels of amino acids stored in the body.

While internal stimuli control food intake (lack of energy and malnutrition), a feeling of hunger occurs to compensate for this lack. On the other hand, external stimuli may lead to uncontrolled food intake.

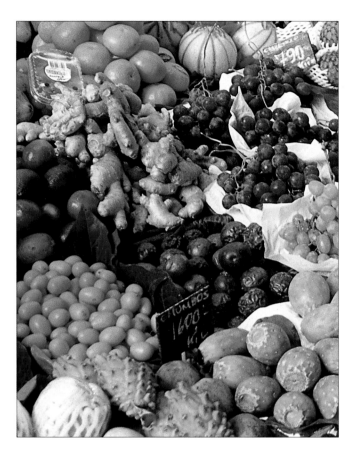

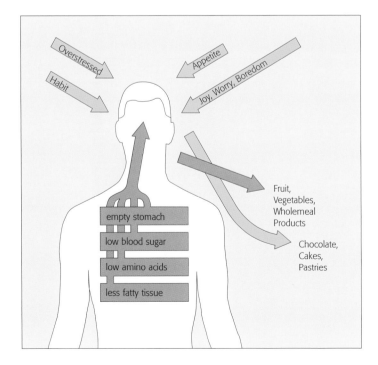

It is presumably a combination of the four factors (stomach content, blood sugar and amino acid levels plus the set-point) which control the internal stimulus to ingest food. By chewing for long enough it is possible, through a reverse mechanism in the brain, to achieve a feeling of repletion. However, this only occurs after about twenty minutes of chewing.

If you think about your favorite food, it becomes clear that ingesting food is not controlled only by your body's needs for nourishment. There is also a multitude of external influences such as appetite, enjoyment, boredom, frustration, solitude, irritation, sociability, etc. If all these external influences did not exist, food science would be superfluous, as the human organism, controlled by internal stimuli, would ingest only the best combination of food. If all the food we needed were available, food intake would be halted when the internal stimulus cut out. Without social and psychological influences, availability of all the necessary foodstuffs would mean that both under- and over-eating would be impossible.

Nutritional Components and Specifics

Even though the average person ingests several thousand different foodstuffs and food products during his lifetime, his food can be very easily analyzed on the basis of its content. On the other hand, this analysis helps us to list foodstuffs on the basis of our requirements. For, in the end, our nourishment is not provided in the form of a pack containing all the relevant individual nutrients we need: we ingest a combination of nutrients in the form of food. In addition to the main nutrients (carbohydrates or sugar, proteins, fats), our food is also made up of essential elements such as vitamins and minerals as well as water. The main nutrients and trace elements are distinguishable by their caloric value, among other things. While vitamins and minerals cannot provide the body with energy directly, energy supply is one of the most important tasks of the main nutrients.

The human organism can only function if it is continuously provided with energy in the form of the main nutrients. It needs this energy to maintain the body temperature and physical processes as well as for work. Energy conversion in the human body transforms about 60 per cent into heat and 40 per cent into chemical energy. The following rates of conversion apply in the human body:

1 g fat	approx 9 kcals or 39 kilojoules (kJ)
1 g carbohydrate	approx 4 kcals or 17 kJ
1 g protein	approx 4 kcals or 17 kJ
1 g alcohol	approx 7 kcals or 30 kJ
1 kcal (kilocalorie) = 4184 kJ (kilojoules)	

Alcohol, however, is not classified as a foodstuff in spite of its high caloric value, and is not a nutrient but a stimulant. If you would like to know how many grams of alcohol a specific alcoholic drink contains, just multiply the percentage figure for that drink (percentage by volume) with the specific gravity of alcohol, that is,

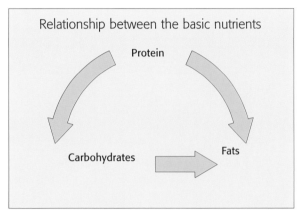

Relationship between the basic nutrients

Protein

Carbohydrates   Fats

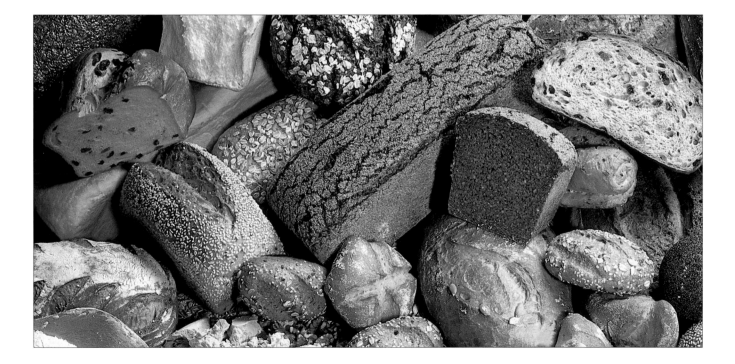

0.79. The result will be the alcohol content of that drink in grams per milliliter. Five hundred milliliters of wine with a 10 per cent volume therefore contains 39.5 grams of alcohol, which alone has an energy content of 276.5 kcals.

Total daily energy requirements depend on many different factors. Most importantly, we mainly have gender, age and the extent and intensity of physical activity.

Guidelines for Energy Intake

	kcals/day male	kcals/day female
10–13 years	2250	2150
13–15 years	2500	2300
15–19 years	3000	2400
19–25 years	2600	2200
25–51 years	2400	2000
51–65 years	2200	1800
65 years and over	1900	1700

The methods used to establish and quantify the energy requirements for one specific individual are very varied. The simplest way is by drawing a table. Recommended guidelines for energy intake, based on the gender and age of individuals in mainly sedentary employment, are supplied in the above table. In addition to these guidelines, the following suggestions can be made with regard to certain professional groupings which cannot be classed as "light physical activity":

- medium to heavy: 600 kcals
- heavy physical work: 1200 kcals
- very heavy physical work: 1600 kcals.

When an attempt is made to classify heavy physical work, it becomes quite clear that general guidelines like these can only give an approximate value for the real energy requirements of a specific individual.

Even the method of assessing energy requirements from the basal metabolic rate plus the performance-related rate and the energy loss through digestion and conversion, only provides an indirect method for calculating the individual metabolic rates of any specific person. This means that standard figures calculated on this basis can only be general in nature.

The only method of analyzing energy requirements so that they correspond to the specific situation for a given individual, is to establish and evaluate nutritional records. This would require a timespan of at least one week, plus a record of all foodstuffs, including drinks, in terms of quantity and caloric value. If the body weight, always measured at the same time and under the same conditions, does not change over the period concerned, the average value of the daily caloric intake forms a reliable basis for, and can be used as, the standard value for energy intake by this specific individual under the living conditions within a specific period. It must be noted that weighing and recording every individual component of every meal over a fairly long period of time also provides several opportunities for error. Eating habits very often change with the awareness that everything being eaten and drunk is recorded in writing. Consciously or unconsciously, less is often eaten than usual. As half a bar of chocolate eaten after ten o'clock at night looks bad in the written records, it is either not eaten or not honestly entered. Apart from this possible source of inaccuracies, a complete record of foodstuffs is expensive and often very difficult to keep when eating away from base.

If you have measured your daily energy requirement by one means or another, the question arises of what you should do with the result. As a twenty-five-year-old woman with a mainly sedentary occupation you have, according to the table, a daily energy requirement of 2200 kcals. We will assume that, although you are regularly involved in some sports activity twice a week, this figure has been corroborated by nutritional records. This means that in the future you can always check that your body is receiving the energy required for its needs – provided that you do not change your lifestyle and measure your daily energy intake by weighing the food on the basis of a nutritional table. However, as very few people have the desire or the possibility to estimate and record the energy content of all the food they eat day after day, the information should be used for other, more long-term purposes. Weighing foodstuffs and calculating the caloric value is an activity which can teach individuals to assess whether the daily food intake is adequate for their needs.

In addition, you can use the standard value for your daily energy intake to calculate how much of any of the main nutrients you should consume. This works as follows: first you calculate your daily protein requirement. According to most recommendations, this is 0.8 grams per 2.2 pounds body weight for adult males and females. If we take a body weight of 132 pounds, the result is a protein requirement of 48 grams with a caloric value of 192 kcals. Of the 2200 kcals energy requirement, after the protein requirement is covered, we still have about 2000 kcals to be supplied by fats and carbohydrates.

For the daily fat intake, the recommendation is either one gram per kilogram bodyweight or 25 to 30 per cent of the total energy intake. In our case, the value relative to the body weight lies just inside the energy percentage range. For a woman weighing 132 pounds we calculate 60 grams of fat which, with a caloric value of 9 kcals per gram, produce 540 kcals of energy. This means we still have about 1460 of the 2200 kcals to be provided by carbohydrates. This means that with a caloric value of 4 kcals per gram for sugar, we need 365 grams of carbohydrates. The 132-pound woman with an energy requirement of 2200 kcals from our example should therefore cover her daily energy requirements with 48 grams of proteins, 60 grams of fats and 365 grams of carbohydrates.

As carbohydrates, fats and proteins are sometimes very different, not only from one another, but also within each group, the following paragraphs show what types of basic nutrients should be used in preference, and in what form.

Carbohydrates

Carbohydrates, or saccharids and sugars are the nutrients which the human organism should consume in the largest proportions. They are formed in plants, from the inorganic compounds formed by energy from the sun through the agency of chlorophyll. Since this process, known as photosynthesis, is the only process in nature where an organic nutrient is produced from inorganic compounds, carbohydrates can be considered the primary products from which fats and proteins are made. Carbohydrates are the classical short- and medium-term energy providers for the human body. To differentiate the various forms of carbohydrates, we use information about how quickly the sugars in foods become available to the body. In the course of the digestive process, all forms of sugars, independent of the length of their chains, are split into simple sugars. The longer the original sugar chain, the longer it takes to have an effect on the blood sugar level.

Simple and binary sugars are quickly assimilated (absorbed) carbohydrates which are quickly detected in the bloodstream. The sugar dissolved in a drink takes about half-an-hour to an hour to be absorbed by the lining in the small intestine, and the sugar in a piece of fruit takes one to two hours before it gets into the blood. In certain cases the effect on the blood sugar level is detected more quickly. If for example, grape sugar or glucose is taken in the form of so-called energy bars, some of the sugar is assimilated through the mouth lining. Since, under normal circumstances, the whole blood supply only contains about 5 grams of glucose, just a few grams of sugar coming into the bloodstream quickly can significantly increase the blood sugar level. As a reaction to the rapid increase in blood sugar, the pancreas excretes the blood sugar regulating hormone insulin into the blood, so that the blood sugar level returns to the normal range (80 – 120 mg %).

Graphically speaking, the insulin closes the door to the body cells, so that the glucose is enclosed within the cells (see illustration on the next page). This causes

Provenance of Different Types of Sugars		
	Types	Foodstuffs
Monosaccharides	Glucose Fruit sugar (Fructose)	Fruit, Honey, Sweets, Fruit Juices
Disaccharides	Beet sugar (Sucrose)	Domestic Sugar, Jams, Sweets, Lemonades
	Malt sugar (Maltodextrine)	Malt Beer
	Lactose	Milk, Yogurt
Oligosaccharides	Maltodextrine	Carbohydrate Concentrates, Energy Drinks
Polysaccharides	Starch	Potatoes, Cereals, Bread, Noodles
	Glycogens	Liver, Muscles (Meat)

the blood sugar level to fall by the relevant amount. Since the response to a rapid increase in the blood sugar level is that of excess insulin being produced, it is perfectly possible for blood sugar levels to fall to a level lower than before the sugar intake because of this counter-measure.

A varied, adequate and balanced diet should therefore include the optimum mix of both rapidly and slowly assimilated carbohydrates, plus indigestible carbohydrates, known as fiber. From a chemical point of view, these indigestible components of vegetable foods belong to the carbohydrates. In fact, some of the fibrous tissues such as cellulose are even almost identical in structure to the starches. Both starches and cellulose consist of very long and complex glucose chains. They are differentiated in the way the individual glucose components are linked with each other. While the starch compounds can be split by the body's own enzyme, mankind lacks the enzyme required to split cellulose compounds. This is why fibrous material is expelled in undigested form from the body. Right until the seventies the fibrous material was considered superfluous. It was only later that a connection was made between the quantities of fiber

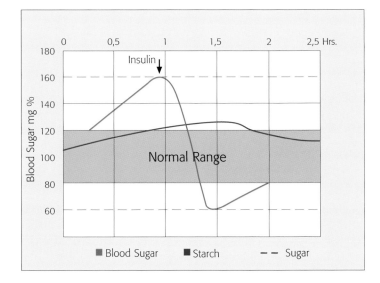

consumed and the appearance of certain diseases. Thus, intestinal diseases such as cancer of the bowel are almost unknown among indigenous populations in South Africa whose food is mainly of vegetable origin and whose intake of fiber is about four times that of the average well-nourished western European. Other differences are also evident here, for instance the Africans have a lower intake of fat and greater physical activity. Thus, we are now certain that the fiber plays an essential role against intestinal diseases and also heart-lung diseases. This is why an intake of 30 grams of fiber a day is recommended.

The main advantage of fiber is its absorbent properties. It absorbs water, which makes the food increase in bulk so that the added volume fills up the stomach and intestines better. Foods rich in fiber remain in the stomach longer but pass more quickly through the intestines through bowel kinetics – the so-called *peristalsis.* This causes an improved satiation effect because the stomach is replete and in consequence the extension receptors in the stomach are stimulated, and there is also a shorter contact time between noxious materials and the intestinal linings. During the digestive process, the fiber is not broken down and absorbed into the bloodstream or the lymph system through the intestinal lining like the individual building blocks from the basic nutrients: it therefore supplies no energy.

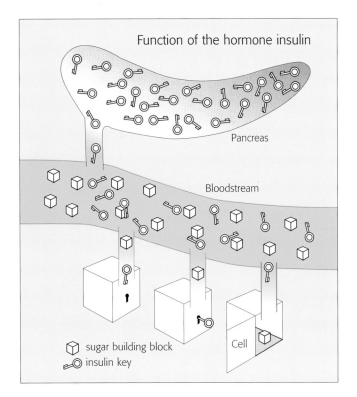

Fats

Fats are generally blamed for weight increase. In fact one gram of fat in foods supplies more than double the energy provided by the same amount of sugar or protein. In spite of this, or for this very reason, fats are very useful to man because of their high energy content, since they form the subcutaneous layer of fatty tissue, an almost inexhaustible energy supply which is used for long-term energy production.

Above and beyond the supply of energy, fats have other vital functions in the human organism. They surround the organs with a protective and insulating layer, they transport fat-soluble vitamins and they are a component of the biological membranes in cell walls. It is important to know that one particular fatty acid is not produced by the body itself: this product, linoleic acid, is necessary to the survival of the human organism. Depending on age, gender and lifestyle, the daily requirement of linoleic acid is between 10 and 30 grams. It is found for example in vegetable oils, nuts and cereals.

Fats, or lipids, are divided into two groups: neutral fats or triglycerides (= alimentary oils) and fat-like substances such as

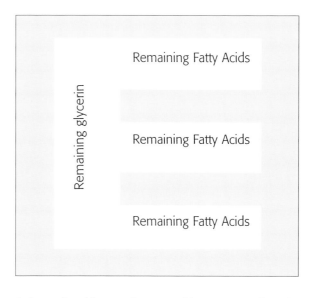

cholesterol and lipoproteins. Neutral fats are not uniform in nature. They consist of a glycerin base and three fatty acids, and are broken down into these individual components during the digestive process.

The different effects of the various fats on the human organism are caused by the different types of fatty acids which form the

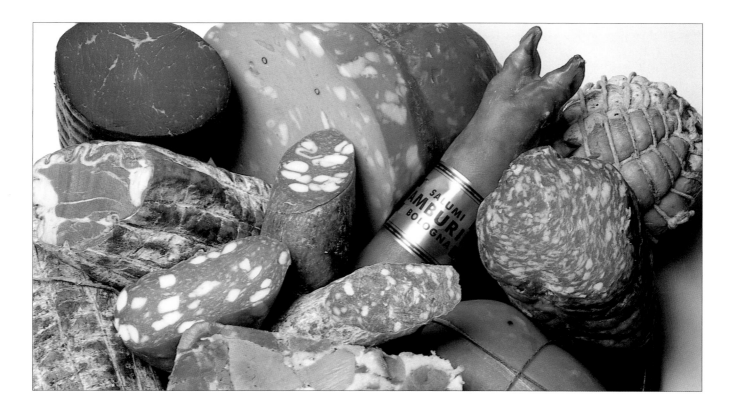

triglycerides. A basic distinction has been made between three types of fatty acids: saturated fatty acids, mono-unsaturated and poly-unsaturated fatty acids.

A fatty acid is described as saturated when all its carbon atoms (C) have been saturated by making the highest possible number of bonds. With a mono-unsaturated fatty acid, not all the carbon atoms are saturated with hydrogen atoms (H), but two of them have free receptors adjacent to each other and these bond with each other through a so-called double bond. If four or more hydrogen atoms are missing and, therefore, at least two double bonds have formed in the carbon chain, these are known as poly-unsaturated fatty acids.

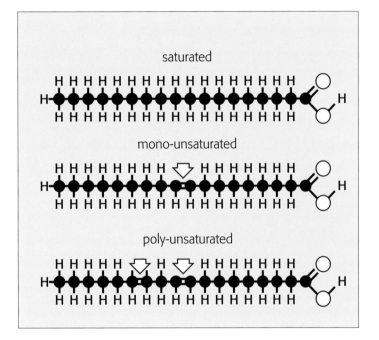

What effects these differently constructed fatty acids have on the human organism only becomes comprehensible when the method of carrying the fatty acids in the blood is explained. The accompanying illustration shows how the different types of fatty acids affect the "transportation" of fats in the bloodstream. In terms of human nutrition, it is important to know that fats from most animal food sources are predominantly saturated fats, while fats from vegetable sources contain predominantly simple and poly-unsaturated fatty acids. It is the animal fats that are often not recognized by the naked eye, such as those in cheese, delicatessen products and meat. This is the "hidden fat" we speak of.

The fats absorbed through the small intestine are not water-soluble. This is why these fats cannot be absorbed by the blood, which consists of more than 90 per cent water. Fats cannot therefore be carried directly by the blood, which means, they need a "carrier." This "taxi" is formed of proteins and fats, so that the protein base becomes the water-soluble carrier of the fats. The "fat carriers" formed are of different sizes, carry varying loads and have various functions within the organism. There are fairly large, not very substantial fat-protein corpuscles, the so-called LDLs (low-density lipoproteins). These can damage the blood vessels, since they lay down cholesterol along the artery walls. This increases the risk of heart and circulatory diseases. Even larger fat-protein corpuscles with even less substance are known as VLDL (very low-density lipoproteins). These also have a harmful effect on the blood vessels, while the small lipoproteins with a higher density, HDL (high-density lipoproteins), help to remove cholesterol from the body by taking superfluous cholesterol from the blood vessels and carrying it to the liver to be broken down and expelled.

◄ ► until now, no effect on the blood has been shown
▲ progressively increases blood density
▼ progressively decreases blood density

Recent research has shown that, for example, the high concentrations of fatty acids in olive oil have a doubly positive effect on the density of lipoproteins in the blood. Not only do they perceptibly increase the concentrations of "good cholesterol" (HDL), but they also lower the concentration of the "bad cholesterol" (LDL). Presumably this is why, for example in Greece, where olive products are very highly rated as everyday foods, the number of fatal heart attacks is very low compared with other European countries.

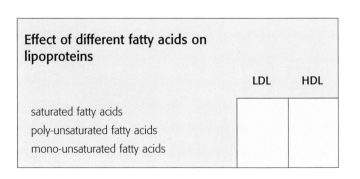

Effect of different fatty acids on lipoproteins

	LDL	HDL
saturated fatty acids		
poly-unsaturated fatty acids		
mono-unsaturated fatty acids		

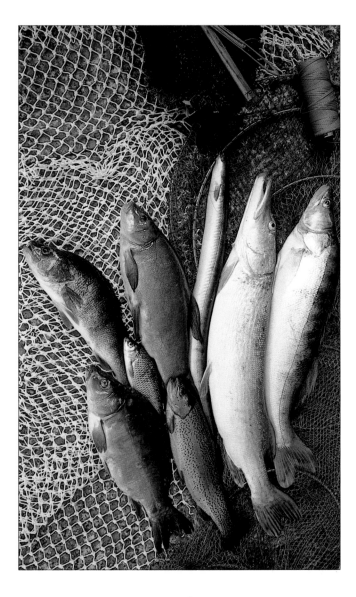

blocks, the amino acids, and then put them back together again in a way that meets their needs. However, plants and a few microorganisms are able (with the aid of bacterial nodules) to transform inorganic nitrogen, as present in the ground, in the form of nitrates or as nitrogen in the air, into organic protein compounds. It is worth noting that all the proteins in the human body are formed from only 20 different basic building blocks, the amino acids. The amino acids form human protein as widely different spatial structures and with a few hundred to several thousand combinations. This is comparable with the alphabet, which in English consists of only 26 letters but with which you can form an unending stream of words, sentences and texts.

Even though the protein ingested with food is again broken down into the different amino acids and double or triple groupings of amino acids (di- or tri-peptides), the origin of the ingested

Animal Protein (Biological Rating)		Vegetable Protein (Biological Rating)	
Whole Egg	100	Soy	84
Beef	92	Green Algae	81
Fish	94	Rye	76
Milk	88	Beans	72
Edam Cheese	85	Rice	70
Swiss Cheese	84	Potatoes	70
		Bread	70
		Lentils	60
		Wheat	56
		Peas	56
		Corn	54

Proteins

Proteins form the highest proportion of all the organic compounds in the human body. The term protein is derived from the Greek "protos," meaning the first. Protein is described as the first, or major substance because it forms the basis for the cells in every living being. Whether muscles, organs, bones, cartilage, blood or skin, every cell contains proteins. Even the structure of enzymes and hormones is only possible because of proteins.

Proteins are formed by plants. Animal organisms are only able to break down the ingested protein into its basic building

protein is important from the point of view of human nutrition. While the human metabolism can construct a few amino acids with the help of others, there are eight amino acids which we cannot produce or construct for ourselves. These so-called essential fatty acids must therefore out of necessity be ingested with our daily food so that a deficiency does not occur.

As the eight essential amino acids are present in different concentrations and in different formats in protein-rich food sources, the value of the various protein sources for human nutrition are given (see table).

One speaks of the biological value of alimentary protein. The ratings attributed to these use the reference value of 100 for the protein content of a whole egg. The degree of convertibility by the human organism of all other proteins is compared against that of egg protein. The eight essential amino acids have a specific distribution in human protein. If only one of the eight essential amino acids is present in alimentary proteins in appreciably lower quantities than in human protein, the biological rating and degree convertibility of the protein for human use is greatly reduced. The amino acids which have a limiting effect on the biological ratings are also called restrictive amino acids. In general, the biological rating of animal proteins is higher than that of vegetable proteins. Nevertheless, it is recommended that no more than one third of the daily protein requirement is taken from animal-based foods. The reason is that, besides the high protein levels, animal-based foodstuffs often contain high levels of unwanted by-products, such as for example purines, cholesterol and fats.

A complementary effect appears when different protein sources with different biological ratings are ingested simultaneously. This means that the restrictive amino acids can also affect a protein source from another protein-rich nutrient if the latter contains a relatively high concentration of restrictive amino acids. If two or more different protein sources are combined, biological ratings of over 100 can even be achieved. The protein ratios indicated in the above table do not refer to the total weight of the foodstuffs used, but to that of the protein extracted from them. For example, this means that with a ratio of 35 per cent of egg protein to 65 per cent of potato protein, you would need to ingest roughly a medium-sized egg with about one pound of potatoes to reach the biological rating indicated.

Protein Combination	Proportion of Protein	Biological Rating
Beans and Corn	52%/48%	101
Milk and Wheat	75%/25%	105
Whole Egg and Wheat	68%/32%	118
Whole Egg and Milk	71%/29%	122
Whole Egg and Potato	35%/65%	137

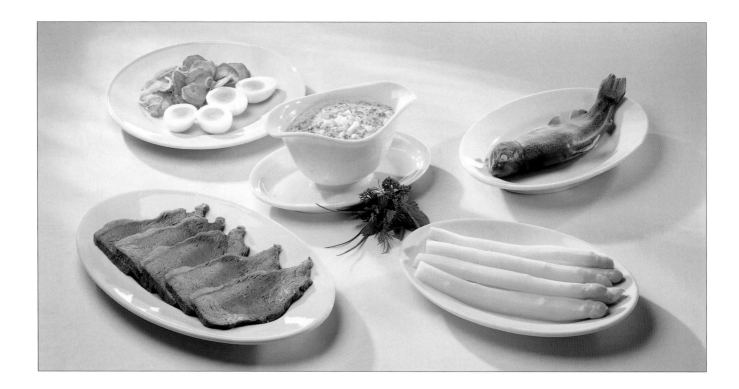

Liquids Management

The human body consists of 58 per cent water. In newborn babies the proportion is 80 per cent of total body weight. For women, the proportion of water is a few percentage points lower. This is explained by the generally higher proportion of fatty tissue in the female organism. While muscles consist of about 77 per cent of water, fat has very little water. If the body loses only 1 per cent of its liquid, a feeling of thirst occurs, and a two per cent loss of liquid reduces endurance performance; a loss of five per cent and upwards leads to an increased heartbeat, apathy, vomiting and muscle cramps, and the human being cannot survive with a liquid loss of over 15 per cent. Water performs several vital functions in the human body. Above all, it is a building block, a solvent, a means of transport and a means of heat regulation. For the organism to have the benefit of these services, it has to have a well-adjusted liquid balance; this means that as the body uses more water, more has to be ingested (see Overview, below). The requirements for liquid can increase considerably, particularly in dry and hot climates and as a result of physical activity. A well-known rule of thumb says that people can survive three weeks without food but only three days without water. Under everyday

Mineral Content (of Human Perspiration)	
Components	**Content (mg/l)**
sodium	1200
chloride	1000
potassium	300
calcium	160
magnesium	36
sulphate	25
phosphate	15
zinc	1,2
iron	1,2

Drinks taken by sports participants during a sports event must to some extent meet other requirements than drinks consumed during the course of a normal day. Above all, they have to replace the liquid lost through perspiration and the minerals dissolved in the sweat. In addition, they have to be made up in such a way that they are absorbed and exploited as quickly as possible by the body. People lose between 2.7 and 3 grams of minerals per liter in sweat (see Overview, above). To compensate for this loss, the liquids consumed must replace the lost minerals. In addition, a trained sports participant sweats more readily than an untrained participant, at a comparable level of exertion, but loses less sodium and chloride with the sweat. The loss of other minerals such as potassium and magnesium remains at the same level per liter of sweat for trained and untrained

Water Intake	ml per Day	Expelled Water	ml per Day
Drinks	1000–1500	Urine	1000–1500
Food	700	Faeces	100
Oxidation Water	300	Skin	500
		Lungs	400
Total	**2000–2500**	**Total**	**2000–2500**

conditions, your body needs at least 1.5 to 2 liters of water a day. If liquid is lost through heat, physical exertion or similar demands, this need may increase to about ten liters a day.

A diet with a high water content is recommended, as demonstrated in the wheel of nutrition (see page 289) to guarantee the liquid intake from foods. With regard to drinks, we should note that some drinks simply provide the body with liquid, without any energy content, whereas others provide liquid as well as energy.

participants. If the liquid consumed during or after sport is to be absorbed at maximum speed, the proportion of substances – such as minerals or sugars – in solution in the liquid consumed should not exceed the proportion of the same substances in the blood (= isoton). Special drinks cater for this. As a rule, an apple juice mix of two or three parts mineral water and one part fruit juice fulfills the same purpose: pure water contains too few parts (= hypotonic) and apple juice contains too many (= hypertonic).

Vitamins and Minerals

Nowadays people are much more familiar with vitamins and minerals as special preparations rather than in their natural form in fruit and vegetables or milk and milk products. Neither vitamins nor minerals supply energy – unlike carbohydrates, fats and protein. Nevertheless, they are included among the essential nutrients, that is, foods that keep you alive. As the body itself cannot produce them, they have to be provided in food we consume. Their main task is to regulate a wide range of metabolic processes. In addition to this, some minerals are used by the body as building blocks.

Functions and Provenance of the Main Minerals

Mineral	Function	Provenance
Sodium	Regulates water management, activates enzymes	Cooking salt, smoked foods, dry sausage, cheese
Potassium	Regulates water management, stimulates nerves and muscles, activates enzymes, glycogen synthesis	Vegetable foods: vegetables, potatoes, pulses, fruit, nuts, dried fruits
Magnesium	Activates enzymes, stimulates nerves and muscles	Green vegetables, potatoes, nuts, fruit, pulses
Calcium	Stimulates nerves and muscles, blood circulation, enzyme activities, building block for bones and teeth	Milk, milk products, egg yolk, vegetables, nuts, fruit
Phosphorous	Found in energy-rich phosphate compounds, building block for bones, teeth and cells	Milk, milk products, offal, meat, fish, egg yolk, pulses, nuts
Chloride	Regulates water management, forms gastric acids	Cooking salt, smoked foods, dry sausage, cheese
Iron	Component of hemoglobin and myoglobin, oxygen circulation	Meat, liver, egg yolk, wholemeal products, pulses, garlic, spinach, brewers' yeast
Iodine	Component of the thyroid hormone	Saltwater fish, eggs, milk, iodine-rich table salt
Zinc	Enzyme activation, component of the hormone insulin	Beef, liver, peas, cereals
Fluoride	Fights the formation of caries	Drinking water, vegetables, tea
Copper	Formation of blood	Offal, fish, eggs, potatoes, pulses, nuts
Selenium	Works with vitamin E	Meat, fish, wholemeal products, fruit, vegetables, yeast products
Manganese	Component of enzymes, skeleton	Liver, cereals, beans, spinach, pulses, fruit
Cobalt	Component of vitamin B12, formation of red blood corpuscles	Liver, cereals, pulses, nuts, root vegetables

Functions and Provenance of the Main Vitamins

Vitamins	Functions	Provenance
Vitamin A	Formation and maintenance of skin and mucous membranes	Butter, margarine, cheese, milk, egg yolk; Carotene: carrots, spinach, apricots
Vitamin D	Formation of bones and teeth, promotes absorption of calcium and phosphorous	Liver, saltwater fish, milk, egg yolk; is formed by the skin in sunshine
Vitamin E	Elasticity in connective tissue and blood vessels, antioxidants in foods, prevents oxidation of multiple fatty acids	Cereal grains, grain oils, nuts, wheat germ, egg yolk, butter, margarine
Vitamin K	Formation of prothrombin (precursor of a blood clotting enzyme), essential for normal blood clotting	Green vegetables, cabbage, green salad; formed in the gut
Vitamin B1	Co-enzyme in carbohydrate metabolism	Wholemeal products, yeast products, pork
Vitamin B2	Component of enzymes in the respiratory system	Yeast products, milk, offal, milk products, green leaf vegetables
Vitamin B6	Co-enzyme in the protein metabolism, formation of red blood vessels	Cereals, wheat germ, yeast, liver, pulses, saltwater fish, nuts, milk
Vitamin B12	Multiple reactions, cell construction, formation of red blood cells, nerve function	Only in animal-based foods: liver, meat, fish, eggs, milk
Vitamin C	Formation of connective tissue, antioxidant, promotes absorption of iron	Fruit, vegetables, potatoes
Niacin	With vitamins B1 and B2, involved in cell reaction for energy release	Yeast products, poultry, meat, fish, pulses, wholemeal products
Pantothenic Acid	Component of the A co-enzyme, plays a part in food metabolism	Wholemeal products, nuts, eggs, yeast products
Folic Acid	Formation of body protein, red blood cells and genetic material	Wheatgerm, yeast products, offal, green vegetables, milk.

The carotinoids listed under Vitamin A are pro-vitamins which occur in plants and from which vitamin A is formed in animals. The antoxidant effect of some vitamins and of selenium is becoming increasingly important to science. They have an important protective role for the cells and thus reduce the risk of heart and circulatory diseases and of cancer.

Ten Rules for Healthy Eating

By "good food" most people mean taste and enjoyment, by "good diet" they mean health and a good figure. However, food and diet are by no means opposites, and health and a good figure can very easily be combined with taste and enjoyment. The following points are based on DGE recommendations:

1. Variety – but not too much

As there are no foods containing an optimum combination of the required nutrients such as fat, protein, minerals, vitamins, water and fiber, the diet must include the required quantities of the various nutrient groups in order to guarantee optimal provision. The wheel of nutrition designed by the DGE provides an easily understandable overview, which combines all the information about the quantities of each foodstuff which should be consumed to achieve a balanced diet. Naturally each group contains some foodstuffs which have a higher rating from the point of view of physiological nourishment, and others which have a lower rating. So, in the group showing cereals and cereal products, we have a slice of wholemeal wheat bread, which is rated higher than a slice of toasted bread made from milled white flour. And a slice of dry turkey sausage is better, because of its lower fat content, than a slice of salami.

2. Less fat and fatty foods

Pay special attention to the so-called hidden fat. This includes for example fat in meat, delicatessen meats, cheese, eggs, nuts, cakes, chocolate, etc. Make sure that this hidden fat amounts to no more than 30 to 40 grams a day. To get a feeling for how much fat is hidden, we recommend that you carry out checks to assess this over a few days. This way, you will have information not just on how high your daily energy intake is and how high your fat consumption is, you will also learn whether the combinations of the main nutrients meets the recommendations.

3. Spicy but not salty

Your sense of taste will very quickly get used to salty food. If you start eating very salty food for a few days you will then find food with a normal amount of salt very tasteless. At the moment many populations use on average twice as much salt as recommended, that is, ten grams of cooking salt instead of five grams per day. There are now questions about whether some people are more susceptible to increased blood pressure and therefore increased risk of heart attacks, possibly as an undesirable side-effect of this high intake of cooking salt. Most cheeses, preserves, prepared dishes, snacks, delicatessen meats, cooking aids such as stock cubes, mustard and concentrates are particularly salty. On the other hand, there is very little salt in milk, yogurt, fresh vegetables, meat and herbs. Use fresh herbs for taste. Only add salt after tasting: if there is an iodine deficiency, the use of iodine salt is recommended since this can help to prevent iodine deficiency. In any case, our sense of taste changes after a few weeks of low-salt diet, so that we will then experience low-salt foods as pleasantly spicy.

4. Not much sweet food

Just as we can form a certain threshold of acceptability for salty food, so too can we for sweet food. A certain dependency on sweet things can develop in this way. While they have a relatively high energy content, sweets have a relatively low nutritional value. Simple sugars and refined sugars are frequently combined with saturated fats. Especially sticky sweets, such as candy, bonbons and pralines, etc., threaten dental health by forming caries. Anyone who eats sweets regularly is absorbing too much energy and is giving up nutritious foods in exchange for sweets with little nutritional value. This, of course, means that the body will be provided with fewer of the nutrients it needs to survive. In addition, sweets offer absolutely no way out of this situation. Even if they contain no energy themselves, they are first of all contributing to raising the level of the sweetness threshold for the sense of taste, and secondly they cannot satisfy the hunger for carbohydrates, because they do not contain any. This is how, when people are hungry and when the blood sugar level is low, they often consume more sweet foods than they actually need for their energy requirements. So if you feel like eating something sweet, you should have some fresh or dried fruit.

5. More wholemeal products

The consumption of products manufactured from milled white flour mainly reduces the quantities of fiber, vitamins and minerals consumed. These elements, contained in the external layers of whole wheat, are mostly lost when it is milled. As the fiber intake of many people is less than the recommended 30 grams, and as the provision of the B-vitamins and certain minerals is not always guaranteed, we should not do without the benefit of wholemeal products in our diets.

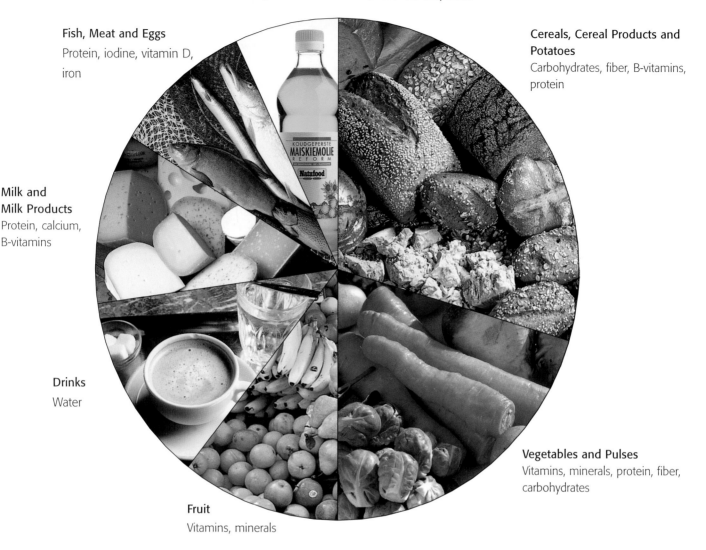

Fats and Oils
Fat, fat-soluble vitamins, essential fatty acids

Fish, Meat and Eggs
Protein, iodine, vitamin D, iron

Cereals, Cereal Products and Potatoes
Carbohydrates, fiber, B-vitamins, protein

Milk and Milk Products
Protein, calcium, B-vitamins

Drinks
Water

Fruit
Vitamins, minerals

Vegetables and Pulses
Vitamins, minerals, protein, fiber, carbohydrates

6. A wealth of vegetables, potatoes and fruit

Fruit and vegetables contain mainly carbohydrates, which are supposed to supply more than half of the energy we consume every day. In addition to this, fruit and vegetables provide the body with fiber, vitamins, minerals and water. The high water and fiber content mean they have a relatively low energy content. Pulses – like potatoes – have, in addition to their particularly high fiber content, a very high protein content, the value of which is enhanced when combined with cereal or milk products. Even deep-frozen fruit and vegetables can be recommended if, as is now common practice, they are quick-frozen immediately after harvesting. This process preserves vitamins which are often lacking

The nutrion wheel shows the various food groups that should fulfil your daily energy needs. The individual segments indicate the recommended energy value of each group.

in fresh fruit and vegetables which have generally spent a few days in storage, which causes volatile vitamins to be lost on their way to the store.

7. Less animal protein

Even though animal protein generally has a higher biological rating than vegetable protein, that is, it is more easily utilized by the human organism, sources of animal protein do not only bring benefits. Apart from providing highly rated protein, meat, delicatessen meats and eggs also give us unwanted by-products such as saturated fats, cholesterol, purines (which can cause gout in high enough concentrations) and salt. This is why meat consumption should be restricted to two or three small portions (maximum 150 grams) per week. Even delicatessen meats (maximum 50 grams) and eggs should not be eaten more than two or three times a week. Instead of eating meat frequently, have saltwater fish twice a week. In addition to having a high protein content, this gives you large amounts of iodine, provided by hardly any other foods. If, in addition to this, you combine your vegetable protein sources with other protein-rich foods such as milk, milk products or cereals in your diet, you need not fear deficiencies in your protein supply, especially if you are involved in strength training.

8. Enlightened drinking

Drinking can provide the fastest energy replacement without any related feeling of satiation. As this energy has no parallel nutritional value, especially when it comes from lemonades and even alcoholic drinks, it is recommended to cut down on this type of drink as much as possible. In particular, alcohol, which in its pure form supplies about 7 kcals per gram, should never be used to quench your thirst. Not only do large quantities of alcohol have a negative effect on the reflexes and coordination, but if taken regularly, leads in the worst cases to an addiction and then also damages the internal organs such as the liver, kidneys, stomach and intestines, as well as the brain. Since about 1.5 liters of your liquid requirement should come from drinks, the ideal is to meet this need with mineral water and fruit teas. Even though they provide no energy, coffee and black tea can only cover the liquid requirement to a limited extent, as they contain stimulants in the form of caffeine and tea bromides, which can lead to a certain dependency. Fruit and vegetable juices should be watered down, where possible (at least 1:1). In this way, you will not only save a lot of energy: juices drunk like this are more easily absorbed by the body.

9. Smaller meals more often

Five smallish meals will not only crank up your metabolism, this will also mean that energy dips during the course of the day have a lesser effect on you (Figure 1). So have a second breakfast and an afternoon snack. But as a result, make your main meals smaller than usual so that your total energy intake does not exceed the required level. If your body weight is normal, you could even allow yourself a little late snack after supper.

10. Make tasty and nutritious food

Cook for as short a time as possible and with little water or fat, to preserve the nutrients and flavor of the food. Vitamins are partially soluble in water and are sensitive to heat, oxygen and

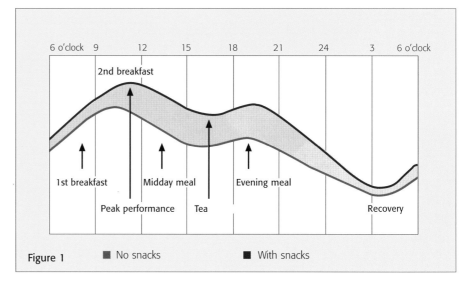

Figure 1   ■ No snacks   ■ With snacks

light. To preserve them, store your vegetables and fruit in a cool, dark place, use them as quickly as possible and never keep them warm for long. In addition, you should wash them before chopping and chop them coarsely so that the surfaces, which can lose nutrients, cover only a limited area. Minerals are also lost in water. Careful preparation not only attains positive results for the nutritional content; it also considerably improves the flavor.

Full Energy Foods

Using the aforementioned ground rules, the concept of full energy foods offers one or two additional ideas which look at nutrition above and beyond simply meeting our needs. Foods are divided into five levels, depending on your current condition. Full energy food is based on the following principles:

- Predominantly egg, milk and vegetable-based dishes.
- Foods from biologically controlled (ecological) farming are preferred.
- Nutritional value should be preserved by minimal preparation.
- Purified and refined products like sugar, refined flours and stimulants should be avoided.
- Specific foods are recommended instead of individual nutrients.

The concept of full energy food was formulated by Werner Kollath in 1942, who, in his book *Die Ordnung der Natur* (Nature's Order), proposed the precept that *food should be as natural as possible.* Kollath's theories were brought up-to-date and expanded by Koerber, Männle and Leitzmann in their book "Vollwert-Ernährung" (Full Energy Food). These basic principles seek to provide the body with all the basic nutritional substances, including some possibly essential nutrients which have not yet been identified. The body should keep healthy because the defense mechanisms against disease are then at their best and the conditions are provided for optimum development of physical and mental capacities. Full energy food aims at an ecologically sound lifestyle by avoiding the waste involved in refinement, by economizing energy and protecting the environmental. This means it is capable of providing long-term support for people following an improved lifestyle in industrial and developing countries – while simultaneously directly reducing costs to health services by reducing food-related diseases.

Food Ratings	
Level I	**Highly Recommended** Unadulterated foods: washed, chilled, hulled grain, peeled fruit
Level II	**Particularly Recommended** Processed foods: chopped, grated, sliced, shredded, milled, hulled, cold-pressed, processed with lactic bacteria
Level III	**Recommended** Heated foods: blanched and frozen, simmered in own juices, boiled, baked, pasteurized, hot-pressed, high-pressure pressed, separated, dried, homogenized, skimmed, smoked
Level IV	**Less Recommended** Processed foods: filtered, sieved (refined flours), polished (rice), fried, roasted, superheated, sterilized, preserved
Level V	**Not Recommended** Refined foods and products, for example, refined sugar.

An example of the waste involved in refinement is that, for instance, to produce animal-based foods like meat and milk, feed is used which could also be used directly to feed people, such as cereals and soy beans and other vegetable products. Currently between 65 and 90 per cent of the food energy and the proteins in vegetable feed plants is lost, since animals do not need most of the food energy for their own metabolism or for building non-meat producing tissue. If at least some of the cereals used for animal feed were used directly for human nutrition, many more people would be fed.

Food Supplements

It is not always easy, in some situations, to meet every nutritional requirement by consuming healthy or full energy foods. A high energy and nutrient requirement, especially in certain competitive sports, may cause serious problems for the competitor. Food intake can lead to serious technical problems, especially in endurance sports, which take several hours everyday over a period of several days.

Basically, there are two areas of application for food supplements. The first is where deficiency occurs. Under certain circumstances, such as during pregnancy or excessive physical exertion, specific individual nutrients or essential elements are provided after a deficiency of these specific substances has been diagnosed. The second area of application is the preventive use of individual nutrients or elements, or combinations of these.

To assess the sense of providing special nutrient compounds, we pose the question of whether a deficiency may not also be remedied by a change in the composition of the foods ingested every day. It is basically true that extra vitamins or minerals do not make a sports hero. Although advertising for these compounds tries to convince us that an excess of specific vitamins does have a particularly positive effect on our performance, the positive influence on performance of any particular substance only occurs when adequate supplies of this substance have not previously been present in the body. The conclusion that the symptoms caused by a deficiency of a specific substance in the body, for instance, tiredness due to a vitamin E deficiency, can be reversed by using a particularly high concentration of this substance is shown to be false, since, to stay with the same example, an excess of vitamin E does not make you particularly intelligent.

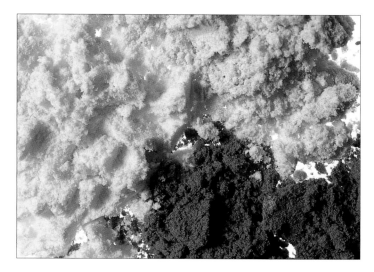

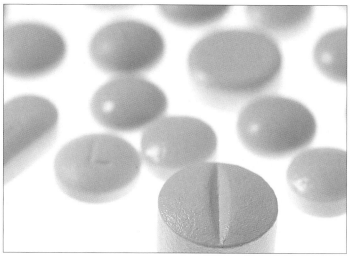

If specific substances are topped up, for example individual amino acids, vitamins, trace elements or minerals, this can prevent the absorption of essential nutrients from later meals and thus inhibit appropriate processing by the body. Thus for example, the essential amino acid tryptophane, which has been isolated and is given in the form of medication, has a tiring effect. However, when it is combined with the other essential amino acids, for instance in a meat dish, this effect is not noticeable. The reason for this is that tryptophane must access the brain through the so-called blood-brain gate in order to have a calming and tiring effect on the human organism. In this respect it acts as a precursor to serotonin. Serotonin is a chemical messenger which creates a relaxed mood and reduces the sensation of pain. But it is not only tryptophane that tries to reach the brain through the blood-brain gate: so do other amino acids which have no comparable biological effect. So long as the amino acids are all ingested together in foodstuffs, the concentration is balanced in such a way that only comparatively small quantities of tryptophane can be transformed into serotonin in the brain. Given in isolation, as medication, tryptophane no longer has competitors when accessing the brain through the blood-brain gate, so a true pharmacological effect becomes possible because of the ingestion of one single essential component of our food. We talk of a pharmacological effect when a different reaction occurs from what was originally intended.

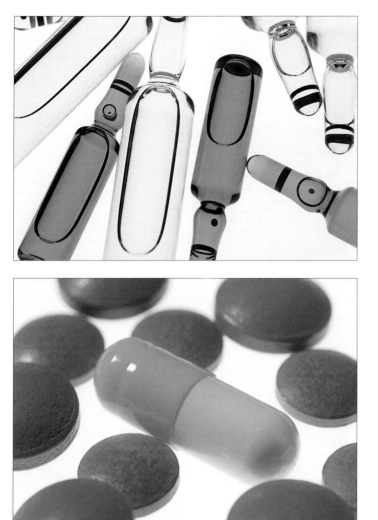

The craving for sweets with a low carbohydrate diet can also be explained by this mechanism. Because of the lack of sugar, very little insulin is released into the blood. This means that not so many of the "competitors" of tryptophane are stored in the cells and that larger quantities of them are available to compete for the blood-brain gate. Relatively speaking, the concentration of tryptophane is therefore lower. This means that in the brain, less serotonin is formed for lack of tryptophane. A serotonin deficiency of this type results in a depressed mood which provokes quite an intense desire for sugar. After a sugar-rich meal the mood improves appreciably, which naturally reflects a psychological as well as a biomedical process: I feel better when I eat something sweet.

As the biomedical effects of the various vital nutrients are only partially known, and biomedical processes generate a multiplicity of links and connections, the supply of isolated nutrients to enhance performance in sport is not to be recommended unless used specifically for intensive endurance trials.

It is only in competitive endurance sport that the use of energy and liquid supplements appears reasonable as current knowledge stands. Replenishing sugar stocks in the muscles and liquid and mineral supplies by means of natural foods is not as effective, especially during endurance trials lasting several hours, as it is with special concentrates. These consist of a combination of carbohydrates containing sugars with different chain lengths, so that absorption is staggered over time and a constant blood sugar level can be guaranteed. These – generally liquid – carbohydrate concentrates may be used to prevent a drop in performance if used before and during endurance trials lasting several hours. On the other hand, the supply of liquids and minerals can be complemented by the use of isotonic drinks.

The hope of achieving a specific performance goal with special dietary supplements has no foundation in science as it stands at present, and certainly not if the participant is already supplied with all the essential nutrients through a balanced, full energy daily diet. The belief that an excess of a specific nutrient reverses the symptoms caused by a deficiency of this substance is unfounded. Basically, a supplement with the specific nutrient can only be advantageous if there was a deficiency of that nutrient beforehand. In any case, this type of deficiency can be avoided by a balanced diet.

An old remedy for disturbed sleep, warm milk with honey, exploits the process by which the pancreas excretes insulin as an immediate response to the ingestion of short-chain sugar. Not only does the insulin enable the blood sugar to enter the cells, but also the long- and branch-chain neutral amino acids competing for entry to the brain through the blood-brain gate. The more these competitors to tryptophane are cleared away, the more serotonin can be formed in the brain from the tryptophane. As milk is naturally high in tryptophane and as honey contains high levels of simple and double sugars, the calming and sleep-inducing qualities of this home remedy are well founded from a biomedical point of view.

Sport, Nutrition and More

What is the use of knowing about the correct sports schedule and healthy, full energy food if everyday problems prevent us from putting them into practice? After a hard day's work many people have their tried and tested ways of finding relaxation and reward for the day's stress. These do in fact have the desired effect, often very quickly and reliably, but rarely lay the foundations for a healthy lifestyle and a good figure. Television and food (often snacks) are at the top of the list of relaxation and reward behavior, both of them happening simultaneously.

First of all, figure and even health problems start appearing, everyday patterns and leisure commitments make it particularly difficult to introduce new activities and a change in diet. Also, the change to a healthy, balanced diet and the introduction of a program of activities involves new obstacles in time management and organization. Planned organization of everyday activities and planned changes to one's usual "habits", therefore, form two more "pillars" for an effective weight reduction program.

Changing Behavior Patterns

The causes of weight problems are as numerous as they are specific: enjoyment, comfort, joie de vivre, sociability – but the search for security and protection can also be included. Some of these motives always have a social element. A change in eating patterns and new sports activities are meant to provide for this social aspect for example, by asking family, friends and colleagues for support but also stimulating them to join in when changing your own behavior patterns.

If you have established a plan to include your knowledge of healthy eating and the right activity into your everyday life, only one thing can now stop you: and that is you. To stimulate you in taking stock of all the small steps needed to embed the intended changes in your activities and eating habits into your everyday life, a few changes in behavior are recommended below. It would be almost impossible for anyone to implement

Organization

Perhaps the most important element of organizing is planning a time schedule. Almost every change to your current diet and activities first requires a change in schedule for your daily life. Whether it involves jogging in the park in the morning or preparing a snack, in every case some degree of planning is needed to change over to your new program. We recommend making a list of all your actions and activities, say for one week, to find out how much time you will have to make. Taking stock in this way could demonstrate to you which of your usual activities you could cut down and which everyday tasks could be passed to someone else – perhaps for payment. During the initial phase it would make perfect sense to include fixed times for the sports program, and also for food preparation. This makes it easier to change over to a newly structured everyday schedule, where sport has a firm place. As already mentioned for the training program at the beginning of the book, when you re-organize all your everyday activities to achieve your new goals, we recommend you set out the current and required status, and make regular checks on your progress (see chapter on *Training Guide*).

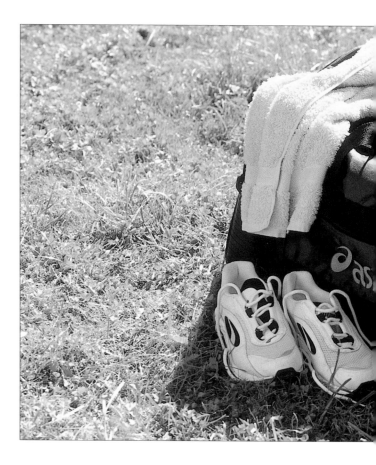

them all – the demands imposed by work, breaks, travelling, etc. are too great and too numerous. But this list can and should be adapted and amended to suit your individual needs:

- Give up using your car as often as possible, and walk or cycle.
- Use the stairs instead of the elevator.
- Plan your meals the day before.
- Never shop when you are hungry and always make a shopping list before you go.
- Only eat at set times.
- Drink a glass of water before your meal to satisfy you first hunger pangs.
- Take small bites and chew thoroughly.
- Have three main meals a day and two snacks between meals (fruit, yogurt, etc.).
- Learn to enjoy your food rather than just "ingesting" it.

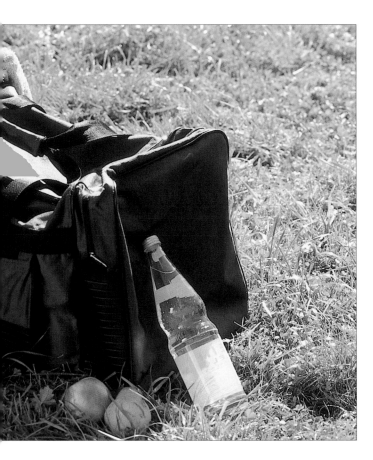

Unfortunately, we are often unaware of the main causes of overeating and excess weight. If, in spite of good intentions, you find it difficult to change your previous eating habits in the long term and to use the tips on changing your everyday habits, you may possibly have a subconscious resistance to this. So here is a final tip:

Do not aim too high, set yourself achievable targets. Do not get discouraged by setbacks, large or small. If weight reduction is very important to you, for health or psychological reasons, you should take the opportunity to seek help and advice from a specialist. A doctor or a dietary advisor may be helpful, or a psychologist, who is trained to recognize subconscious behavior patterns and to help you change them.

Weight Reduction – Conclusion

- Stimulate your metabolism by general physical activity, regular meals and muscle building.
- Be sure to observe the four principles of organization, nutrition, sport and psychology.
- If you are not in average condition for endurance training, exercise initially on the basis of pulse of 180 minus age, to improve your endurance performance.
- Continue your endurance training long enough to burn off fat (at least half an hour), at a uniform pace and not too intensively, that is, training at a pulse rate of 160 minus your age if your aerobic fitness is average.
- Plan a maximum body fat loss of about one pound per week, and to do this, reduce your energy intake by only about 500 kcals a day.
- Follow a mixed, low-fat, low-salt diet with not many sweets and more wholemeal products, vegetables, fruit and reduced animal protein, and have smaller meals. Have low-energy drinks and prepare tasty and nutritious meals.
- Cook your food as little as possible and only use food supplements in situations of extreme physical stress, for example during endurance trials lasting several hours.
- Plan your day in advance, so that you give yourself enough time for sport and preparation of your meals.

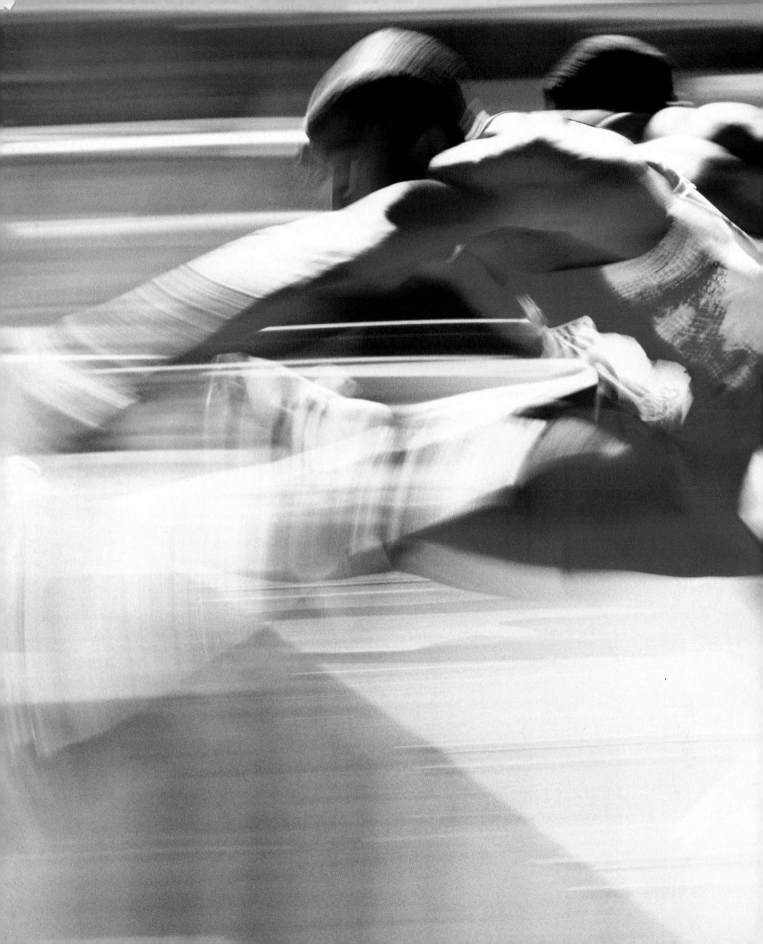

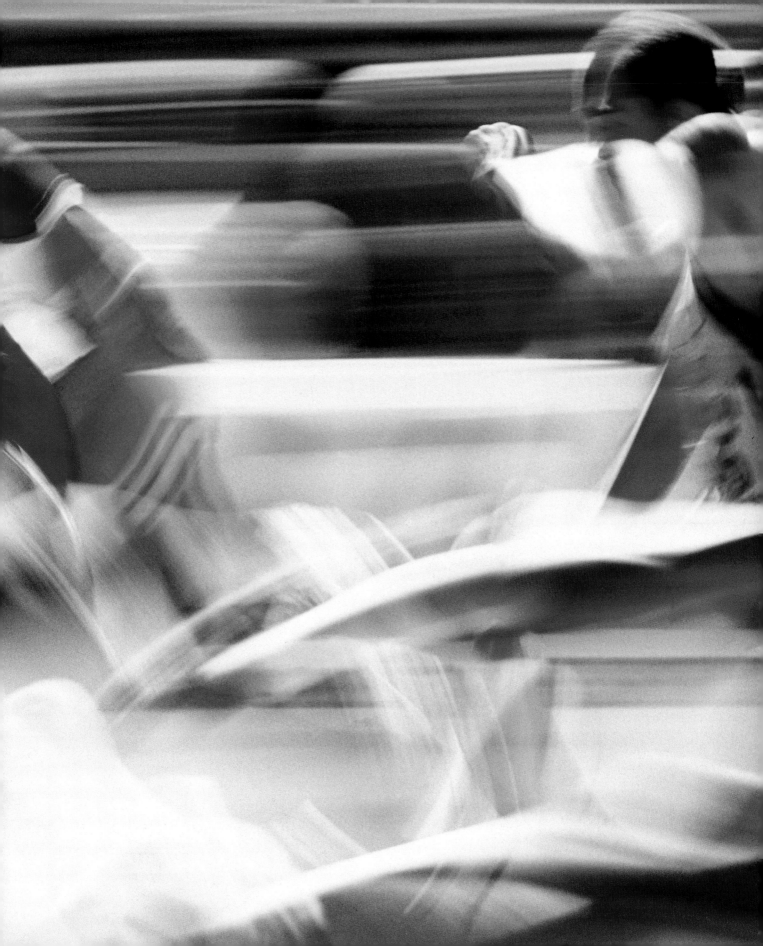

Anatomy

Besides improving the performance of various organs, the main reason people start fitness training is the desire to improve their external appearance. Of course, many characteristics of our appearance, such as body size or constitutional type, are determined by hereditary factors (see the chapter *Training Guide*), but nonetheless adults can change their appearance considerably through specific training. The outward signs of this are both a reduction in body fat and development of muscles.

Even though a fitness manual such as this cannot replace a competent trainer, and is not intended to, this chapter may help you to evolve your own functional understanding of the physical restraints involved in movement. In the long term, a basic grasp of them will make it easier not only to optimize your exercise technique but also to avoid applying effort incorrectly. This goes for strength exercises as much as for exercises which serve to improve mobility. Bearing that in mind, the outline of anatomy in this chapter is limited solely to the body parts of movement. First, the structure and function of the skeletal musculature and striated musculature are explained. Following that is an overview of the skeleton and description of the structure of the joints in a functional context as they relate to the knee joints and spinal column. Finally, selected basic biomechanical laws are explained by way of examples, to give the reader some idea of the forces involved in the body parts of motion.

Human Muscles

The special characteristic of muscle cells is their ability to contract. The skeletal musculature, also called the striated muscles, can be controlled voluntarily whereas the two other types of muscle tissue, the cardiac and smooth muscles, are not subject to brain control. The capacity of the muscle cells to contract is a result of the particular structure of muscles (see Fig. 1). The smallest elements of muscle cells, that is, the protein filaments, crowd together as they do.

The skeletal muscles that are important for motion in an adult make up about 40 to 45 per cent of total body mass; in other words a man weighing about 155 pounds carries around 66 pounds in muscle. As we age, the proportion of muscles to total weight

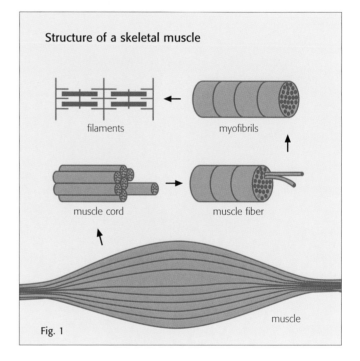

Structure of a skeletal muscle

filaments

myofibrils

muscle cord

muscle fiber

muscle

Fig. 1

changes, to the disadvantage of the muscles. Thus a 70-year-old man has a muscle weight of only 50 pounds. This degeneration of the muscles is more likely the consequence of inadequate use, including insufficient training stimuli, than of hormonal changes.

The functions of the motor muscles

Back and abdominal muscles form a muscular corset that helps stabilize the vertebral column and make an erect posture possible. It is quite obvious that this requires correspondingly powerful muscles. The functions of the motor musculature include stretching the spinal column as well as moving the shoulder blades and shoulder girdle. Other functions of the motor musculature include moving the upper extremities, bending sideways, rotating and curling up the trunk.

Functional units

As shown in the section on exercises for strength training, most movements involve several muscles. Human muscles can accordingly be divided up into a number of overlapping functional units. These units comprise:

- the arm and shoulder area
- the vertebral column in the head, neck and dorsal areas down to the fifth *thoracic vertebra*
- the dorsal vertebral column from the fifth to the twelfth thoracic vertebra and the lumbar-pelvis-hip area
- the lower part of the lumbar vertebral column and the joints of the hips, small of the back, ilium and legs.

Muscles of the arms, chest and shoulder are involved in movements of the arms (bending and stretching at the elbows, moving them sideways, fowards and backwards, lifting, dropping and rotating them). The leg and buttock muscles are especially important for pelvic posture, relieving strain on the hips and stabilizing the knee joints, for bending and stretching the hips and bending and stretching the knees. Lateral movements of the leg are also one of their functions, as is standing on tiptoes.

Consumption of energy

Whereas muscles need only a fifth of the energy you consume in a rest position, at the peak of sporting effort they can take up to 90 per cent of the total energy used. Sports training is therefore the option to choose not only to maintain mobility but also to control your weight. This is due to the fact that if

muscle tissue is increased by training, such as in weight training, this has an increased activation effect on your metabolism, even in a rest position.

Overview of the skeletal muscles

The following is only a small selection of over 400 skeletal muscles and is no way comprehensive. The assignment of the muscles described on the following pages is not always clearcut, as several of the muscles depicted are attached to several joints, that is, at least two joints. A selection of the muscles depicted is explained with their origin, insertion and function.

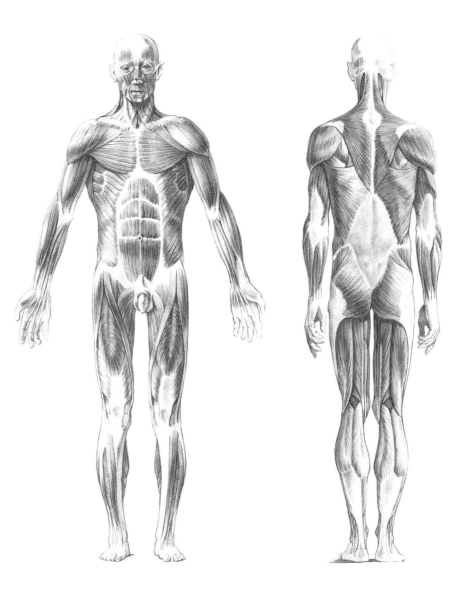

Muscles of the Shoulder Joint

1 M. latissimus dorsi
- Origin: Originates over lumbo-dorsal fascia on the spines of lower six thoracic vertebrae and lumbar vertebrae, small of back and iliac crest.

- Insertion: Intertubercular sulcus of humerus.
- Functions: Lowers raised arm, turns dangling arm inwards and pulls it backwards. Also adducts arms in *lateral hold* position.

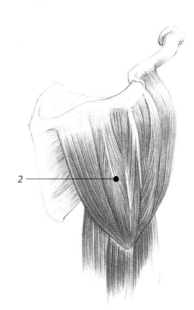

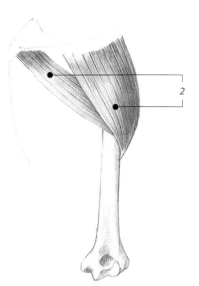

2 Deltoid muscle – *m. deltoideus*
- Origin: Divided into three parts which originate from the collar bone, top of shoulder and shoulder blade.
- Insertion: Deltoid tuberosity of humerus.
- Functions: The front part of the deltoid muscle raises the arm forwards and rotates it inwards. The rear part raises the arm backwards, the center part lifts the arm sideways. Besides these dynamic functions, the deltoid muscle helps substantially towards stabilizing the shoulder joint.

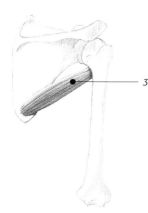

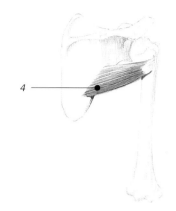

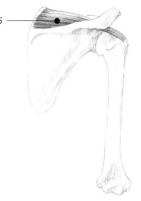

3 M. teres major

- Origin: Lower outer third of shoulder blade.
- Insertion: Intertubercular sulcus of humerus.
- Functions: Teres major adducts the arm, turns it inwards and pulls a raised arm downwards and backwards.

4 M. teres minor

- Origin: Shoulder blade.
- Insertion: Greater tubercle of humerus.
- Functions: Teres minor adducts the humerus, rotates it outwards and pulls a raised arm downwards and backwards.

5 Supraspinous muscle –
m. supraspinatus

- Origin: Supraspinous fossa in shoulder blade.
- Insertion: Greater tubercle of humerus, upper facet of outer rotator flap.
- Functions: Extends arm and rotates it outwards from rear.

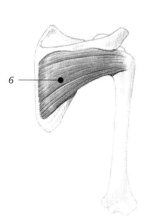

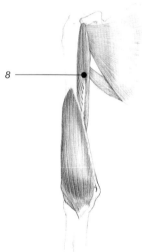

6 Infraspinous muscle –
m. infraspinatus

- Origin: Infraspinous fossa of shoulder blade.
- Insertion: Greater tubercle of humerus.
- Functions: Extends the arm with its upper fiber parts and draws it in with the lower ones. Also rotates arm outwards.

7 Subscapular muscle –
m. subscapularis

- Origin: Rib side of shoulder blade.
- Insertion: Lesser tubercle of humerus.
- Functions: Rotates humerus inwards and draws raised arm downwards. Abducts the humerus with upper fiber parts, and adducts it with the lower ones.

8 Coracobrachial muscle –
m. coracobrachialis

- Origin: Coracoid process of shoulder blade.
- Insertion: Front and inner proximal base of humerus.
- Functions: Adducts the raised arm and rotates it inwards.

Muscles of the Shoulder Joint

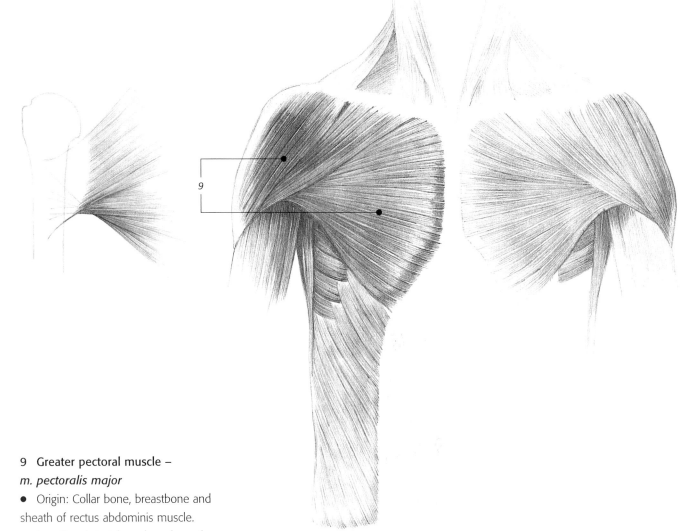

9 Greater pectoral muscle –
m. pectoralis major

- Origin: Collar bone, breastbone and sheath of rectus abdominis muscle.
- Insertion: Intertubercular sulcus of humerus.
- Functions: Enables forward movement of arm raised laterally backwards. Also causes arm to rotate inwards.

Muscles of the Shoulder Girdle

10 Rhomboid muscles – *m. rhomboideus*

- Origin: Most originate from spines of top four dorsal vertebrae, while the rest originate from the spines of the lower two cervical vertebrae.
- Insertion: Inner margin of shoulder blade.
- Function: Draws shoulder blade upwards to vertebral column.

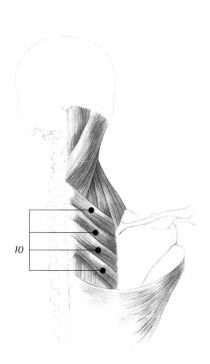

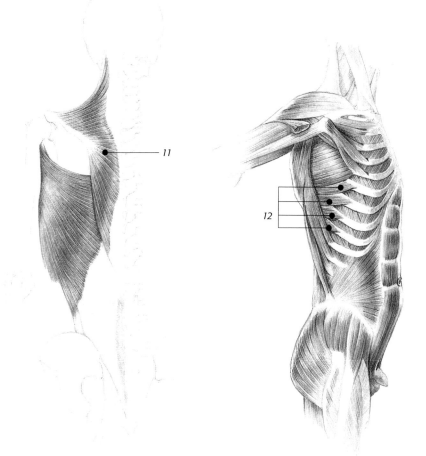

11 M. trapezius

- Origin: Occipital bone, spines of cervical and dorsal vertebrae.
- Insertion: Collar bone, top of shoulder, spine of shoulder blade.
- Functions: The upper part of the trapezius draws the shoulders upwards, lifts the collar bone, and in the case of unbalanced contraction turns the head towards the opposite side. It also supports the rotation of the shoulder blade. The medial oblique part pulls the shoulderblades together towards the spine, while the lower part lowers the shoulders and rotates the shoulder blade.

12 Anterior serratus muscle – *m. serratus anterior*

- Origin: Ribs 1–9.
- Insertion: Inner margin of shoulder blade and upper and lower shoulder blade angle.
- Functions: Attaches shoulder blade to trunk. The upper part serves to lift the shoulder blade, while the lower part draws the lower shoulder blade angle forwards. With a locked shoulder blade, anterior serratus muscle supports breathing by lifting the ribs.

Elbow Muscles

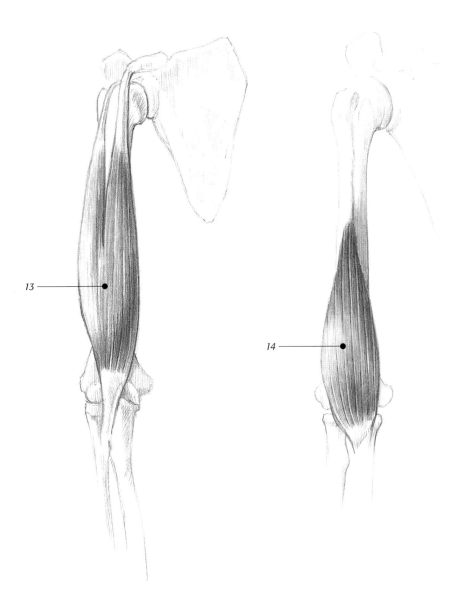

15 Brachioradial muscle –
m. brachioradialis

- Origin: Lateral ridge of humerus.
- Insertion: Lower end of radius.
- Function: Bends the arm at the elbow.

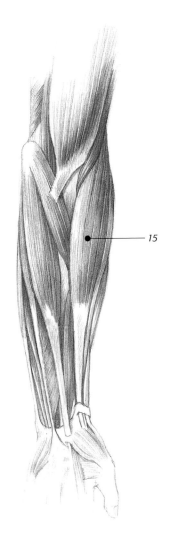

13 Biceps muscle – *m. biceps brachii*
- Origin: The short head of the biceps (arm) muscle originates at the tip of the coracoid process of the shoulder blade, the long head at its supraglenoid tubercle.
- Insertion: Tuberosity of radius.
- Functions: Bends the arm at the elbow, rotates the under arm outwards and moves the arm forwards at the shoulder joint.

14 Brachial muscle – *m. brachialis*
- Origin: Distal anterior aspect of humerus.
- Insertion: Coronoid process of ulna.
- Function: Bends the forearm at the elbow.

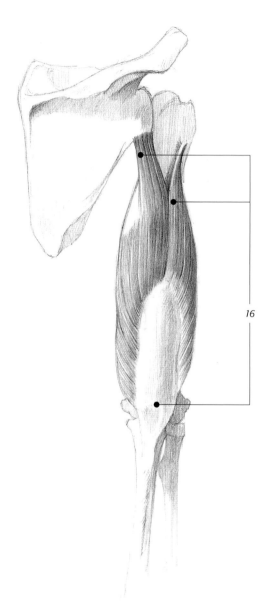

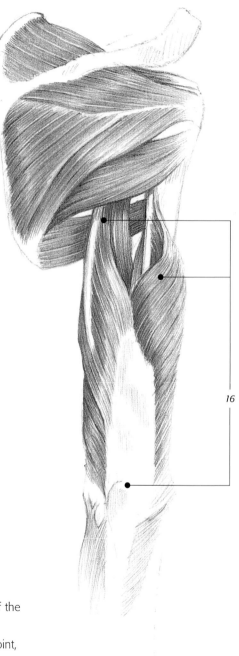

16 Triceps – *m. triceps brachii*
(left: lower layer, right: medial layer)

● Origin: The long head originates at the tubercle under the shoulder joint socket, the lateral and medial heads at the rear aspect of the humerus.

● Insertion: Large upper process of the ulna.

● Functions: Stretches the elbow joint, and with the long head moves the arm backwards in the shoulder joint.

The Wrist Muscles

17 Radial flexor muscle –
m. flexor carpi radialis,
18 Ulnar flexor muscle –
m. flexor carpi ulnaris

- Origin: Radialis originates at the inner epicondyle of the humerus, while ulnaris originates as a two-headed muscle, with one head at the inner epicondyle of the humerus, the other at the large upper process of the ulna.

- Insertion: Radialis at the base of the metacarpal of the index finger, ulnaris at the base of the metacarpal of the little finger.
- Function: Main function is to flex the wrist.

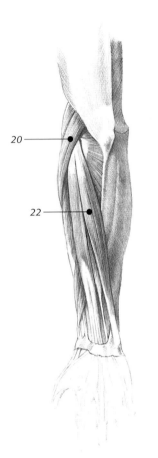

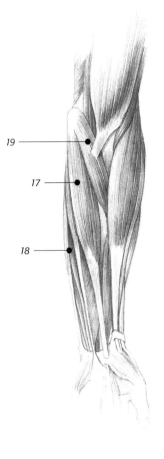

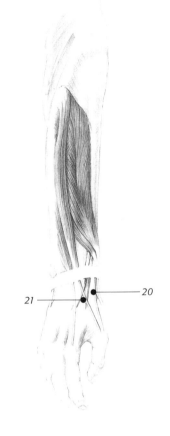

19 M. pronator teres
- Origin: Originates at the joint epicondyle of the humerus and the coronoid of the ulna.
- Insertion: Medial third of the radius.
- Functions: Supports the flexing of the arm at the elbow and rotates the forearm inwards in turning the flat of the hand downwards and the back of the hand upwards.

20 Long radial extensor muscle –
m. extensor carpi radialis longus,
21 Short radial extensor muscle –
m. extensor carpi radialis brevis,
22 Ulnar extensor muscle –
m. extensor carpi ulnaris
- Origin: Radialis longus, radialis brevis and ulnaris originate on lateral epicondyle of humerus.

- Insertion: Longus at the base of the index finger metacarpal, brevis at the base of middle finger metacarpal and ulnaris at the base of the little finger metacarpal.
- Functions: Besides extending the wrist, they draw the thumb side of the hand towards the radius – they abduct the hand to the radius.

Muscles around the Vertebral Column

23 Internal oblique abdominal muscle –
m. obliquus internus abdominis
- Origin: Iliac crest, inguinal ligament, lumbodorsal fascia.
- Insertion: Ribs 9–12, linea alba.
- Functions: When fully contracted, supports the trunk in bending forwards; when laterally contracted, turns the trunk sideways, tensing one side.

24 Straight abdominal muscle –
m. rectus abdominis
- Origin: Pubis.
- Insertion: Rib cartilages 5–7, xiphoid process of sternum.
- Functions: With locked pelvis, rectus abdominis draws the trunk forwards; with the thorax locked, it lifts the pelvis.

25 Quadrate lumbar muscle –
m. quadratus lumborum
(not illustrated)
- Origin: Iliac crest.
- Insertion: Rib 12, oblique processes of lumbar vertebrae.
- Functions: Draws the trunk backwards if it tenses overall. If only one side contracts, it bends the trunk to the side.

26 Oblique external abdominal muscle –
m. obliquus externus abdominus
- Origin: Exterior aspect of ribs 5–12.
- Insertion: Iliac crest, inguinal ligament, pubic tubercle, linea alba.
- Functions: When fully contracted, supports the trunk in leaning forwards, when contracted only on one side, twists the trunk to the opposite side, i.e. the right oblique external abdominal muscle turns the trunk to the left, and vice versa.

The Hip Joint Muscles

27 M. iliopsoas
- Origin: Consists of the psoas muscle, which originates at the last thoracic vertebra, lumbar vertebrae 1–4 and the rib processes, and the iliac muscle, which originates at the iliac fossa and sacrum.
- Insertion: Lesser trochanter of femur.
- Functions: Bends the hips, i.e. moves the leg forwards, inwards and rotates it outwards.

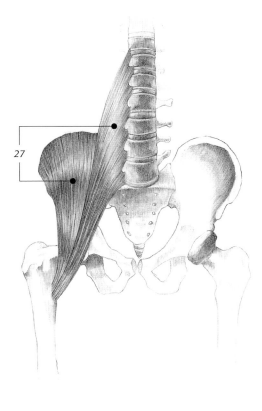

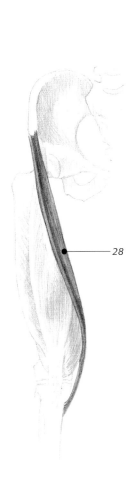

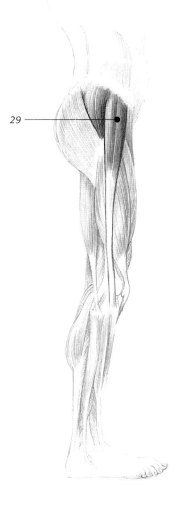

28 Tailor's muscle – *m. sartorius*
- Origin: Anterior inferior iliac spine.
- Insertion: Inner margin of shinbone tuberosity.
- Function: Sartorius flexes both at hip and knee joints. It extends the thigh and rotates it outwards. When the knee joint is bent, it also bends the lower leg inwards. At approximately one foot seven inches in length, it is the longest human muscle.

29 M. tensor fasciae latae
- Origin: Anterior upper iliac spine.
- Insertion: Iliotibial tract.
- Functions: The tensor flexes the hips and extends the thigh.

30 M. pectineus

- Origin: Pubic crest.
- Insertion: Pectineal line of thigh.
- Functions: Pectineus draws the thigh inwards and helps with flexing and rotation of hip joint.

31 Short adductor muscle –
m. adductor brevis

- Origin: Lower pubic ramus.
- Insertion: Proximal part of linea aspera.
- Functions: Draws the thigh to the middle and rotates it outwards.

32 Long adductor muscle –
m. adductor longus

- Origin: Below the pubic tuber.
- Insertion: Middle third of medial linea aspera.
- Functions: Adducts the thigh and helps to bend the hip joint.

33 Greater adductor muscle –
m. adductor magnus

- Origin: Ischial ramus and lower margin of ischial tuber.
- Insertion: Partly to medial labium of linea aspera, partly to inner femur tuber.
- Functions: Adducts the thigh and rotates it inwards.

34 M. gracilis

- Origin: Margin of lower pubic ramus.
- Insertion: Inner margin of tibia.
- Functions: Draws the thigh to the middle and helps with bending the knees and inwards rotation of thigh.

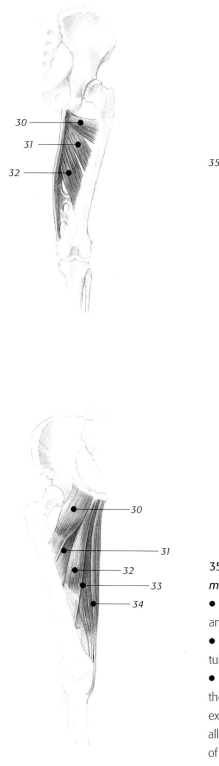

35 Greatest gluteal muscle –
m. gluteus maximus

- Origin: Ligament of ilium, small of back and coccyx.
- Insertion: Fascia of thigh, gluteal tuberosity of femur.
- Functions: The main function is to stretch the hip joint. Also, upper part of muscle extends leg, lower part draws it in. Additionally it rotates the thigh outwards. It is one of the most powerful human muscles.

The Knee Muscles

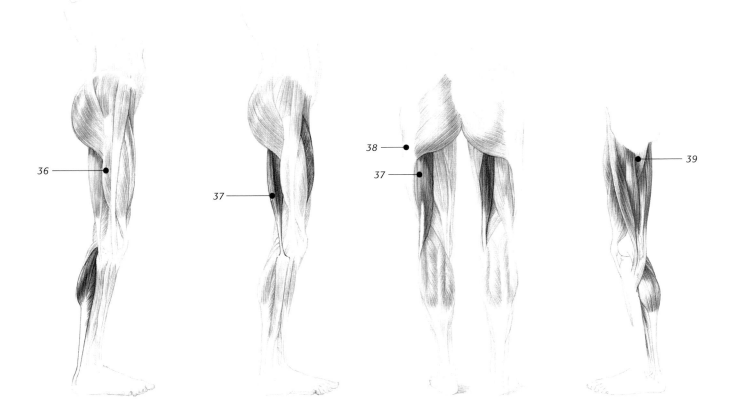

36 Large extensor thigh muscle –
m. quadriceps femoris
- Origin: One part *(m. rectus femoris)* of the four-headed quadriceps femoris originates at the anterior lower iliac spine and anterior margin of the hip joint socket. The three other parts *(Mm. medialis, lateralis and intermedius)* originate at different locations of the thigh.
- Insertion: Over the patella into the tubercle of the tibia.
- Functions: Extends the knee joint and flexes with the rectus femoris and also the hip joint. This muscle counts as the largest and most powerful human muscle.

37 Biceps muscle of the thigh –
m. biceps femoris
- Origin: The long head starts at the ischial tuber, the short head at the linea aspera of the femur.
- Insertion: Head of fibula.
- Functions: When the leg is stretched out, it supports the flexing of the hips, bends the knee joint and rotates the bent lower leg outwards. Together with *m. semitendinosus* and *m. semimembranosus, m. biceps femoris* forms a group of muscles called ischiocrural muscles.

38 M. semitendinosus
- Origin: Ischial tuber.
- Insertion: Medial aspect of tibial tuberosity.
- Functions: When leg is outstretched, supports bending of the hip, bends the knee joint and twists the bent lower leg inwards.

39 M. semimembranosus
- Origin: Ischial tuber.
- Insertion: Medial condyle of tibia.
- Functions: Supports bending of hip when leg is outstretched, bends the knee joint and twists the bent lower leg inwards. *M. semimembranosus* lies beneath *m. semitendinosus* and is somewhat stronger.

Ankle Muscles

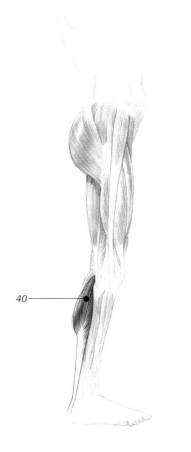

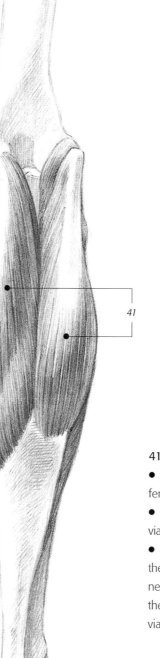

40 M. soleus

- Origin: Fibula head, rear aspect of tibia and fibula.
- Insertion: Posterior surface of calceneus via Achilles tendon.
- Functions: Flexes the ankle.

41 M. gastrocnemius

- Origin: Lateral and medial condyle of femur.
- Insertion: Posterior surface of calceneus via Achilles tendon.
- Functions: Flexes the ankle and bends the knee joint. Together with soleus beneath it, it is also known as triceps sirae, as the insertion of both is at the calceneus via the Achilles tendon.

The Human Skeleton

The human skeleton is made up of more than 200 bones (see below) which are joined by elastic connective tissue. Together with the muscles and ligaments, the human skeleton gives the body support and stability. At the same time, it also makes mobility possible, providing leverage for the inserted muscles. In addition, the protective function of certain bones is immediately obvious, as for example in the protection of the brain by the skull.

The vertebral column

Thanks to its double S-curve, the vertebral column of the human body, as seen from the side, operates like a huge shock absorber (see bottom right). And that is precisely what constitutes the main function of the in-and-out curves of the vertebral column. The vertebral column consists of 24 mobile vertebrae that have grown together, and nine or ten vertebrae ossified together. The basic structure of a vertebra cannot be distinguished in the vertebrae of the small of the back and coccyx, which have firmly grown together, but is clearly visible in the area of the five lumbar, twelve dorsal and seven cervical vertebrae.

The vertebral bodies, between which the intervertebral disks lie, are continued to the rear in the vertebral arches. Whereas the vertebral bodies form the pillars of the spinal column, the vertebral foramen between the vertebral arches and vertebral bodies provides space for the nerve fibers of the spinal cord. The vertebral arch goes right and left into the two transverse processes and to the rear into the spine process (see left cross-section, opposite page).

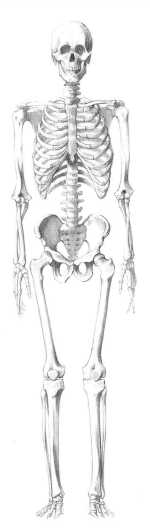
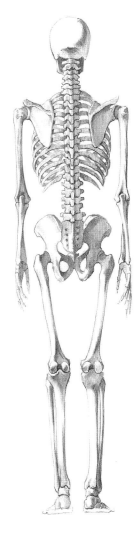
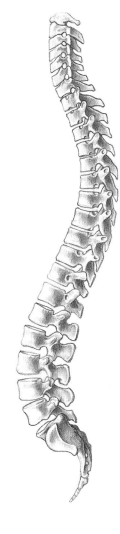

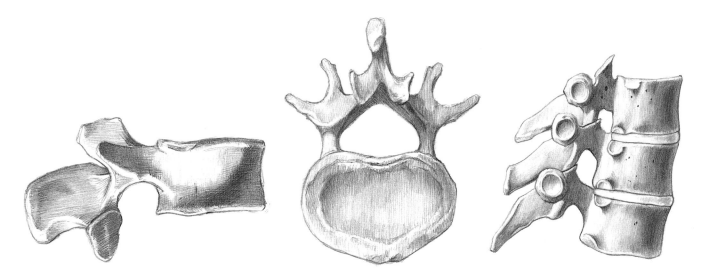

The insertion of the various muscles of the back extensors is in these processes, which is how they support the active mobility of the vertberal column. The intervertebral foramina are formed between the proximal vertebral arches of two superimposed vertebral bodies, to serve the passage of the spinal nerves (see above). If the intervertebral foramina are constricted by damage to the intervertebral disks or by changes to the bone structure induced by illness or injury, this can result in injuries to or disorders in the protruding nerves, which can take the form of lumbago or sciatica.

The intervertebral disks in the spinal column constitute especially striking structures (Fig. 2). They are fibrocartilageous disks containing a jelly-like core, which moves aside under any pressure exerted unequally on the disk from above or below. The intervertebral disks can withstand great forces exerted on the axis of the vertebral column. However, if a great load is exerted in a round back posture, the core of the disk is pressed strongly backwards, in the direction of the spinal cord. In this posterior area high tractive forces arise (T) whereas in the anterior area proximal to the abdomen the fiber rings of the intervertebral disks can be highly compressed (C). The worst consequence of such misdirected effort is a slipped disk. This involves a rupture of the fiber rings of the disk in the posterior area near the spinal cord such that the core of the disk presses on the spinal cord. For this reason, doing strengthening exercises with a round back is always insistently advised against. Only in the natural fluid pose on its normal axis can the vertebral column accept even great loads without difficulty. Deviations from the "normal" shape of the vertebral column – or variants from the norm – should be watched for in training, just like illnesses involving the vertebral column. If your mobility system shows chronic problems, you should consult a doctor and physiotherapist before starting training, to discuss how far particular exercises are sensible, worth concentrating on or are to be avoided. Only when no more problems crop up should you plan your training on your own.

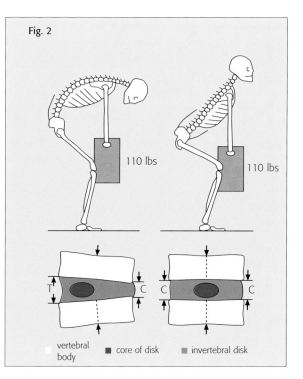

Fig. 2

110 lbs

110 lbs

T   C   C   C

vertebral body   ■ core of disk   ■ invertebral disk

The Joints

Bones that are firmly linked preserve the stability of the skeletal system. They have no, or very little, influence on the mobility of the body. Such firm links between two bones are found for example between the tibia and the fibula, in the form of very taut cartilage, or between the two halves of the pubic bone in the form of fibrous cartilage, or between the sacral vertebrae and the coccyx as ossification.

The joints, as moving interfaces between two bones, are especially important for an appreciation of movement and the functional links. Distinctions are made between joints having one, two or three axes and a varying range of movement. Ignoring the multiplicity of forms and greatly differing range of movement, all real (i.e. moving) joints display a certain basic type (Fig. 3).

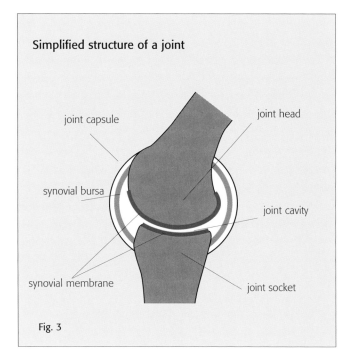

Simplified structure of a joint

joint capsule

joint head

synovial bursa

joint cavity

synovial membrane

joint socket

Fig. 3

The synovial membrane serves not only as a buffer in the case of compressive forces, but also considerably reduces the friction between the two moving ends of the bones. The synovial fluid, which fills up the joint cavity between the two opposed membranous layers as lubrication, is formed in the synovial bursa of the joint capsule. It is soaked up by the membrane, particularly in the alternation between pressure and suction forces, thus thickening the buffer zone and nourishing the cartilaginous tissue.

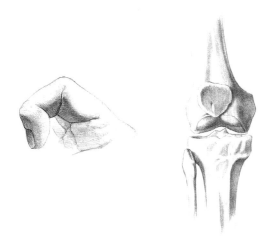

Functional Movements

From a health point of view, the functionality of movements should be watched in any sporting activity. This means keeping in mind what movements the joints can make, what the muscles involved are for and what the exercise is intended to achieve. Muscular dysbalances resulting from changes should also be taken into account. Moreover, the biomechanical structure of the muscles should be considered: as one group of muscles is intended more for active movements whereas another is mainly for support purposes, this orientation should be borne in mind in the choice of training methods. The inappropriate matching of dynamic structures and discrepant training methods always represents a health risk just as much as ignoring functional connections. This should become apparent in the following description of one particular joint.

The Knee Joint

We generally only become aware of a particular joint when it demands our attention in some painful way or other. The knee joint is the most common offender in this respect. It is not only the largest and most complicated joint in the human body, but also the most sensitive. Within the knee joint, there are a number of unique structures that distinguish it from the basic type of joint. The most obvious of these are the kneecap and the menisci. The following explanation should enable you to treat this important joint with the consideration it needs, because, like the spine, it can be at risk from badly executed exercises.

The special structure of the knee joint is a result of the two different functions it has to fulfill. On the one hand, it has to ensure the stable support function of the leg in an outstretched position, while on the other hand it has to facilitate mobility in a bent position. As in the former outstretched position where over 90 per cent of the body's weight rests on the knees, the special structure of the knees ensures a particularly large contact surface between the femur and the tibia, in order to distribute the pressure over as large a surface as possible. It is in this outstretched position that the importance of the menisci becomes most apparent. Connected with the tibia, they even out the unevenness of shape between the femur and the tibia. As a thick fibrous wedge of cartilage, the menisci represent an outstanding additional buffer between the two joint ends. In view of the great weight imposed on the knee joint from above, they make a substantial contribution towards sparing and relieving the synovial membrane. From the outstretched position, the knee can only be stretched or bent, which provides the additional stability required.

In the bent position, the contact surface of the knee joint is clearly reduced by the sharp curve in the posterior area of the synovial membrane of the femur. In the bent position, the knee can be not only bent or stretched but also rotated. This appears sensible because the knee does not usually have to carry the weight of the body in bent position, and such a great freedom of movement is here an advantageous replacement of high stability.

The kneecap (patella) constitutes the most striking peculiarity of the knee joint. It is a bone firmly embedded in the femoral extensor tendon, and serves important functions beside the mechanically protective one. Thus the force of the femoral extensor muscles is provided with goal-oriented guidance, as the kneecap fits very closely in the indentation between the lateral and medial condyle of the femur. Likewise the corresponding leverage for the force of the femoral extensor is improved by the kneecap, as the insertion tendon of the muscle is moved further from the point of rotation of the knee joint thereby.

The kneecap also forms an important factor in stopping a knee-bending movement, in which it acts like a brake block (Fig. 4). The greater the force the femoral extensor exerts on the kneecap, or the more abruptly a movement is braked, the greater is the force between the inside of the kneecap and condyle of the femur. This of course puts the cartilage under greater pressure. An

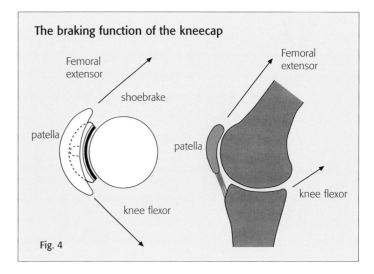

The braking function of the kneecap

Femoral extensor

shoebrake

patella

knee flexor

Femoral extensor

patella

knee flexor

Fig. 4

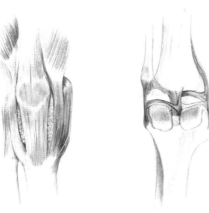

additional factor is that, if the knee is bent at more than 90 degrees, the kneecap largely loses contact with the medial condyle, so that practically all the pressure is now distributed between the lateral part of the kneecap cartilage and the cartilage of the exterior joint condyle. This, and the circumstance that the braking force of the kneecap at an angle of over 90 degrees is effected wholly in the joint, whereas with smaller angles the effect is carried past the joint, leads to the conclusion that in strengthening exercises involving knee stretch – as for example in exercises S43–S46 described in *Strength Training* (Knee Bend, Frontal Knee Bend, Leg Press-Ups, Leg Stretch – an angle of 90 degrees should not be exceeded.

Biomechanics

Every sporting movement involves numerous different forces which are subject to certain laws. A rough grasp of, and taking due note of, these laws will ensure that not only your strength training is easy on your joints but your endurance training is energy saving. It will also help you to recognize to some extent unusual strains exerted on the passive motor system during certain lift techniques and thereby avoid incorrect movements.

The diagram below shows how expenditure of energy is determined by the proximity of the weight to be lifted from the initial position. The forces are shown as arrows, which also indicate the size and direction of the force. A weight of roughly 22 pounds is thus subject to a gravity of about 100 Newtons. The Newton unit is a measure of force, and when directed vertically downwards the force expressed in Newtons is always ten times the relevant weight. If a force operates on a point from a given distance, torque is exercised on it. The torque is thus the product of the effective force and the length of the lift. If two forces from opposite directions operate on a point, they stand in balance if the product of the length of the lifting arm and the force is equal.

As the torque with an unchanged load and longer lift gets greater and greater, the load on the structures concerned also increases. The consequence for both strength and endurance training is that weights moved or parts of body moved should be as close to the body as possible, partly in order not to overstrain the kinesthetic system and partly to save energy.

In an erect, immobile body there are a multiplicity of levers and forces which must ultimately be in balance so that the body does not move. In every immobile body there is a point where it can be hung up so that, however it is rotated from this point, it will always be in balance. This is the center of gravity. The upper body's center of gravity lies in its dynamic effect line in front of the spinal column, which, depending on the type of physique, is more or less far in front of the hip joint. This means that, to stand erect, the back extensor muscles and gluteal muscles are needed to generate an immobile balance (Fig. 6). If the center of gravity moves forwards when the upper body is bent forwards at the hip joint, the forces required to maintain balance rise to a multiple of the original value.

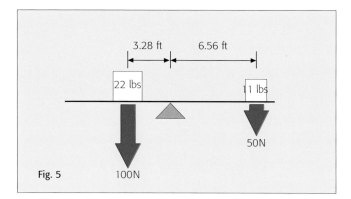

Fig. 5

Above: The balance of forces of two different loads. Being at different distances from the pivotal point, they develop different torque. The product (force × distance from pivot) is equal, e.g. 100 Newtons × 3.28 ft = 50 Newtons × 6.56 ft.

Right: The energy used by the back muscles for establishing balance at the center of gravity: if the center of gravity of the upper body as pivot is thrice as far from the vertebral bodies as the distance of the back muscles behind the pivotal point, the tractive power of the back muscles must be thrice as large as the weight of the upper body.

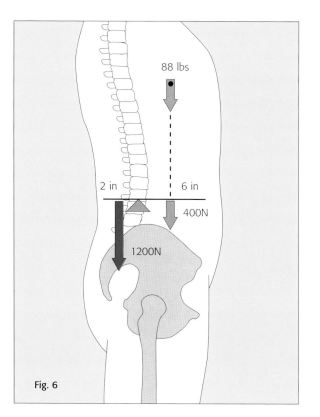

Fig. 6

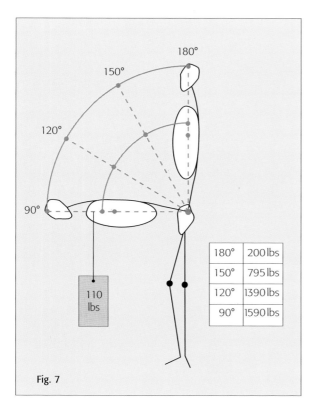

180°	200 lbs
150°	795 lbs
120°	1390 lbs
90°	1590 lbs

Fig. 7

Above: The load on the lumbar vertebral column when holding a weight at various angles of the spinal column.

Below: Sundry joint loadings on the shoulder and elbow with various lift techniques following a shift in the center of gravity of the weight.

To be able to judge which muscles are greatly or less greatly involved, biomechanical awareness is necessary as well as an understanding of the insertion and origin of musculature. Particularly central to the former are the concepts of torque and center of gravity presented here, together with the laws of lifting derived from them. If for example one lifts a weight by bending the forearm at the elbow, the strength with which individual muscles are involved in the movement varies according to the technique used to lift the weight. If the elbow moves backwards while lifting the load (Fig. 8a), the load arm between the dynamic effect line of the weight (passing directly under the shoulder joint) and the pivotal point in the elbow is shortened. In this lifting technique, the arm-bending muscles are less strained by the relatively shorter lift as in the diagram beside it (Fig. 8b.). In the latter case, not only is the lift clearly longer between the elbow and the weight, the strain on the shoulder joint is also clearly higher because a longer load arm lies between the center of gravity in the weight and the pivot in the shoulder, whereby greater torque is effected in the shoulder joint. In the first picture on the other hand, the center of gravity of the weight lies just beneath the pivot of the shoulder, so that the torque, and therefore also its load, is virtually zero. If on the other hand the upper arm rests on an inclined cushion (Scott-curl), the arm flexor muscles are indeed maximally loaded, but at the same time the shoulder muscles and joint are relieved by locking the body and body support (Fig. 8c). As this example shows, a biomechanical understanding can help the trainer, when comparing other exercises as well, choose the exercise best suited for the given training task.

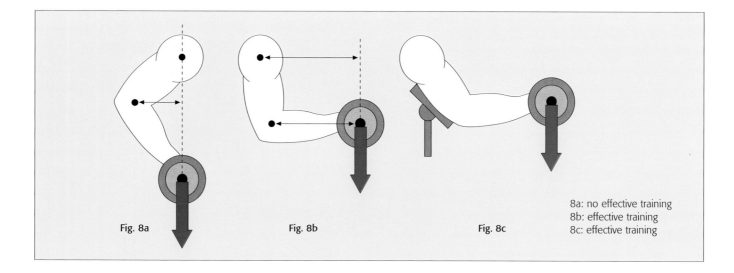

Fig. 8a   **Fig. 8b**   **Fig. 8c**

8a: no effective training
8b: effective training
8c: effective training

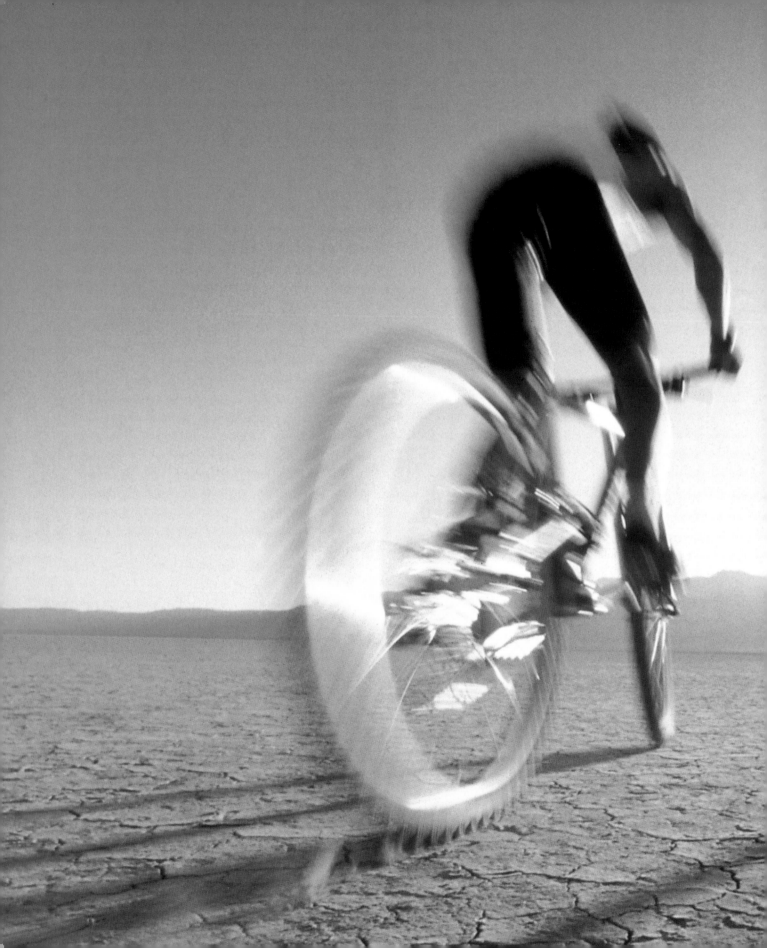

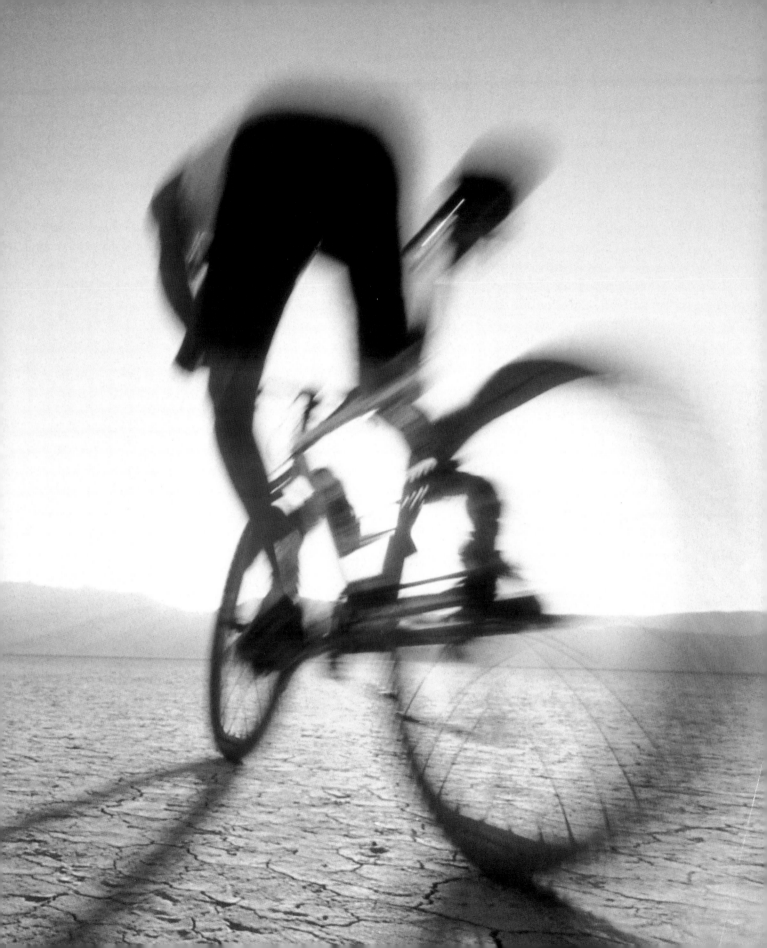

Programs

Target Setting

The following programs are being proposed to stimulate you into actually turning your own long cherished, good intentions into actions. The general outlines of the training schedule suggested in the chapter *Training Guide* were specially designed for weight training, based on the IPC method. The advice of a well-trained, experienced trainer would, of course, always be useful. The schedules cover three areas:

Macrocycle – long-term training schedules
Mesocycle – medium-term training schedules
Microcycle – short-term training schedules

The meso- and the microcycles are always shown together on the same table. This is a table in the classic style of a training schedule, that is, you go to your training session with the mesocycle table, which includes the microcycle as a separate training section, and you can see exactly what you have to do from start to finish. There is no need to plan a macrocycle for the introductory level, since this training schedule lasts altogether only four to six weeks. Basically, with a weight training mesocycle of four to six weeks, you can work primarily on improving your strength and muscular endurance, and stimulating muscular growth.

General Approach

Plan your training in the long term so that you regularly alternate between the various areas involved: endurance, hypertrophy and strength training. If you put together a macrocycle for the next six months or a year of training, your overall targets will determine how often and in what order the separate mesocycles can best be implemented. If you are mainly interested in muscle growth for example, it would be logical in a later mesocycle (for advanced work) to include two hypertrophic cycles followed by a strength cycle and an endurance cycle, as this gives more scope for promoting increased muscle volume. If you are looking for uniform improvement in all areas, the following sequence of separate mesocycles could be scheduled within the macrocycle:

1. Endurance
2. Hypertrophy
3. Strength

The metabolic adaptations targeted by each of the cycles are built up one after the other during this sequence. First of all the lactic acid storage capacity of the muscle is improved during the endurance cycle. Then, during the hypertrophic cycle, the work rate is raised to as high and uniform a level as possible, without hyperacidity occurring in the improved buffer muscle; finally, the

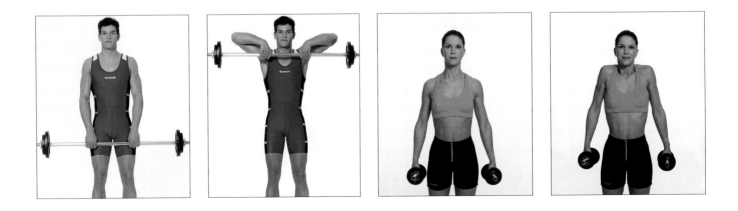

strength cycle encourages the enhanced muscle tissue to coordinate better with the nervous system. If you complete all three mesocycles within four to six weeks each, you can start again with endurance training. Because of the different metabolic requirements, a different general approach should be used in each mesocycle.

Endurance mesocycle

Repetitions: 15–20. Rest between sets: 90 seconds – 2 minutes. Approach: auxotonic or isotonic. Pace: slow to steady and smooth. Range of exercises: optional mixture of equipment and dumbbell training.

Hypertrophic mesocycle

Repetitions: 10–12. Rest between sets: 45–90 seconds. Approach: isotonic, that is, as uniform as possible and without any loss of tension. Pace: slow and smooth. Range of exercises: preferably equipment-based involving exocentric work or individual movements such as concentration curls or dumbbell kickbacks.

Strength mesocycle

Repetitions: 5–8. Rest between sets: 3–5 minutes. Approach: auxotonic (similar to the "usual" training pace with short rest periods at the end of each movement). Exercises carried out with explosive energy: the test is to snatch the weight from the lowest point; as soon as the movement speeds up through improved leverage, control is applied again to prevent it from swinging; steady and smooth overall. Range of exercises: preferably dumbbell work, equipment using pulleys such as in the lat machines, on several joints.

Introductory Level

Duration in months: 0–1.5
Training: whole body
Sessions per week: 2–3
Exercises per muscle group: 1–2
Sets per exercise: 1–2
Repetitions per set: 10–12
IPC workload level: low, which means that you will be using light weights so that by the end of each set, you would be able to repeat the exercises a few times. Choice of weights for the training session is not subject to IPC tests.

How does this work? No improvement in performance is expected for these initial weeks of training. The idea really is that you get used to regular training sessions, get to know and try out a few basic exercises and learn to use the steady, controlled movements and the right breathing techniques. One exercise is used for each of the major muscle groups (for example, legs, back, chest), while the small muscle groups are indirectly exercised by one of the basic exercises for the large muscles. This is where you will get to understand "Exercises per muscle group" – either one muscle is being targeted by a specific exercise and will be doing most of the work or it is used to support another muscle group which is being targeted in the training session. In this way the whole body can be trained with six to eight exercises during the introductory level and the beginner level sessions. For the four to six weeks that you train during the introductory level, it would be preferable to ask a trainer to give you regular checks and correct the way you do your exercises.

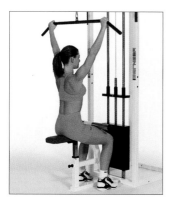
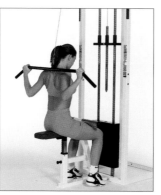
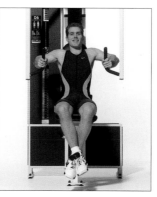
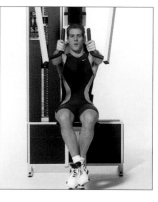

Beginner/Entry Level

Duration in months: 1.5–6
Training: whole body
Sessions per week: 2
Exercises per muscle group: 1–2
Sets per exercise: 1–2
Repetitions per set: minimum 8, maximum 15
IPC workload level: 50–70%

How does this work? At this stage you will for the first time receive an individual performance chart. Special attention should therefore be paid to carrying out the test correctly. Do the test thoroughly and only after warming up well with the aid of a partner or a trainer. It would be logical to use the same exercises in the first mesocycle that you used in your introductory level. It is particularly the beginner level participants who have the feeling of underachieving during the first weeks of training. The muscle strength available would generally allow heavier loads than those allocated by the tests for the first months of training. At this point, to stifle any false pride, it is important to recall once more the different speeds of adaptation for muscles and the passively nourished tissues like tendons, ligaments and cartilage. Only after you have allowed these more slowly nourished elements of the joints an opportunity to gradually get used to the stimulus of the training sessions and the increasing workload are you assured of continued progress with your training, without breaks for injury. During the first months of training that you spend at the beginner level, you will also develop a feeling for the different types of movement (isotonic, auxotonic and explosive), as well as increasing the range of your training sessions.

Intermediate Level

Duration in months: 6–12
Training: whole body or two-way split
Sessions per week: 2–3
Exercises per muscle group: 2
Sets per exercise: 2
Repetitions per set: minimum 8, maximum 20
IPC workload level: 50–70%

At the intermediate level, with at least six months experience of training, it is now possible, and under certain circumstances desirable, to break down your program and use a split-routine for your training. Splitting the work like this is recommended mainly if you decide on a third training session per week. The demands from your training sessions could be too much, particularly for the larger muscle groups like the legs or the back. In this case, full recovery and the principle of supercompensation no longer apply. Spreading the load over different muscle groups on different days means that recovery time is considerably extended. However, if you work through your bodybuilding program in only two sessions a week, splitting does not make sense as all the muscle groups would then only work out once a week each. You should ask an experienced trainer for help in planning a logical spread of all muscle groups over two sessions on different days each week. With a three-day training program, it is advisable to keep the biceps separate from the dorsals and the triceps from the pectorals and humerals. In this way, the smaller muscles, which recover more quickly, train more often every week than the larger muscle groups, which require longer to recover.

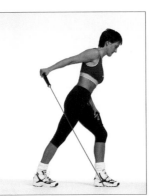
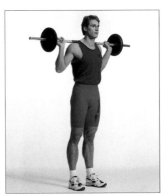
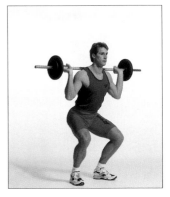

Advanced Level

Duration in months: 12–36
Training: two-way split
Sessions per week: 3–4
Exercises per muscle group: 2–3
Sets per exercise: 2–3
Repetitions per set: minimum 5, maximum 25
IPC workload level: 70–90%

If you have been training regularly for at least a year using the IPC method, your passive kinesthetic system has been taken through the adaptation process needed for the muscle groups now to work to full capacity. At the advanced level, this always happens in the final weeks, when the workload reaches 90 per cent of the maximum for your individual performance profile. It could, however, be that you cannot handle the increased training weights programmed for the last week or two for all the repetitions in every exercise. There are various possibilities if this happens. The simplest thing is to complete only as many repetitions as you can using the correct technique. It is more effective if your training partner can give you the right amount of help with the remaining repetitions to enable you to complete the full set. To do this, your training partner should be positioned so that the dumbbell, the bar on the equipment or your body itself receives the required support. On the other hand, even if you find that this so-called intensive repetition is very effective, please do not attempt to extend these intensive workouts for longer than originally planned. The result could be over-training. You should remember that continued improvement does not follow a direct trajectory, but has peaks and troughs.

Competitive Training Level

Duration in months: 36 and over
Training: two-way or three-way split
Sessions per week: 4–6
Exercises per muscle group: 2–4
Sets per exercise: 3–4
Repetitions per set: minimum 5, maximum 25
IPC workload level: 80–100%

Once you have reached the level of competitive training, you are the best person to manage your training. This is because, after at least three years of regular training during which your strength has improved considerably, you have developed an excellent knowledge of the exercises and the recovery rates that suit you. At this level, you will experience prolonged periods of performance plateaus. This is when you can take the opportunity to experiment and deviate from the *Training Guide* schedule so as to encourage further development in your performance. However, the IPC method of training still provides a solid basis even at this level and it will provide measurable improvement time and again. At this stage, the extent to which you increase the workload over the last few weeks of training depends only on your own capacities. In principle, you can increase the workload in each training cycle to the point where you can no longer perform the required number of repetitions for every exercise. Generally, this happens at 90 to 95 per cent of your individual performance chart. It is, of course, also possible to move up to the competitive training level even if you do not want to or cannot work out four to six times a week and do not intend to compete in power sports or bodybuilding.

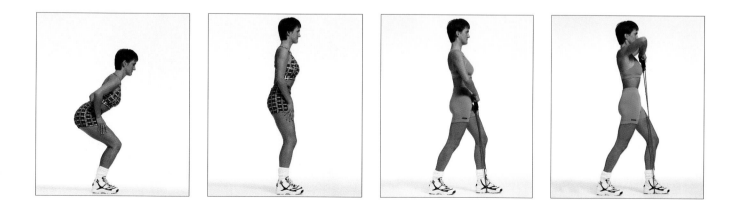

Planning Your Training

The following examples should make this method a little clearer for you – try to continue carrying out the instructions on the basis of the fundamental points given in this chapter and to set out your own macrocycle. Remember that:

Before the weights used for each of the training weeks can be assessed, an IPC test must be carried out for each of the exercises. This will give you a current training performance (number of repetitions) for the specific training requirement and therefore also for the specific demands on the metabolism. It is on the basis of this result that your training levels for each exercise, over the next four to six weeks (mesocyle), are calculated. Before doing the IPC tests, remember to warm up thoroughly generally and specifically. Then carry out each of the exercises, using a weight you believe you can do precisely the required number of repetitions with. To help you to calculate the test results, we repeat below the general schedule for the Training Guide using the IPC method.

+ Whole body training exercises all the large muscles in the body directly and indirectly, in one training session.

* Not all the muscle groups in the body are exercised during a split training session. Instead, they are divided between two or more sessions. In this case, program A and program B are established for a two-way split and programs A, B and C for a three-way split. This means that with four sessions a week, advanced training will have a two-way split with, for example program A for stomach, legs, back, biceps, and program B for the lower back, chest, shoulder and triceps. With a three-way split, the distribution could be as follows: program A covers stomach, legs; program B covers the whole back and the arms; program C covers chest and shoulders.

The level of work does not describe a single, one-off maximum effort, but the maximum performance in terms of repetitions for that session.

Rough schedule for the optimum training schedule according to IPC method

	orientation stage	beginners	experienced	advanced	serious athletes
time level in months	up to 1.5	1.5–6	6–12	12–36	36 and more
training system	whole body +	whole body +	whole body + and split in two*	split in two*	split in two and three*
training frequency	2	2	2–3	3–4	4–6
number of exercises per muscle group	1–2	1–2	2	2–3	2–4
number of sets per exercise	1–2	1–2	2	2–3	3–4
repetitions per set	10–12	min. 8, max. 15	min. 8, max. 20	min. 5, max. 25	min. 5, max. 25
intensity in % of IPM	low	50–70 #	60–80 #	70–90 #	80–100 #

Advanced Level Macrocycle

	Mesocycle 1	Mesocycle 2	Mesocycle 3	Mesocycle 4	Mesocycle 5
Duration of mesocycle	4 weeks	4 weeks	4 weeks	4 weeks	4 weeks
Training objective	hypertrophy	hypertrophy	maximum strength	endurance	hypertrophy
Training system	two-way split*	two-way split*	two-way split*	two-way split*	two-way split*
Sessions per week	3 – 4	3 – 4	3 – 4	3 – 4	3 – 4
Exercises per muscle group	2 – 3	2 – 3	2 – 3	2 – 3	2 – 3
Sets per exercise	2 – 3	2 – 3	2 – 3	2 – 3	2 – 3
Repetitions per set	12	10	5	15	10
Rest interval	2 mins	2 mins	2 mins	2 mins	1 min
Workload as % of IPC	70 – 90 #	70 – 90 #	70 – 90 #	70 – 90 #	70 – 90 #
Approach	auxotonic	isotonic	auxotonic	auxotonic	isotonic
Pace	smooth and steady	slow and steady	explosive, smooth and steady	slow and steady	slow and steady

The above sample macrocycle for advanced training can be applied to any other level using the information about the IPC method from the general schedule.

Remember that the conditions for the performance levels are taken from a general schedule. There may be reasons that make it reasonable or even necessary to deviate from these guidelines. For example, people who have been training for many years in another type of sport may well go through the performance levels more quickly, while others may never even aspire to train four or six times a week. Rational planning of your resistance training based on the general grid and using the IPC method will mean you can exploit the basic principle of performance improvement through supercompensation to optimum effect. But to do this, it is important not only to keep to the correct pattern of training sessions but also, and above all, to apply the gradually increasing workload week by week.

Sample Programs

The adjacent table gives an example of how to set up an IPC test for the beginner level. Below, the test has been applied using basic data from the general schedule, to produce a training program for several weeks. Below this you have an example of split sessions for advanced training for a six-week period.

Level: beginner women
Period: 17 July–26 August
Mesocycle no.: 2
Workload as a % of IPC: 50–70%
Training session no.: 1
Repetitions per set: 10–12
Training sessions per week: 2
Sets per exercise: 1–2
Rest: 1 minute
Approach: isotonic
Pace of work: slow, smooth

Sample IPC-Test

	Exercise No.	Name	Weights used	No. of Repetitions per Test
Stomach	S37	Crunches Machine	65 lbs	10
Lower back movements	S42	Rear Torso Bends	*no additional weight*	12
Legs	S45	Leg Presses	175 lbs	10
Leg adductors	S49	Leg Adduction	55 lbs	11
Leg abductors	S50	Leg Abduction	45 lbs	12
Leg flexors	S48	Seated Leg Curls	55 lbs	10
Back	S9	Front Lat Machine Pulldowns	55 lbs	11
Chest	S14	Vertical Chest Press	45 lbs	12

Beginner Level Training Schedule

	Exercise No.	Name	1st Week	2nd Week	3rd Week	4th Week	5th Week	6th Week
Stomach	S37	Crunches Machine						
Lower back movements	S42	Rear Torso Bends						
Legs	S45	Leg Presses	*50%= 90 lbs*	*52,5%= 95 lbs*	*55%= 100 lbs*	*60%= 105 lbs*	*65%= 110 lbs*	*70%= 115 lbs*
Leg adductors	S49	Leg Adduction						
Leg flexors	S48	Seated Leg Curls						
Back	S9	Front Lat Machine Pulldowns						
Chest	S14	Vertical Chest Press						

In the above sample IPC test, the test subject could not carry out the same number of repetitions for all the exercises because of the different levels of difficulty. This means that, for these exercises, she will have to do the number of repetitions she managed to do during the test over the next six weeks of training. The weights used for each of the exercises are also based on the weights used during the test, and are rated as 100% (see the example of the leg presses). Before you begin your training using the IPC method, the test results for the selected exercises should be established as described and entered on the training schedule.

Below you will find a training schedule for advanced work, with a two-way split:

Period: 17 July–26 August
Level: advanced women
Mesocycle no.: 1
Workload as a % of IPC: 70–90%
Training session no.: A + B
Repetitions per set: 10–12
Training sessions per week: 3–4
Sets per exercise: 2–3
Rest: 2 minutes
Approach: auxotonic
Pace of work: brisk, smooth

We include some sheets for you to copy after this section so that you can draw up your own training schedules.

Advanced Level Training Schedule: Two-Way Split, Schedule A

	Exercise No.	Name	1st Week	2nd Week	3rd Week	4th Week	5th Week	6th Week
Stomach	S35	Floor Crunches						
Legs	S43	Squats						
Leg flexors	S47	Lying Leg Curls						
Leg adductors	S51	Multi-hip Adductor						
Back	S9	Front Lat Machine Pulldowns						
Back	S8	Lat Machine Pulldowns Behind the Neck						
Triceps muscle	S24	Pulley Pushdowns						

Advanced Level Training Schedule: Two-Way Split, Schedule B

	Exercise No.	Name	1st Week	2nd Week	3rd Week	4th Week	5th Week	6th Week
Lower back movements	S40	Machine Lower Back Movements						
Stomach	S36	Twisted Crunches						
Chest	S13	Incline Presses						
Chest	S17	Flat Bench Dumbbell Flyes						
Shoulder	S1	Dumbbell Side Laterals						
Shoulder	S3	Dumbbell Bent-Over Laterals						
Biceps	S19	Seated Dumbbell Curls						

Use the examples we give here only as a basis. As you complete each mesocycle you will gain experience, which you can then draw on for planning your future training schedules. Remember that, with any weight training, you should complete a general warm-up cycle of eight to 12 minutes and cool down afterwards, and that you should also complete your endurance training and your mobility training. We recommend that you record these on your training schedule as well as the exercises with weights, so that they become an automatic feature of your sessions. When selecting stretching exercises make sure that the muscles you exercised with the weights are the ones you stretch.

Alternatives to Equipment-Based Training

If you do not have the opportunity to use a fitness or training center with modern equipment, you can also achieve good results with physical strengthening exercises (P-Exercises). However, in this case, there are only limited possibilities of producing an individual performance chart, as resistivity cannot be measured as accurately as on exercise machines with adjustable weights or with barbells and dumbbells. However, the flexible resistance training bands or tubes give you a choice of certain levels. With exercises which use only body weight or parts of the body, a certain degree of control over the workload is possible through the number of repetitions required. If, for example, you are at the advanced level and manage 20 full push-ups (P8), you will do three sets of 14 repetitions (= 70%) of this exercise during the first week, 15 in the second, 16 in the third, 17 in the fourth and finally, in the fifth week, 18 repetitions per set (= 90%). Also remember to observe the ground rules of strength training during the physical strengthening exercises: for instance, slow, controlled exercises and correct breathing. Make sure you adopt the basic position as described, and carry out the instructions correctly. When using physical strengthening exercises,

we recommend between one and 25 repetitions for endurance training. Strength training using between five and eight repetitions and with correspondingly high resistance is not a practical proposition with physical strengthening exercises. The overview below provides an alternative for resistance training from the range of physical strengthening exercises. For most exercises you will need a tube or other aid such as a step, hand weights, band or wrist weights.

●[1] *Exercises P23–P29 can only be completed with a partner.*
●[2] *With this exercise, the alternative only partially delivers the effect of the S-exercise*
●[3] *There are no alternatives to endurance exercises S35, S36 and S39, since these are already physical strengthening exercises. Alternatives to S37 and S38 are only found among the endurance exercises, but can be carried out as strengthening exercises without aids.*

Muscles of the Shoulder and Pectoral Girdle, Elbow Muscles

		P1	P2	P3	P4	P5	P6	P7	P8	P23	P24	P25	P27
S1	Dumbbell Side Laterals	●								●[1]			
S2	Dumbbell Alternate Front Raises		●										
S3	Dumbbell Bent-Over Laterals			●									
S4	Seated Dumbbell Overhead Presses		●										
S5	Seated Overhead Presses		●										
S6	Upright Rows				●								
S7	Dumbbell Shrugs				●								
S8	Lat Machine Pulldowns behind the Neck					●					●[1]		
S9	Front Lat Machine Pulldowns					●					●[1]		
S10	Machine Rows						●						●[1]
S11	One-Arm Dumbbell Bent-Over Rows						●						●[1]
S12	Bench Presses							●	●				
S13	Incline Presses							●	●				
S14	Vertical Chest Presses							●	●				
S15	Pullover					●[2]		●[2]					
S16	Pec Deck Flyes							●[2]				●[1]	
S17	Flat-Bench Dumbbell Flyes							●[2]				●[1]	

Muscles of the Elbow Joint

	P7	P8	P9	P10	P11	P12	P13	P14	P17	P18	P19	P20	P21	P22	P26	P27	P28	P29
S18 Barbell Curls			●			●												
S19 Seated Dumbbell Curls			●			●												
S20 Standing Dumbbell Curls			●			●												
S21 Scottcurls			●			●												
S22 Concentration Curls			●			●												
S23 Preacher Curls			●			●												
S24 Pulley Pushdowns				●		●												
S25 One-Arm Dumbbell Triceps Extensions				●		●												
S26 Dumbbell Kickbacks				●														
S27 Bench Presses, Narrow	●[2]	●[2]			●													
S28 Machine Dips					●													
S29 Lying Barbell Triceps Extensions				●		●												
S30 Lying Dumbbell Triceps Extensions				●		●												

Wrist Muscles

	P7	P8	P9	P10	P11	P12	P13	P14	P17	P18	P19	P20	P21	P22	P26	P27	P28	P29
S31 Barbell Wrist Curls, Palms Facing Up			●[2]															
S32 Dumbbell Wrist Curls, Palms Facing Up			●[2]															
S33 Barbell Wrist Curls, Palms Facing Down			●[2]															
S34 Dumbbell Wrist Curls, Palms Facing Down			●[2]															

Muscles supporting the Spinal Column

	P7	P8	P9	P10	P11	P12	P13	P14	P17	P18	P19	P20	P21	P22	P26	P27	P28	P29
S35–S39[3]																		
S40 Machine Lower-Back Movements						●	●	●										
S41 Back Hyperextensions						●	●	●										
S42 Hyperextensions Reversed						●	●	●										

Muscles of the Hips, Knees and Ankle Joint

	P7	P8	P9	P10	P11	P12	P13	P14	P17	P18	P19	P20	P21	P22	P26	P27	P28	P29
S43 Squats									●								●[1]	
S44 Front Squats									●								●[1]	
S45 Leg Presses									●								●[1]	
S46 Leg Extensions									●[2]		●[2]						●[1/2]	
S47 Lying Leg Curls											●[2]					●[1]		
S48 Seated Leg Curls											●[2]					●[1]		

Muscles of the Hip Joint

	P7	P8	P9	P10	P11	P12	P13	P14	P17	P18	P19	P20	P21	P22	P26	P27	P28	P29
S49 Leg Adduction Machine												●						●[1]
S50 Leg Abduction Machine													●					●[1]
S51 Multi-Hip Adductor												●						●
S52 Multi-Hip Abductor													●					●
S53 Multi-Hip Gluteal Exercise										●	●							

Muscles of the Ankle Joint

	P7	P8	P9	P10	P11	P12	P13	P14	P17	P18	P19	P20	P21	P22	P26	P27	P28	P29
S54 Standing Calf-Machine Toe Raises														●				

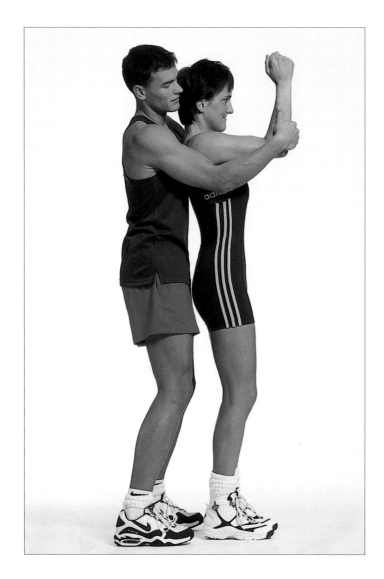

Working with a Partner

A training schedule based on the establishment of an individual performance chart only makes sense if you can grade the workload with precision. This is not possible either with exercises using bands or tubes, or with exercises using your own body weight or parts of the body. These also include exercises P23–P29 in the list, using a partner. Training with a partner is of course not only possible with physical strengthening exercises, but also with the exercise machines and dumbbells in a fitness club or at home. The difference is that you should not do these exercises simultaneously, as with the partner exercises, but one after the

other. This is an important advantage since you can help each other whenever the weights are too heavy.

It is, nevertheless, difficult to establish a training program for two very different people where as much as possible of the same program is to be carried out together. Optimum consideration cannot be given to individual strengths and weaknesses or targets. This is why the ideal situation for this type of training is where two partners share the same training objectives and, best of all, have similar strengths and weaknesses.

In any case, your motivation will benefit from training with a partner. With a training partner, it is much more difficult to miss a session you have planned. Encourage each other during training and after the session and enjoy the relaxation period together.

Complementary Training for Other Sports

For many people, fitness training as described in this book, has become a sport in itself. Others see fitness training as a complement to their "real" sports training. This applies mainly to the various ball games like football, basketball, handball and volleyball, as well as to tennis, squash, badminton and golf. Athletes who compete in any of the ball games listed run the risk of some form of mobility problems through unbalanced development without complementary or compensatory exercise. The result in the worst case could be overstrain or injury. The muscular imbalances already described are particularly liable to occur if no compensating action is taken.

Complementary training is usually undertaken in competitive sport to provide further enhancement to performance-related factors. However, imbalances may be further aggravated by this. For example, this can occur when one half of the body becomes dominant because of performance in one sport and then special exercises are used to strengthen it further. In comparison with the methods usually applied in competitive sport, rationally delivered compensating training will attempt to bring the weaker half of the body to the same level as the stronger. The same happens when certain muscle groups are worked harder than others, for example the leg muscles for football players. In this case the upper body is given training to compensate for the different demands placed on it.

Ideally, the mobility of the muscle groups which the ball games listed before tend to shorten should be tested by an experienced trainer, concentrating mainly on the hip flexors and the long femoral muscles, the thigh tensor muscle and, except for football, the chest muscles. If a trainer is not available, you can test yourself for possible mobility problems with the help of your training partner and the muscle function tests described in the chapter *Training Guides.*

Enjoy Your Training

Perhaps you have already tried out some of the exercises we have shown; perhaps you even went a stage further and have already established a training schedule based on your own personal requirements and targets. However, it is also possible that you did not want to start your training until you had read this book completely. If you are interested in long-term, long-lasting improvements in fitness, you should enjoy your training sessions. Unlike the various ball games and other sports such as martial arts, fitness training is not about measuring your strength in some way against that of your opponent. The only opponent you have to overcome in fitness training is your "inner monster." Fitness training in particular has one element of motivation very rarely found in the same way in other sports: continuing improvements in basic motor performance and, more importantly, a visible improvement in external appearance.

If your motivation is to last more than the first few weeks, you will find it helps a lot to enjoy the movement and the physical activity. In addition to resistance training, try the various endurance sports as well, and decide on whichever of these you enjoy most. If training gets boring, try something new. Mix the exercises for strength and mobility improvement regularly every four to six weeks, to create a new program. In endurance training, vary the use of endurance and interval training. You may also enjoy small-scale competitions with others to try out your strength. Even in endurance training you can compare performance with your training partner. But do not substitute this for a planned training session. If your motivation starts to fall, take a break from training for one or two weeks. Use the knowledge you have gained from this book to organize your life dynamically and to make fitness a life work. To learn something and not act on it means you have learnt nothing at all!

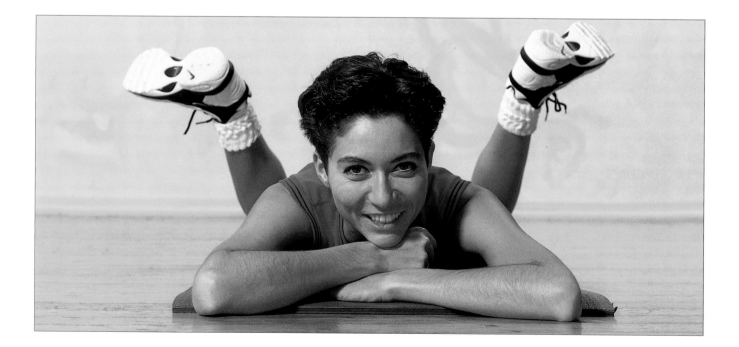

Sample Sheet

IPC Test			
Exercise No.	Name	Test Weight	No. of Repetitions

Training Schedule – Strength Training							
Exercise No.	Name	1st Week	2nd Week	3rd Week	4th Week	5th Week	6th Week

Workout Diary

Date [   ]   Body Weight [   ]

Workout

Muscle Area	Exercise	Sets	Repetitions	Weight per Set			

Workout Duration [   ]

Aerobic Activity

Exercise Machine/Sport	Duration	Workload (Wattage/Level)	Initial Pulse Rate	Mid-Term Pulse Rate	Final Pulse Rate	Pulse after Recovery

Total Workout Duration [   ]

Rest Intervals

From	To	Duration	Comments
	Total		

Glossary

Arms Sideways Arms are placed slightly bent at the sides of the body at shoulder height as an extension of the shoulder axis.

Abduction Movement of the leg away from the median axis of the body.

ABEC Quality standard for ball bearings. Classified by ABEC 1–9. The higher the ABEC number, the higher the quality of the ball bearing.

Adduction Movement of the leg towards the median axis of the body.

Adenosine Triphosphate (ATP) Major source of energy for the muscles. The burning up of ATP releases energy that is used by the muscle cell for contraction.

Adhesive Wax Allows a skier to climb without slipping. The wax must be highly adhesive but not hinder or slow down the skier in the sliding phase.

Adrenaline Hormone that is increasingly secreted in response to stress or higher muscular activity. Raises heart rate and blood pressure.

Aerobic Energy Production In combination with oxygen the decomposition of glucose or fat leads to a production of energy.

Agonist Muscle that adds to a certain movement by active contraction.

Air-cushioning Special air-cushioning system in shoes. The structure of the material resembles a sponge or honeycomb construction. The cavity is filled with air or gas.

Amplitude Unit of measurement for the maximum scope of a swinging body movement, e.g. how deep the leg is carried under the water surface when crawling.

Anaerobic Energy Production Production of energy in the course of burning up carbohydrates without oxygen. In addition, ATP lactate is produced. At first, it leads to a hyperacidity of the muscle and finally to the termination of the muscular activity.

Antagonist Any muscle that opposes the action of another muscle (agonist).

Aqua-Running Various types of jogging in water. It can take place in ankle-deep water on the beach, or in the deep end of a swimming pool without any contact to the bottom. In this case, people wear a special vest that enables them to stay in an upright position. This sort of exercise, which takes the strain off the joints, is especially used for rehabilitation.

Atrophy Muscular degeneration.

Autogenic Training (AT) Relaxation technique using autosuggestion.

Auxotonic Muscular Tension/ Contraction While the muscle length decreases, the muscle tension increases.

Basal Metabolic Rate Minimal metabolic activity during rest phase.

Beat Beat in music. In aerobics each step corresponds to a beat. Exception: "Funk Aerobics."

Bending Line The overall flexibility of a ski from the tip to the bottom. Flexibility optimizes the distribution of weight and propulsion pressure.

Beta-Blocker Drug for lowering blood pressure as well as stabilizing and reducing the heart rate. Impedes the effect of adrenaline and noradrenaline. Included in the doping list.

Bio-Impedance Analysis (BIA) Analysis to determine the body fat percentage. A weak current runs through the body. The velocity of the current and the resistance that builds up determine, through the use of special formulas, the body fat percentage.

Body Fat Percentage The total body fat in relation to body weight.

Body Mass Index (BMI) Standard for assessing the physique on the basis of body surface and body weight.

Booties Special sliding socks that people slip over their sneakers to enable sliding.

BPM BPM stands for "beats per minute." The BPM figure indicates the tempo of the music and thus the speed and intensity of the exercise. In step aerobics, music with 118–122 BPM should be used.

Broca Formula Formula for the calculation of the optimum and ideal body weight depending on height.

Broca, Paul French physician (surgeon and anthropologist), 1824–1880. Developed a formula for the determination of the ideal body weight.

Capacity of Oxygen Uptake Quantity of oxygen that can be absorbed by the organism, measured in liter per minute.

Cam Individually shaped discs for weight training. They balance out the muscular tension created through lifting. Thus, the tension is equally distributed during the training instead of constantly changing as it does during the body's natural movement.

Capillarisation Development of the hairline blood vessels that are the smallest connections between the arteries leading to and from the heart.

Cardiopulmonary System Refers to the cardiovascular system, its connection to the lung and its vascular connections to and from the heart.

Cardiovascular System Consists of the vessels that supply the cardiac muscle with oxygen-enriched blood. It is the first to branch off from the aorta.

Center of gravity or mass The center of gravity or mass is a fixed point from where, if a body was hung, it would always remain in balance, irrespective of how it moved and turned.

Centrifugal Force Force away from the center of a turning motion outwards.

Choreography (Greek) dance notation. Laying down single steps and postures of a dance or its creation.

Citycruiser Bike for use in the city (shopping, errands, etc.). Features: completely equipped according to the respective traffic regulations, including headlight, carrier, fender, etc.

Civilization Disease Diseases that occur due to behavioral patterns or environmental influence, e.g. degenerative diseases of the cardiovascular system, high blood pressure or cardiac infarction.

Competition Method One-off, tournament-like excursion with maximum intensity.

Concentric Muscle Working/ Positive Phase of Movement The muscle shortens under increasing tension when overcoming a resistance – the positive phase of movement or lifting of the weight.

Contraction Shortening of the muscles through tension.

Contralateral Transfer Describes the effect of an exercising strain on the respective structure of the opposite side of the body. This effect is especially relevant to physiotherapy because immobile parts of the body can be strengthened by putting strain on the healthy opposite side of the body. In stamina training it results in a general increase of the aerobic stamina fitness, provided that at least one-sixth of the total muscle mass works aerobically. This improvement, however, is not a contralateral transfer according to the original meaning of the word.

Cooper, Kenneth "Father of aerobe exercise." Physician in the US Air Force. Developed a performance test named after him and an endurance training program – e.g. for astronauts – to prevent cardiovascular diseases.

Coordination Cooperation of the nervous system and the skeletal muscles within a deliberate process.

Creatine-Phosphate Energy reserve supply of the body that is used for the creation of ATP.

Crossrobic Stationary whole-body training equipment for effective endurance training.

Curl Bending movement, e.g. arm or leg bend.

Diabetes Mellitus Disorder of the carbohydrate metabolism.

Deuserband Elastic rubber band available in various degrees of elasticity. Used for gymnastic exercises.

Duration Training Method Regular and lengthy stamina training carried out without breaks and which is particularly effective.

Durometer Degree of hardness of the roll.

Dynamic Muscular Working Muscular contraction. The muscle works by contracting and stretching again.

Eccentric Muscle Work/Negative Movement Phase Muscle contraction. The muscle lengthens while building up tension; the downwards or negative movement in a bodybuilding exercise.

Endurance (Stamina) An athlete's bodily and mental resistance against fatigue in conjunction with his/her ability to recover.

Enzyme Protein units which accelerate chemical reactions in the body. Ergostat fixed heart and circulation training machine which trains only the arms and shoulders.

Eutonia (Greek) *eu* = well-being, *tonus* = tension. A western method (created by Gerda Alexander) that views the human body as a whole. Eutonie is a dynamic process that must be repeated constantly in order to achieve a permanent effect. Through minimal movements one can perceive and experience their body. Blockages can be identified and dispersed of.

Extensive Long training with a low level of intensity (60–80 % of the MHF).

EZ-Barbell A zigzag curved barbell that allows different holding positions when exercising the upper arms and thus relieves the strain on the wrists.

Fat Calipers Devise for measuring the skin-thickness; through the use of special formulae the body fat percentage can be calculated.

Fat Caliper Measurement Method of calculating the body fat percentage. Using calipers, the thickness of skin layers, for example on the biceps, triceps, stomach or waist is measured. Using a table, the percentage of body fat can be calculated.

Feldenkrais, Moshe Jewish physicist and engineer, 1904–1984. Founder of the self-healing method *Wahrneh-*

mung durch Bewegung, self-awareness through movement. For improvement of posture, to enhance awareness of superfluous muscle tension, and *Funktionelle Integration,* functional integration of treatment.

Fixx, James F. In 1977 brought out the bestseller *The Complete Book of Running* and thus established himself as the "jogging guru." He was 52 years old when he died on June 20, 1984 whilst jogging. His death attracted world-wide attention.

Flexibility Ability to perform movements of high amplitude in one or more joints by your own doing or by means of external forces.

Four-Feet Posture To crouch on one's hands and knees with a straight back.

Frame Frame or track for a running conveyer belt.

Frequency of Movement Movements, e.g. steps per unit.

Glucose The muscle's energy source. It can be broken down with or without oxygen. How the body supplies energy depends on the amount needed and the length of the endurance need.

Golgi Apparatus The sensory organ of the tendons. It registers the current tension in the nerves as well as observing changes.

Hays Diet Dietary principle that carbohydrates and proteins should not be consumed at the same meal. Currently in various forms that can be credited to the original Hays diet. No scientific evidence.

Hardboots Shoes with a hard outer shell and a removable inner shoe.

Heart Rate (HR) Number of heartbeats per minute.

Heel Stop Slowing down with the back brake.

Hg Mercury. The unit of measurement *millimeter mercury column* (mm Hg) is used for specifying the blood pressure.

High Impact High impact movements develop a higher strain on the joints. Typical movements are e.g. running and jumping. High impact movements can be identified by the fact that both feet leave the ground for a moment (flying phase).

Hydrostatic Lift The lift of water is a force that counteracts the weight of the body. It enables people to float on the water surface.

Hypertension An unhealthy rise of blood pressure.

Hyperosmotic Solution Contains more osmotic particles than blood.

Hypertrophy Enlargement of cellular tissue, e.g. of the muscle cells. Leads to a general enlargement of the muscle.

Hypotension Low blood pressure.

Hypotonic Solution Contains fewer osmotic particles than blood.

Infrared Measurement Determination of the body fat percentage through infrared rays.

Insertion Link of the muscle with the moveable bone that is normally situated further away from the median axis of the body.

Intensive Repetition When an athlete is unable to complete an exercise cycle alone, a training partner helps to ensure the correct completion of the exercise.

Interval Method Alternating systematically between strain and relief. During the rest interval only an incomplete recovery takes place. The heart rate is the decisive factor.

Isometric Muscle Tension The muscle length remains the same, the muscle tension increases.

Isotonic Muscle Tension Muscle shortening under constant tension.

Isotonic Solution Contains the same osmotic particles as blood.

Jab In boxing a straight punch with the leading hand. This punch is meant to keep the opponent busy and at a distance.

Jacobson, Edmund Internist, 1885–1976. Developed the progressive muscle relaxation method which he presented at Chicago University in 1938. Published a number of scientific papers and books on the effect of psychological tension on the body, e.g. *Progressive Relaxation in Theory and Practice.*

Jell Cushioning Special shoe-cushioning system using fluid.

Kicking Style The foot is put down ball first when walking.

Kilocalorie (kcal) Unit of measurement for the energetic value of food. Also used for work, energy, heat. One calorie is the quantity of heat that is necessary to heat up e.g. one liter of water from 14.5 to 15.5 degrees Celsius.

Kilojoule (kJ) Unit of measurement for caloric value. Has not gained acceptance in everyday usage in comparison to *kilocalorie.* Conversion factor: 1 kilocalorie is about 4.186 kilojoules.

Lactate Salt of the lactic acid that develops when carbohydrates are decomposed in absence of oxygen. It accumulates in the muscles. As a result, the hyperacidity of the cells stops the chemical reactions that create energy and thus the physical effort has to be terminated.

Lactic Acid A by-product produced by the metabolism when saccharose is not fully burnt up with too little oxygen. The over-production of acid in the cells curbs the chemical processes meant for generating energy and thus terminates the physical strain.

Long-Term Endurance Stamina strain between seven and 30 minutes are described as long-term endurance I, between 30 and 90 minutes as long-term endurance II, and more than 90 minutes as long-term endurance III.

Loss of Energy Due to incomplete exploitation of nutrient media during digestion, part of the energy stored in food is lost.

Low Impact Low impact refers to a very joint-friendly strain. In low impact movements, at least one foot remains on the ground, e.g. walking in place.

Macrobiotics Alternative dietary system which classifies food into ten groups. Originates from Zen Buddhism.

Macrocycle Long-term training schedule of at least six months. It is composed of several mesocycles.

Maximal Strength The highest possible power that can be exerted against another force.

Maximum Pulse Rate Maximum value of the heart rate which should be 220 beats per minute minus the respective age of a person.

Medium-Term Endurance Stamina strain between two and ten minutes.

Mesocycle Part of the training schedule that lasts four to six weeks.

MHR Maximum heart rate.

Microcycle Shortest part of an exercising schedule that consists of one unit, with up to one week of exercise.

Mitochondria Volume Mitochondria are small cell organs that contain mainly the enzymes for energy production with oxygen. They are called *power stations of the cell*.

Mountain Bike Special bike for sports use in forests and difficult terrain. Features: low frame, sturdy tubes, small wheels with wide tires and large handlebars.

Muscle Cell The muscle cell corresponds to the muscle fiber and, from the mechanical point of view, has the ability to contract.

Muscle Cross Section Surface of the muscle when cut across the fibers.

Muscle Fiber Basic unit of the skeletal muscle. The muscle fiber corresponds to the muscle cell and has the mechanical ability to contract.

Muscle Filament Protein chain of the muscle.

Muscle Imbalance Imbalance of the antagonistic muscles of a joint, due to weakening and shortening of the muscles involved.

Muscle Spindle Sense organ of the muscle that recognizes the length and length alterations of the muscle.

Muscle Tone Active state of the muscle.

Muscular Apparatus In addition to the skeletal musculature that is subject to will and joins two flexibly connected bones, the unstrained musculature and the cardiac muscles exist which cannot be influenced by will.

Nerves Nerves or the nervous system together with hormones coordinate all the organs and their functions in the human body.

Newton Unit of measurement for gravity.

Noradrenaline Hormone that resembles adrenaline in structure and has some similar effects, e.g. increasing the blood pressure, but also has weaker or even the opposite effect, e.g. lowering the pulse rate.

Origin The link of the muscle to the bone that is rigid and normally nearer to the body center.

Over-Training If, between two exercising phases, insufficient rest is taken, the whole organism is weakened. Over-training can be identified by an increased pulse rate and a drop in performance.

Pacing Style The foot is put down heel first when walking (heel walk).

Paddles A type of fin for use on the hands. They have various functions when used in swimming. The plastic discs increase the size of the hands which leads to an improvement in technique as the feel for an efficient pushing away is trained. In addition, swimming with paddles requires more power and leads to an improvement of drive.

Passive Locomotor System Includes bones, cartilage and ligaments. Static and stabilizing function.

Pedaling The technical ideal is a steady, vertical pull and pressure on the pedal while cycling. This increases the effectiveness of the pedaling motion.

Performance Improvement Through the Circular Method Variation of the endurance levels between low, medium and high to avoid stagnation in performance.

Performance Transformation Energy required in addition to that needed for the maintenance of the basic metabolism and body temperature.

Peristalsis Waves of involuntary muscular contraction of the intestine that transport food and waste products.

Phasic Muscles Their main function is to execute dynamic movements. In case of wrong or lack of usage, the muscle tension is lowered and the muscle becomes weaker.

Phosphaic Compounds Chemical compounds that contain energy. The energy is released when a phosphate is decomposed.

Physiognomy The individual expression and features of a face.

Physiological Natural physical functions.

Power (Strength) In the physical sense defined as mass × acceleration. In terms of sport, it refers to the ability of the muscle to cope with resistance – by holding, overcoming or yielding.

Prevention, Preventive Measures to prevent disease – Prophylaxis, prophylactic.

Progressive Muscular Relaxation (PM) Developed by physician Edmund Jacobson, 1885–1976. Relaxation technique that can easily be learned and makes it possible to relax intensely by active contraction and subsequent deliberate relaxation of the muscles. The perception of the body helps to detect tension at an early stage and to get rid of it quickly and effectively.

Protein Chain The protein components, so-called amino acids, chains themselves together in order to perform certain tasks.

Pull-Buoys Light foam rubber buoys. They are placed between the thighs and provide a horizontal and stable position of the body in water. When exercising in water, the focus can be placed on arm work.

Punch A straight strike with the leading hand.

Purines Purines from food are transformed into uric acid within the body. They settle in the kidneys, joints and tendons and can cause kidney stones and gout, when highly concentrated.

Racing bike Special bike for cycle racing. Features: narrow tires, lighter but sturdy rigid frame, and sporty seat.

Radial In the direction of the spoke.

Raised Arms Position The arms are over your head, turned upwards and slightly bend. Shoulders are normally down.

Reflex Contraction Automatic contraction of the muscles caused by a signal of the muscle spindle via the spinal cord.

Regeneration Recovery of power and the ability to cope with strain on the organism.

Repetition Single lifting and lowering of an object.

Repetition Method Repeated intensive stamina training with complete breaks in-between.

Respiratory minute volume The quantity of air that is inhaled and exhaled per minute.

Rockering Adjustable roller height.

Rubberband Ring of rubber used to intensify the effort required for certain physical exercises. Available in various strengths.

Set Repeated lifting and lowering of a weight without long breaks. For fitness training the number of repetitions per set is normally between five and 25.

Shadow An evasive action in boxing.

Sheldon, William Herbert American physician and psychologist. Born November 19, 1899 in Warwick. Professor at Columbia University in New York and (from 1946) director of the Constitution Laboratory. Developed a constitutional typology of three physical dimensions corresponding to three types of people.

Short-Term Endurance Endurance training lasting between 35 seconds and two minutes.

Ski Hardness Influences the sliding and pressure behavior of the ski. The suitable ski hardness depends on body weight, the intensity of the leg propulsion and the size of the ski. The correct classification is found out by means of tables and tests. Classification: soft, medium or hard.

Ski Wax The use of ski wax minimizes friction. Specialty shops offer a range of waxes for different snow conditions. The consumer can use a wax table to choose the correct wax.

Slide The slide board is a sliding board made of plastic or resin polymer.

Softboots Solid shoes made of nylon or imitation leather which are very comfortable to wear.

Speed Ability to react to a stimulus or signal as fast as possible. Ability to perform movements at various levels of difficulty as quickly as possible.

Speed-Strength Ability to create the strongest possible impact as fast as possible.

Static Muscle Working The muscle flexes against resistance without shortening.

Step Platform for stepping up and down, variable in height.

Stepper Stationary whole body training equipment for building up stamina. A sort of climbing movement is simulated.

Strength Endurance Ability to resist fatigue while using at least one third of the body's maximum strength and fitness.

Super-Compensation Strengthening and improving of the organism's functions through the stimulus of exercise.

Supination Outward turn, e.g. the lower arm is turned palm upwards and the back of the hands downwards.

Synergist Companion of the working muscle. Two muscles create the same movement in a joint by contracting and thus supporting each other.

Systemic Circulation Part of the blood vessel system that supplies the whole body, with the exception of the lung. It is called circulation because it starts and ends at the heart.

Synovia Synovial fluid of the joint that is secreted by the membrane lining of the articular capsule, the bursa and the tendon sheath.

Thoracic Vertebra Breast vertebra.

Tights Tightly fitting sports trousers.

Tonic Muscles Their main task is to hold upright. When used wrongly, e.g. over-use, the muscle tension is increased and thus the muscle is shortened.

Training Heart Rate Pulse rate at which an endurance strain workout takes place.

Trekking Bike These *hybrids* are extremely suitable for daily use on the street as well as on country lanes and in forests. Features: big frame, bigger and narrower wheels than a mountain bike.

Tube Rubber band with handles on both ends. Available in various strengths.

Ulnar In the direction of the ulna.

U-Posture Arm position whereby the upper arms are parallel to the ground and the lower arms are at a right angle to the upper arms, so that they form a U.

Uppercut A punch from below, upwards.

UV Light Ultraviolet radiation. The natural ultraviolet radiation (UV-A, UV-B) reddens and tans the skin.

Vegetarianism Special diet without meat. The so-called ovo-lacto vegetarians include animal products like milk, dairy products and eggs. Vegans avoid these products as well as honey.

Vegetarian Ovo-Lacto Diet The vegetarian ovo-lacto diet includes vegetables as well as eggs, milk and dairy products.

Visualization Imagining real or future events in your mind's eye.

Vital Substances Active substances necessary for the vital functions of the body, e.g. vitamins, hormones, essential fatty acids and amino acids.

VO$_2$max Maximum oxygen absorption. Gross criterion for stamina efficiency.

V-Slip A V-shaped aerobic movement.

Waist to Hip Rate Relationship between the waist and hip measurements.

Water of Oxidation While burning up carbohydrates, fat and protein, the cells release water. In a balanced diet about 2,500 kcal usually produce about 300 ml of water. The water results from splitting and transformation of the basic nutrients into their single components.

Watt Unit of measurement for power.

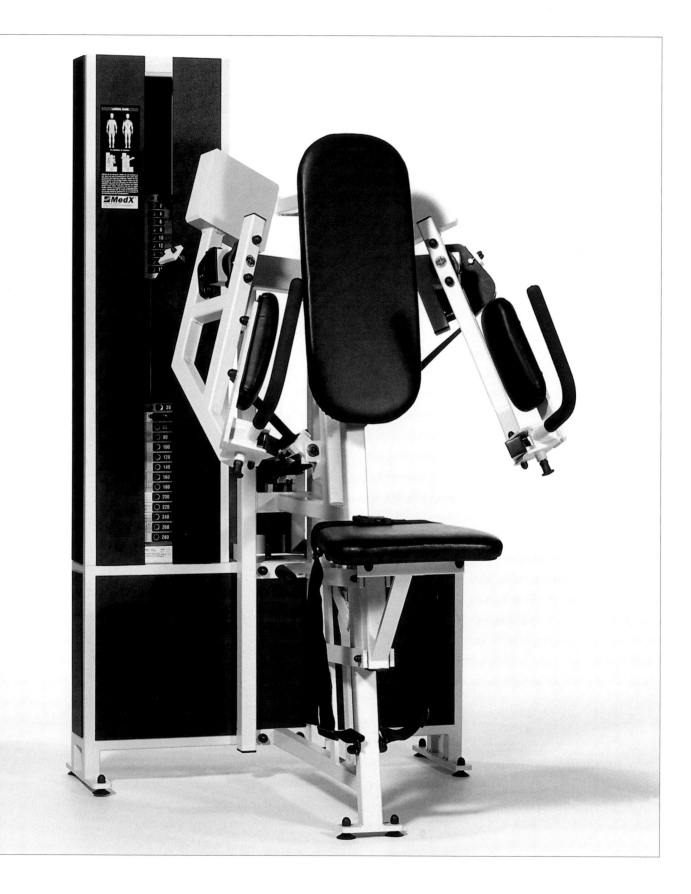

343

Index

Bibliography

Fitness, weight training and physical strengthening

Baechle, Thomas R. and Roger W. Earle. Fitness Weight Training. Champaign, IL: Human Kinetics Pub, 1994.

Bompa, Tudor. Periodization of Strength: the New Wave in Strength Training. Champaign, Il: Human Kinetics Pub, 1999.

Fahey, Thomas D. Basic Weight Training for Men & Women. Mountain View, CA.: Mayfield Publishing Company, 1996.

Fine, Judylaine. Conquering Back Pain. New York: Prentice Hall Press, 1987.

Fleck, Steven J. William J. Kraemer. Periodization Breakthrough!: The Ultimate Training System. Ronkonkoma, NY: Advanced Research Press, 1996.

Grymkowski, Peter, et al. The Gold's Gym Training Encyclopedia. Chicago: Contemporary Books, 1994.

Hochschuler, Stephen, et al. Treat Your Back Without Surgery: The Best Non-Surgical Alternatives to Eliminating Back and Neck Pain. Alameda, CA: Hunter House Publishers, 1998.

Maharam, Lewis G. A Healthy Back: A Sports Medicine Doctor's Back-Care Program for Everybody. New York: Henry Holt (paper), 1998.

Pearl, Bill. Getting Stronger: Weight Training for Men and Women: Sports Training, General Conditioning, Bodybuilding. New York: Random House,1990.

Reynolds, Bill. Bodybuilding for Beginners. Chicago: Contemporary Books, 1983.

Schlosberg, Suzanne. Fitness for Dummies. Foster City, CA: IDG Books Worldwide, 1996.

—. Weight Training for Dummies. Foster City, CA: IDG Books Worldwide, 1997.

Schwarzenegger, Arnold et al. Encyclopedia of Modern Bodybuilding. New York: Simon and Schuster, 1987.

Sobel, Dava, et al. Backache: What Exercises Work. New York: St. Martin's Griffin, 1996.

Sprague, Ken, John Bauguess. Sports Strength: Strength Training Routines to Improve Power, Speed, and Flexibility for Virtually Every Sport. New York: Putnam, 1993.

Yessis, Michael. Kinesiology of Exercise: A Safe and Effective Way to Improve Athletic Performance. Indianapolis, IN: Masters Press, 1995.

Endurance

Brant, Richards. The Fantastic Book of Mountain Biking. Brookfield, CT: Copper Beach Books, 1998.

Brems, Marianne. The Fit Swimmer: 120 Workout and Training Tips. Chicago: Contemporary Books, 1984.

Brown, Richard L. Fitness Running. Champaign, IL: Human Kinetics Pub, 1994.

Burfoot, Amby (ed.) Runner's World Complete Book of Running: Everything You Need to Know to Run for Fun, Fitness and Competition. New York: Rodale Pr., 1997.

Burke, Edmund R. Serious Cycling. Champaign, IL: Human Kinetics Publ., 1994.

Carmichael, Chris, Edmund R. Burke. Fitness Cycling. Champaign, IL: Human Kinetics Publ., 1994.

Cazeneuve, Brian. Cross-Country Skiing: A Complete Guide. New York: W. W. Norton & Company, 1995.

Chris Edwards. The Young Inline Skater. New York: DK Publishing, 1996.

Counsilman, James E. Complete Book of Swimming. New York: Macmillan General Reference, 1979.

Crowther, Nicky. The Ultimate Montain Bike Book: The Definitive Illustrated Guide to Bikes, Components, Technique, Thrills and Trails. Osceola, WI: Motorbooks International, 1996.

Cuthbertson, Tom. Anybody's Bike Book. Berkeley, CA: Ten Speed Press, 1998.

Elling, Mark, et al. The All-Mountain Skier: The Way to Expert Skiing. 1997.

Evans; Jeremy, Brant Richards. Pro Mountain Biker: The Complete Manual of Mountain Biking-Bikes, Accessories, and Techniques. Osceola, WI: Motorbooks International, 1996.

Fenton, Mark, Seth Bauer. The 90-Day Fitness Walking Program. New York: Berkley, 1995.

Forester, John. Effective Cycling. Cambridge, Mass.: MIT Press, 1993.

Gaskill, Steven E. Fitness Cross-Country Skiing. Champaign, IL: Human Kinetics Pub, 1997.

Glover, Bob, et. al. The Runner's Handbook: The Best-Selling Classic Fitness Guide for Beginner and Intermediate Runners. New York: Penguin USA, 1996.

Gordon, Herb. Essential Skiing: A Bible for Beginning Skiers. New York: The Lyons Press, 1996.

Higdon, Hal. Hal Higdon's Smart Running: Expert Advice on Training, Motivation, Injury Prevention, Nutrition, and Good Health for Runners of Any Age and Ability. New York: Rodale Pr, 1998.

Hines, Emmett W. Fitness Swimming. Champaign, IL: Human Kinetics Pub, 1998.

Katz, Jane, Nancy Pauline Bruning. Swimming for Total Fitness: A Progressive Aerobic Program. Garden City: Dolphin Books, 1981.

Lebow, Fred (ed.) The New York Road Runners Club Complete Book of Running and Fitness. New York: Random House, 1992.

Malkin, Mort. Aerobic Walking, the Weight-Loss Exercise: A Complete Program to Reduce Weight, Stress, and Hypertention. New York: John Wiley & Sons, 1995.

Micheli, Lyle J. Healthy Runner's Handbook. Champaign, IL: Human Kinetics Pub., 1996.

Miller, Liz (ed.) California In-Line Skating. San Francisco, CA.: Foghorn Pr., 1996.

Moynier, John. The Basic Essentials of Cross-Contry Skiing. Merrillville, IN.: ICS Books, 1990.

Older, Jules. Cross-Country Skiing for Everyone. Mechanicsburg, PA: Stackpole Books,1998.

Powell, Mark, John Svensson. Inline Skating. Champaign, IL: Human Kinetics Pub, 1993.

Richards, Brant, Steve Worland. The Complete Book of Mountain Biking. New York: Harper Collins Pub, 1997.

Sleamaker, Rob, Ray Browning. Serious Training for Endurance Athletes. Champaign, IL: Human Kinetics Publ., 1996.

Strassman, Michael A. The Basic Essentials of Mountain Biking. Merrillville, IN.: Ics Books, 1989.

Thomas, David G. Advanced Swimming: Steps to Success. Champaign, IL: Human Kinetics Pub, 1990.

van der Plas, Rob. The Bicycle Fitness Book; Cycling for Health and Fitness. San Francisco, CA.: Bicycle Books, 1989.

Stretching, mobility, relaxation

Alter, Michael J. Sport Stretch. Champaign, IL: Human Kinetics Pub, 1997.

—. Science of Flexibility. Champaign, IL: Human Kinetics Pub. 1996.

Black, Sara. The Supple Body: The Way to Fitness, Strength, and Flexibility. New York: Macmillan General References, 1997.

Brennan, Richard. The Alexander Technique Manual: A Step-By-Step Guide to Improve Breathing, Posture and Well-Being. Boston: Journey Editions, 1996.

Gordon, Neil F. Breathing Disorders: Your Complete Exercise Guide (The Cooper Clinic and Research Institute Fitness). Champaign, IL: Human Kinnetics Pub, 1993.

Jacobson, Edmund. You Must Relax. National Foundation for Progressive Relaxation. London: Souvenir Press, 1977

Kurz, Thomas. Stretching Scientifically: A Guide to Flexibility Training. Island Pond, VT: Stadion Publishing Co, 1994.

Ries, Andrew L. (ed.) Shortness of Breath: A Guide to Better Living Breathing. St. Lois, MO: Mosby-Year Book, 1995.

Sauna Society of American Staff. Sauna. N. p.: Commercial Associates, 1994.

Smolley, Laurence A., et al. Breathe Right Now: A Comprehensive Guide to Understanding and Treating the Most Common Breathing Disorders . New York: W. W. Norton & Company, 1998.

Tobias, Maxine, John Patrick Sullivan. Complete Stretching: A New Exercise Program for Health and Vitality. New York: Knopf, 1992.

Virtanen, John O. The Finnish Sauna: peace of mind, body, and soul: a modern guide to sauna usage, planning, and building for full sauna enjoyment. Portland, OR.: Continental Pub. House, 1974

Wharton, Jim, et al. The Wharton's Stretch Book: Featuring the Breakthrough Method of Active-Isolated Stretching. New York: Times Books, 1996.

Wu, K.K. Therapeutic Breathing Exercise. Hongkong: Hai Feng Publ. Co., 1984.

Nutrition

Berning, Jacqueline R., Suzanne Nelson Steen. Nutrition for Sports and Exercise. Gaithersburg, MD.: Aspen Publishers, 1998.

Coleman, Ellen. Eating for Endurance. Palo Alto, CA: Bull Publ. Co., 1997.

Coleman, Ellen, Suzanne Nelson Steen. The Ultimate Sports Nutrition Handbook. Palo Alto, CA: Bull Publ. Co., 1996.

Epps, Roselyn Payne (ed.) The American Medical Women's Association Guide to Nutrition and Wellness. New York: Dell Publ., 1995.

Fischer, Lynn. Lowfat Cooking for Dummies, Healthy Eating On-The-Go for Dummies. Foster City, CA: IDG Books Worldwide, 1997.

Landis, Robyn. Bodyfueling: The Groundbreaking Approach to Eating for Health, Energy, Fitness and Fat Loss. New York, N.Y.: Warner Books, 1994.

Peterson, Marilyn S. Eat to Compete: A Guide to Sports Nutrition. St. Louis: Mosby-Year Book, 1996.

Ratzin Jackson, Catherine G. Nutrition for the Recreational Athlete. Boca Raton: CRC Pr, 1995.

Rinzler, Carol Ann. Nutritional for Dummies. Foster City, CA: IDG Books Worldwide, 1997.

Simopoulos, A. P. Nutrition and Fitness for Athletes/Nutrition and Fitness in Health and Disease and in Growth and Development. New York: Karger, 1993.

Anatomy, physiology, sports biology

Baker, Arnie. Bicycling Medicine: Cycling Nutrition, Physiology, and Injury Prevention and Treatment for Riders of All Levels. New York: Simon and Schuster, 1998.

Douillard, John. Body, Mind, and Sport: The Mind-Body Guide to Lifrlong Fitness and Your Personal Best. New York: Harmony Books, 1995.

MacAuley, Domhnall. Sports Medicine: Practical Guidelines for General Practice. Boston: Butterworth Heinemann1998.

Netter, Frank H. Atlas of Human Anatomy. Summit, NJ: Ciba-Geigy Corp, 1998.

Safran, Marc. R., Douglas McKeag (eds.) Manual of Sports Medicine. Philadelphia: Lippincott-Raven Publishers, 1998.

Sherry, Eugene, Stephen Wilson. Oxford Handbook of Sports Medicine. New York: Oxford University Press, 1998.

Weineck, Jürgen. Functional Anatomy in Sports. Chicago: Year Book Medical Publ., 1990.

Acknowledgements

The editor extends his sincere thanks to:
Heide Ecker-Rosendahl, owner of the Club Heide Rosendahl, who allowed the necessary access for the work involved in this book, and to the staff at the club for their supportive commitment in her absence. Johannes Marx, owner of the BSA Academy, for his support in every respect, and to my colleagues at the academy for the major contribution they made. Irmgard Elsner and Jürgen Schulzki for the intuitive understanding they demonstrated in their photography.

I would also like to thank the following: my wife, Kerstin, my son, Timo, and the rest of the Mutschka family, Frank, Jürgen, Natasha, Sascha and Ulla; Erika Busch-Ostermann, Alex Morkramer and my friends Gunnar and Tina, Justyna, Susanne Haag and Klaus Grochowiak.

The publishers, editor and photographers wish to thank the following individuals and companies for their cooperation and support with the photography:
Adidas, Herzogenaurach – Antje Baron, Cologne – Barbara Siever, Cologne – Bodyshop, Cologne – Competition Line GmbH, Detmold – Falke Gruppe, Schmallenberg – Frank Herlet, Cologne – Haleko GmbH, Hamburg – Kaiser Training, Cologne – Künzler Sportgeräte GmbH, Winterbach – Life Fitness, Unterschleissheim – Move In, Cologne – Nike International, Mörfelden – Olaf Wull Nickel, Kürten – Omega Sports, Cologne – Pedale Radsport, Etzbach – Polar Radfieber, Cologne – Reebok Deutschland GmbH, Oberhaching – RSH Maschinenbau GmbH, Dieburg – Ruprecht Stempell, Cologne – Sportesse, Essen – SSZ Cologne Wahn e.V. Abtl. Bogenschiessen, Cologne – Stage 24, Cologne – Sülztal Familiensauna, Lohmar – TAG Textilausrüstungs-Gesellschaft Schroers GmbH & Co, KG, Krefeld – Tanita Europe GmbH, Sindelfingen – TSD GmbH, Willich – Veloladen, Bergisch Gladbach.

In addition, the publishers would like to thank:
Jürgen Wolf, Cross-Country Ski Diploma trainer and proprietor of the Rehazentrum Neckar-Odenwald, for valuable advice on cross-country skiing; Silke Greuel, Teacher for Physical Education and Data-Manager, for valuable advice on fitness terminology in English; and Lilian Bernhardt for proofreading.

Contributors

Oliver Barteck (born 1967), advanced diploma in nutritional science, has since his youth been involved in the theory and practice of fitness training. When fitness was still primarily a matter of weight training, he had already recognized the value of additional compensatory endurance and mobility training. As a result of this, he has, for the past eight years, been collaborating in the establishment of several multi-functional health clubs. In addition to club management, Oliver Barteck has also been working on a degree-level training qualification for the BSA teaching center, an educational center aimed at the fitness training sector in Europe. He also acts as a collaborator and advisor for the *Bodylife Trainer* journal, and is a consultant to national conferences on fitness training.

Erika Busch-Ostermann (born 1956) is a teacher for physical education and gymnastics at a German high school, a moderator for sports development courses and a health and nutrition advisor. Her considerable achievements include designing and implementing health and continuing education projects, and publishing in various media. She contributed to this book as a specialist editor and consultant.

Knuth Kröger (born 1965) studied Sports Science at the University of Saarbrücken and then trained with the Chamber of Industry and Commerce as a fitness center manager. Since 1993 he has been involved with the BSA Academy as a teaching associate, and also acts as a consultant to international conferences and pharmaceutical companies. As the author of a textbook and an independent trainer in fitness maintenance and competitive aerobics training, he contributed to this book by writing the section on endurance training.

Alex Morkramer (born 1967), MA in English, German and Education, with several years of theoretical and practical experience in the fitness training sector, is currently completing a professional qualification as a trainer at the BSA teaching center. She contributed the sections on mobility, flexibility and cooling-down.

Simon Oswald (born 1969) studied Sports (specializing in swimming and soccer) and Mathematics at the university of Freiburg, and at the Technical University for Sport in Cologne. He is currently a student teacher at a German high school. He contributed the section on swimming.

Dr. Gunnar Wöbke (born 1967), advanced diploma in nutritional science, concentrated mainly on the relationship between sports and nutrition for his studies and doctoral thesis. He was an active German league basketball player until 1995. Since 1997 he has been the director of a sports marketing agency. Gunnar Wöbke wrote the section on nutrition.

Illustrations

The overwhelming majority of photographs, which are not listed individually,
are all new shots by the photographic team of Irmgard Elsner and Jürgen Schulski.
Other graphic material was kindly made available or produced for us by:

© Food Foto, Cologne: p. 4, bottom
© Mark Gamba, Origon: pp. 6/7, pp. 40/41, pp. 162/163, pp. 208/209, pp. 266/267,
    pp. 296/297
© Jump, Hamburg: pp. 200–204
© Könemann Verlagsgesellschaft mbH, Cologne/Photos: Ruprecht Stempell:
    p. 269, p. 272, pp. 274/275, p. 289 (2); Photos: Günter Beer: p. 276 top,
    p. 277 top, p. 281 bottom, p. 289 (3); Fuis & Büschel GbR/Photos: Büschel:
    p. 283, p. 289 (2) from: *Arbeitsbuch zum Diabetiker-Lehrprogramm* (Workbook for a
    Diabetics Study Program), Mainz, 1985
© Novo-Nordisk, p. 280.
© Horst Müller Pressebilddienst GmbH, Düsseldorf, p. 8
© Schwinn International, p. 171

Pictograms: Claudia Faber: pp. 167–209
Drawings: Claudia Faber: p. 308 left; András Szunyoghy, pp. 299–307,
p. 308, center right, to p. 313, top, p. 314, top right, p. 315 bottom left
(all: © Könemann Verlagsgesellschaft mbH, Cologne).

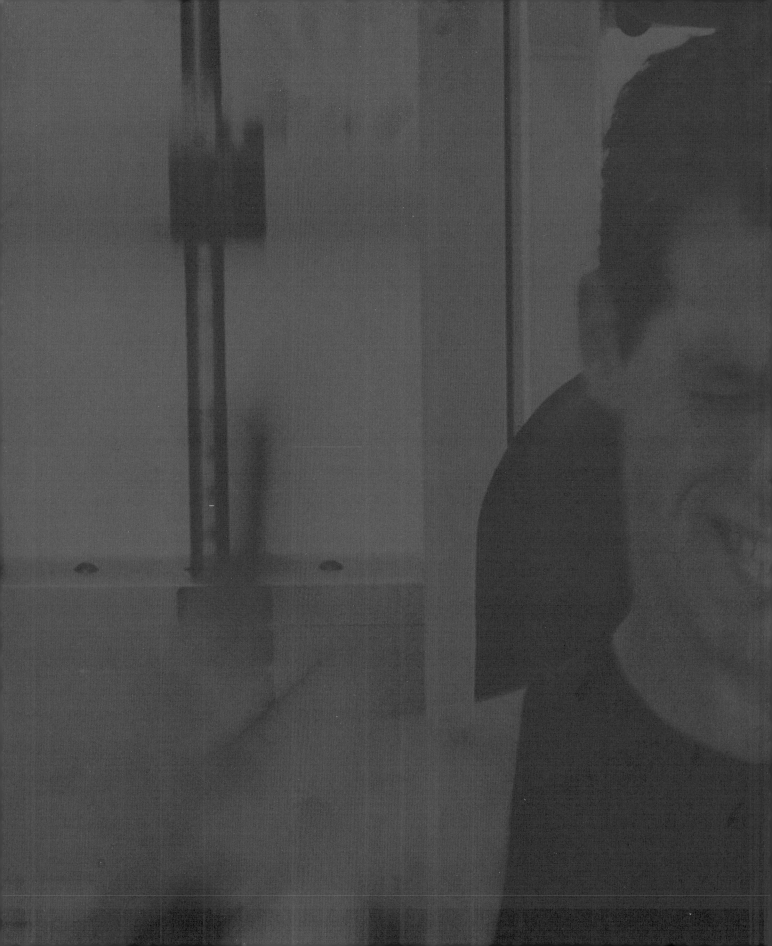